The Neuropsychology
of Vision

The Neuropsychology of Vision

Edited by

Professor Manfred Fahle

Director, Institute of Brain Research
University of Bremen
Germany

Professor Mark Greenlee

Department of Psychology
University of Oldenburg
Germany

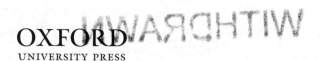

OXFORD
UNIVERSITY PRESS

OXFORD

UNIVERSITY PRESS

Great Clarendon Street, Oxford OX2 6DP

Oxford University Press is a department of the University of Oxford.
It furthers the University's objective of excellence in research, scholarship,
and education by publishing worldwide in

Oxford New York

Auckland Bangkok Buenos Aires Cape Town Chennai
Dar es Salaam Delhi Hong Kong Istanbul Karachi Kolkata
Kuala Lumpur Madrid Melbourne Mexico City Mumbai Nairobi
São Paulo Shanghai Taipei Tokyo Toronto

Oxford is a registered trade mark of Oxford University Press
in the UK and in certain other countries

Published in the United States
by Oxford University Press Inc., New York

A catalogue record for this title is available from the British Library

British Library Cataloguing in Publication Data

Library of Congress Cataloging in Publication Data

(Data available)

ISBN 0 19 850582 5

10 9 8 7 6 5 4 3 2 1

Typeset by Newgen Imaging Systems (P) Ltd., Chennai, India
Printed in Great Britain
on acid-free paper by
T. J. International Ltd, Padstow

Foreword

Glyn Humphreys,

University of Birmingham.

Intuitively, vision seems to be a simple process, occurring automatically and with such little effort that it is difficult not to recognise objects even when it would pay us not to! Yet, like many apparently simple processes, it turns out that vision is extremely complicated—so much so that, after nearly thirty years of intensive study and investment, we still do not have artificial vision systems that can approximate anything like the human ability to recognise objects and to use vision to negotiate the world. Some important insights into the complexity of vision can be gained by studying its break down after damage to our visual system, and hence the study of the neuropsychology of vision, directed at understanding such break downs, plays an important role in our scientific endeavours. In this excellent book, Fahle and Greenlee bring together state-of-the-art summaries of basic research into vision, providing a background in basic visual physiology to clinical studies of patients with disorders of object and colour processing, to studies of neuropsychological recovery and rehabilitation. The work covers studies at the single cell level to studies of sub-system behaviour measured through brain imaging. It reviews studies that use fine-grained time-based analyses of vision (electro- and magnetoencephalography) through to long-term recovery from brain lesion. This coverage is important for grounding our knowledge of why particular forms of neuropsychological deficit occur, and is vital if we are to develop practical applications – for patient recovery, but also for useful, artificial vision systems. By bringing together this breadth of work, this book provides one useful step along this path.

Preface

Understanding symptoms and predicting outcomes in visual neuropsychology

What always fascinated me about neuropsychology is that the subject has such far reaching implications for so many different areas of science, medicine, and, as I believe, even for the social sciences.

For medical implications, consider, for example, the large number of patients who, after cortical stroke, trauma, or tumours, suffer from symptoms that are highly disquieting and strange for the patients themselves, their friends and/or families, or even the patients' physicians. This fact alone certainly provides a strong motivation for continued, interdisciplinary research and for teaching in neuropsychology and its related fields, aimed at improving both diagnosis and treatment of these patients.

Most general practitioners and, more often than not, most ophthalmologists do not have an intimate knowledge of neuropsychological symptomology. An important aim of this book is to provide knowledge about **visual perception symptoms** emanating from damage to the 'visual' brain and thus to explain these symptoms based on up-to-date knowledge about the normal function of this part of the (human) brain.

The better we understand the function of the intact brain, the better we will be able to diagnose defects, relate such defects to functional units within the brain, and eventually find 'workarounds' for these defects. At the very least, we will be able to reassure patients that they are not 'mad' but that the hallucinations or other strange perceptual phenomena they are experiencing are caused by 'anomalies' or 'not their fault' defects in certain parts of their brains.

Moreover, we will be better able to predict the outcome or prognosis, at least in terms of symptomology, and its effects. For example, by being able to more correctly classify varying symptoms as belonging to a specific entity or syndrome, we will be better equipped to foresee how the symptoms will develop over time based on the experience gained from other patients suffering from the same syndrome. Often, there is a good chance that 1) the symptoms may spontaneously disappear or at least alleviate in months to come or 2) the syndrome can be treated effectively via syndrome-specific methods (see, for example, Chapter 11).

Knowledge of brain physiology helps to classify symptoms

A great challenge in neuropsychology is the variability of symptoms in general and that a patient's apparent presentations usually are influenced, especially some time after the defect or insult has occurred, by his or her way of dealing with the problem. Patients try to at least partly compensate for the symptom-generated disability, a compensatory plasticity similar to that found in perceptual learning (see Fahle and Poggio 2002).

Needless to say that in real life, as opposed to 'textbook life', many patients present with *not* classical textbook symptoms that often differ among patients suffering from the same syndrome but that indicate a similar future course and final outcome. (For example, the size and extent of cortical lesions differ considerably—bleedings and damage in general tend to differ among patients. So it is little surprise that symptoms differ more strongly among neuropsychological patients than they do among patients suffering from most other 'illnesses' such as diabetes or common cold, and even patients with these diseases show marked inter-patient symptom differences.)

Knowledge about brain physiology can greatly help in understanding symptoms deviating from the classical syndromes. I firmly believe that knowing the general rules of visual information processing in the visual brain allows the therapist to better understand the root, cause, and etiology of a patient's symptoms, especially when said symptoms are atypical for a certain syndrome. Hence mere memorizing of symptoms without any knowledge about the underlying neuronal processes is a severe handicap in dealing with neuropsychological patients.

To bring the reader up-to-date with present knowledge about the normal functioning of the visual cortex, the opening chapters by Rainer and Logothetis and by Bullier provide insights into the basic aspects of the neuronal processes underlying visual perception, e.g., the general anatomy and physiology of the normal visual system in humans and primates.

Modern methods of visualizing brain function

There are several highly elucidating methods for studying the cortex, including recording from single nerve cells or small groups of neurons. But these methods simply cannot be used in humans except under very restricted conditions. Thus, a large part of present knowledge about the neuronal processes underlying visual perception comes from our nearest relatives in the animal kingdom, the (primate) monkeys.

Fortunately, the advent of modern imaging techniques such as Computed Tomography (CT) and (functional) Magnetic Resonance Imaging (MRI) now allow us to precisely visualize a patient's structural cortical defects (which earlier could be determined, if at all, only by autopsy after the patient's death). These methods moreover allow us to more closely evaluate the changes in cortical activity resulting from different stimuli and to visualize the neuronal activity associated with the visual brain when dealing with different perceptual tasks.

These exciting new methods open up greater possibilities for the researcher to visualize the processes taking place during visual perception in an almost non-invasive way and with high spatial resolution that seemed completely unthinkable twenty years ago. Electrophysiological methods in addition offer analysis of electrical activity produced by the cortex with temporal resolution in the millisecond range by means of recordings through the intact skull. The basics of these methods are presented in Chapter 3 by Munthe and Heinze, while those of functional MRI (fMRI) are explained in Chapter 4 by Greenlee.

These methods, which can be applied to both man and monkey, allow better correlation of the results obtained in single neuron studies in monkeys with the results from the more traditional neuropsychological investigations in human patients. The information about the neuronal basis of visual perception and the methods employed to study perception supplied by the first four chapters, allows the reader to better categorize the symptoms of a patient presenting with unusual combinations of symptoms and, thus, to *understand* and *discern*, rather than to merely *memorize*, at least some of the symptoms caused by lesions in different parts of the brain.

Lesion studies in animals and humans: experimental neuropsychology

The chapter by Merigan and Pasternak then continues by elegantly bridging the gap between basic science and patient studies, describing the deficits of visual perception caused by lesions in primate visual cortex, e.g., lesions caused by ablation experiments in monkeys and by relating these symptoms caused by the lesions to the physiology of the visual system. Ellison and co-workers, in Chapter 6, subsequently demonstrate that short lasting, reversible functional lesions can be safely generated in healthy humans, too, by means of transcranial magnetic stimulation (TMS). Hence, TMS constitutes a novel method to correlate animal studies with those on patients and to create a new discipline, experimental neuropsychology, in humans.

Brain function based on cortical specialization and parallel processing

A generally accepted view of specialization in the visual brain is emerging, albeit slowly. Neuropsychological studies in patients and animals, single neuron recordings in animals, and human and animal fMRI studies have made it increasingly clear that there is not just one visual cortex or even five of them devoted to different aspects of visual perception (see Cowey 1994, for review), but that there are more than 40 discernible cortical areas in the occipital, parietal, and temporal lobes involved with different aspects of visual perception (see van Essen, Andersen, & Felleman 1992). These areas together seem to use up almost one-third of the cortical machinery of our brains, thus indicating that humans are most certainly *visual* animals.

Most of these visual areas seem to represent the entire visual field, and several of their representations are ordered in a topological fashion (e.g. V_1, V_2, V_3). That is, neighbouring points in the outer world are represented by neighbouring neurons in the cortex. This duplication, or rather multiplication, of the *representation* of the visual surroundings suggests that different cortical areas analyse different aspects of visual scenes, leading to a functional specialization as opposed to a duplication of *function*.

Vision, it appears, therefore is not just one holistic unit, but quite to the contrary, visual perception is the 'holistic' subjective correlate of neuronal activity in different cortical areas that analyse different aspects of visual stimuli partly independently from each other *in parallel* (see Chapters 7 and 10). And even sub-functions of visual perception such as colour or motion perception seem to be divided into still further sub-units such as detection of colour borders, achievement of colour constancy, and form identification based on colour to name a few (see Chapter 8).

Functional specialization of cortex leads to specificity of symptoms

Let us consider the consequences of functional specialization of cortical areas for neuropsychology. Clearly, processing of moving stimuli relies at least partly on specific areas that differ from those more specialized for the processing of colour. While certain cortical areas seem to be more important than others for certain sub-aspects of vision, such as V_4 for colour and V_5 for motion, it would certainly be too simplistic to assume that each sub-function of vision is subserved by one and only one cortical area.

In conclusion, we are left with a highly segregated visual cortex with many sub-areas subserving, probably in well-defined cooperation between areas, the different computations that together constitute the astonishing precision and speed of human object recognition. The most important aspect of this insight for neuropsychology is that a defect in each of these areas will produce a deficiency of visual perception, some of which are profound and debilitating for the patient while others are so subtle that they escape our present clinical tests. The different sub-aspects of perceptual deficits relating to, for example, colour (Chapter 8) or motion (e.g. Chapters 5 and 7) are described in detail in specialized chapters herein.

Learning from neuropsychological patients

Unfortunately, we do not know exactly which of the specialized cortical areas subserve which sub-functions of visual perception. This lack of knowledge is partly due to the fact that cortical physiology is still incompletely known. We still do not know exactly the elements or building blocks of visual perception. As a consequence, we still do not fully understand how the brain analyses or processes visual scenes with such astonishing success (outperforming even the most advanced computers).

A large portion of our current knowledge is based on the insights gained from the testing of neuropsychological patients in combination with the knowledge gained from the studies of animals and normal subjects. These tests have become far more detailed and sophisticated than they were in the past. The improvement is due both to a better (if incomplete) understanding of cortical physiology and to the availability of personal computers with tremendous graphical capabilities that allow performing, on a single device, a large number of sophisticated tests each of which would have required an often voluminous opto-mechanical instrument in the old days.

Probably the best-known example of how patients suffering from a (limited) disorder of vision helped expand an understanding of the basic principles of visual perception is the study of patients presenting with colour deficiencies. Patients with such symptoms provided clues, including the inability to discriminate between certain hues while clearly discriminating others, which were absolutely crucial for the early (here used historically) development of theories on colour perception.

Investigating the perceptual deficits of neuropsychological patients will undoubtedly improve knowledge about the function of the intact human brain. It is reassuring that many neuropsychological patients have a quite positive attitude toward the testing of their deficits; they often better accept their handicaps when knowing that the testing and exploration thereof somehow contributes to the improvement of knowledge about the functioning of the brain and its disorders.

So the transfer of knowledge works both ways: Basic science improves understanding of neuropsychological symptoms, and testing neuropsychological patients leads to insights about brain physiology, especially for 'higher level' disorders of visual perception, such as agnosias (see below).

A hierarchy of processing levels and of associated visual disorders

The emerging picture on cortical physiology is consistent with the assumption that different aspects of visual scenes are computed in parallel by a number of cortical pathways or channels as indicated above. Within each of these channels, processing aims to reduce redundancy of the input signal by extracting important features and eliminating all signals less crucial for adequate analysis of the outer world. More specifically, borders or contours are extracted while areas of constant appearance are largely neglected, as both single cell recordings and psychophysical experiments in normal observers indicate. Disturbances on this level prevent patients from detecting contours based on say, colour, or direction of motion, and I would like to propose the term 'visual indiscriminations' for this class of defects.

As a next step, figures or objects are separated from their surroundings by combining the contours belonging to the same object through a process of binding. Defects on this level may lead to apperceptive agnosias.

Thirdly, this representation of an object is categorized via comparison with stored representations. A disorder on this level seems to underlie at least some forms of associative agnosias.

Lastly, semantic knowledge or 'comprehension' is bound to this representation via a word or phrase, and a deficit on this level leads to optic aphasia. Deficits may occur on each of these sequential steps, leading to sometimes dramatic symptoms that differ largely from patient to patient depending upon the processing level involved. Hence, symptoms range from complete blindness to agnosia or aphasia.

Several chapters deal with the symptoms of these more 'cognitive' forms of visual defects and categorize the symptoms within the framework of the normal function of the visual system (see Chapters 7 through 10), proceeding from the basis of the knowledge on 'early' perceptual processes and their deficits, as outlined in the earlier chapters.

Visual perception as interplay between image analysis and synthesis

This process of sequential analysis is not fully determined by the input, but in a usually iterative process with strong feedback, a representation is synthesized rather than determined by a pure analysis of the retinal image. Agnosias represent, according to this view, defects on different levels of both *analysis* of objects and *synthesis* of object representations. Patients suffering from so-called apperceptive agnosias are able to react to visual stimuli but cannot bind together the contours they perceive to coherent objects and, as a result, cannot copy even simple line drawings (cf. Chapter 10). Patients with associative agnosias, on the other hand, are able to copy line drawings in a line-by-line way but are unable to describe—verbally or otherwise—what object they just copied. But even defects restricted to the 'higher' processing levels should, according to this new view, deteriorate processing on the lower levels due to lack of top-down influences, hence associative agnosias should impair binding of contours under certain conditions.

Blindsight and neglect: seeing without perceiving?

Finally, two phenomena in neuropsychological patients are presented and discussed that are generally considered to be related to still more cognitive aspects of visual perception. The first, blindsight, reveals that at least a limited analysis of visual signals continues in some patients even in those parts of their visual field for which they are subjectively blind (see Chapter 9). The second phenomenon, neglect, demonstrates the overwhelming importance of attentional processes for conscious visual processing. Patients will not consciously perceive, and thus not react to, stimuli in the contralesional half of the world, in spite of subconsciously analysing at least certain aspects of these stimuli. (See Chapter 7 which also supplies a general overview of all types of patient studies.)

Aims of this book

The initial chapters reviewing the insights gained by basic science on the structure and function of the visual system, as contributed by physiology, anatomy, and imaging studies together with the subsequent chapters on more classical neuropsychological patient studies, provide a clear picture of our present knowledge about the cortical processing of visual signals (mundanely called 'seeing') and about its possible disorders. Together, the information presented in these and subsequent chapters should make it evident that not only can therapists treating patients benefit from a deeper and more complete knowledge of the neuronal mechanisms underlying normal visual perception but that also researchers in basic science can gain important insights on the functioning of the normal visual system from the symptoms presented by neuropsychological patients.

An outlook

In conclusion, I would like to draw the reader's attention to the fact that neuropsychology, more than other disciplines, forces us to realize that the brain is the substance, or organ, underlying our subjective experience of the outer world as well as the inner 'world' of ourselves. In this respect, neuropsychology has implications for philosophical and theological questions central for the understanding of consciousness and of our own 'nature'. These metaphysical questions, however, have not been dealt with in the present book. Instead, this book attempts to bring closer together the patient- and science-based approaches to the function of the (human) brain. (Perhaps we will add a chapter on the philosophical, theological, and, if you will, metaphysical issues in a later edition.) It is hoped that the present text will prove a useful tool for all those involved with patients suffering from visual disorders caused by cerebral deficits, and for most of those studying brain function.

References

Cowey, A. (1994). Cortical Visual Areas and the Neurobiology of Higher Visual Processes. In *The Neuropsychology of High-Level Vision* (eds. M.J. Farah and G. Ratcliff). Lawrence Erlbaum, Hillsdale, New Jersey.

Fahle, M. and Poggio, I. (2002). *Perceptual Learning.* MIT Press.

van Essen, D.C., Anderson, C.H., and Felleman, D.J. (1992). Information processing in the primate visual system: an integrated systems perspectives. *Science.* **255**(5043), 419–23.

Manfred Fahle
2003

Contents

Contributors

Jean Bullier
Centre de Recherche Cerveau et
Cognition, CNRS-UPS UMR 5549,
31062 Toulouse Cedex, France

A. Cowey
Department of Experimental
Psychology, University of Oxford,
Oxford OX1 3UD, UK

Amanda Ellison
Department of Psychology, Science
Laboratories, University of Durham,
Durham DH1 3LE, UK

Manfred Fahle
Department of Human Neurobiology,
University of Bremen, 28211 Bremen,
Germany

Martha J. Farah
Department of Psychology, University
of Pennsylvania, Philadelphia,
Pennsylvania, USA

Mark W. Greenlee
Cognitive Neuroscience, Department of
Psychology, University of Oldenburg,
26111 Oldenburg, Germany

Hans-Jochen Heinze
Department of Neurology II,
Otto-von-Guericke University,
39112 Magdeburg, Germany

C.A. Heywood
Department of Psychology, Science
Laboratories, University of Durham,
Durham DH1 3LE, UK

Nikos K. Logothetis
Department Logothetis, Max-Planck
Institute for Biological Cybernetics,
72076 Tübingen, Germany

William H. Merigan
Departments of Ophthalmology,
Brain and Cognitive Sciences, and
Center for Visual Science, University of
Rochester, Rochester, New York
14642, USA

Thomas F. Münte
Department of Neuropsychology,
Otto-von-Guericke University, 39112
Magdeburg, Germany

Tatiana Pasternak
Departments of Neurobiology and
anatomy, Brain and Cognitive
Sciences, and Center for Visual
Science, University of Rochester,
Rochester, New York 14642, USA

Gregor Rainer
Department Logothetis, Max-Planck
Institute for Biological Cybernetics,
72076 Tübingen, Germany

Lauren Stewart
Institute of Cognitive Neuroscience,
London WC1N 3AR, UK

Vincent Walsh
Institute of Cognitive Neuroscience,
London WC1N 3AR, UK

L. Weiskrantz
Department of Experimental
Psychology, University of Oxford,
Oxford OX1 3UD, UK

Josef Zihl
Department of Psychology/
Neuropsychology, University of
Munich and Max-Planck Institute of
Psychiatry, Munich, Germany

Part 1

Physiology and anatomy of the visual system: single cells

Chapter 1

Vision, behaviour, and the single neuron

Gregor Rainer and Nikos K. Logothetis

Introduction

The single neuron is the fundamental computational element of the brain. By correlating the activity of single neurons with sensory and behavioural events, vast amounts of knowledge about different brain areas and their function in cognition have been gathered. It has proved possible to uncover neural representations of sensory stimuli such as oriented line segments, moving patterns, or complex objects. Neural correlates of cognitive operations such as short-term memory, attention, and planning have also been found. In this chapter we will begin by describing some of the historical developments that represent the origins of single-neuron recording and first attempts to relate the observed neural activity to behaviour. We will then outline more specifically the progress that has been made in our understanding of different regions of the monkey brain by recording the activity of single neurons. In many cases, single neurons signal task-relevant information at levels comparable to the behavioural performance of the monkey, and there exist remarkable parallels between neural and behavioural performance parameters. While much has been accomplished there remains a lot of work to be done, in particular in terms of providing mechanistic accounts of how the observed phenomena arise. The incorporation of knowledge from other areas of neuroscience such as human neuropsychology and brain imaging, *in vitro* physiology, or computational modelling promises further progress in unravelling how single neurons underlie cognitive functions and ultimately our mental life.

Historical origins of single-neuron recording

Neurons transmit information to each other by sending unitary events called action potentials down their axons. The action potential was discovered by Edgar Adrian in 1919, working on a preparation consisting of a muscle mechanoreceptor and the associated sensory neuron in the frog. He described properties of the action potential that are still central to our interpretation of neural activity today. Adrian found that stimulation of the receptor caused a series of action potentials to be transmitted down the axon of the associated nerve fibre. Stronger stimulation did not change the properties of individual action potentials, but rather caused more of them to be transmitted. This is known as a rate code, because information about stimulus intensity is represented by how many action potentials are transmitted (the firing rate of the neuron). Although we have realized since then that the precise timing of action potentials can and does play a role in information transmission and encoding, the idea of the rate code is still a central concept of systems neuroscience today. Adrian also noticed that neurons sometimes emitted action potentials in the absence of any sensory stimulation. He called this background activity, and such activity also represents a general property of neurons in the mammalian brain.

When examining the activity of peripheral sensory neurons, we can be sure that their action potentials represent activations of the corresponding receptors. The question as to what sensory attributes neurons represent becomes more difficult to answer as we enter the central nervous system. In vision, the concept of the receptive field introduced by Halden Hartline (1938) represents a major advance. Recording from neurons in the optic nerve of the frog, Hartline defined the receptive field of a neuron as that area of visual space where stimulation leads to an increase in the neuron's firing rate. The receptive field remains an important concept today, and much has been learned about the functions of different areas by comparing the receptive fields of their neurons. The receptive field can be thought of as a window through which a neuron has access to information in the visual field. However, it provides only a basic characterization of a neuron's response properties. Neurons are also selective for features, in that their firing rate will vary as a function of which particular stimulus is presented in their receptive field.

In the 1950s, pioneering work on feature selectivity was carried out by Horace Barlow (1953) and Jerome Lettvin and colleagues (1959). Recording from frog retinal ganglion cells, they put forward the idea that neurons actually communicate information about behaviourally relevant features and not merely about local differences in illumination. For example, they described direction-selective ganglion cells that might be used by the frog to detect flies. This represents perhaps the first attempt to relate the response of single neurons to behaviour, an enterprise that has been a major focus of systems neuroscience since then. Unlike in the frog, retinal ganglion cells in mammals are not direction-selective and code only for local differences in illumination. In mammals, the vast majority of these neurons project to primary visual cortex via the thalamus. A breakthrough in our understanding of primary visual cortex came when, in 1959, David Hubel and Torsten Wiesel discovered that oriented line segments or bars appeared to be the features represented by the primary visual cortex. Working on anaesthetized cats, they found that a given neuron will respond vigorously to a bar oriented in its preferred orientation, but not to an orthogonally oriented bar. Different neurons are optimally activated by bars of different orientations so that across a population of neurons many different orientations are represented. Primary visual cortex can thus be viewed as a filtering device that extracts edge information from the retinal input. This represents the first and best-understood feature extraction process of the cortical visual system.

Meanwhile, Barlow continued to study the retina and did some of his most influential work on the quantification of neural responses in the retina of the cat (Barlow *et al.* 1971), using a similar approach to that which Vernon Mountcastle had employed in the somatosensory system (Werner and Mountcastle 1963). Barlow and colleagues were interested in how well single retinal ganglion cells signalled small differences in illumination (Fig. 1.1). To do this, they employed receiver-operating-characteristic (ROC) analyses. Conceptually, ROC analyses provide an estimate in the form of a single number (called the ROC area) of how different the activity of a single neuron is between two conditions. One proceeds by collecting the firing rate of a given neuron for each of two conditions A and B. Because neural activity is characterized by large variability, firing rates will in general not be identical on different trials. Instead, one observes distributions of firing rates for each condition. The ROC area provides an assumption-free measure of how different these distributions are. A value of 0.5 means that they are completely overlapping, whereas a value of 1 means that the distributions are disjoint. The importance of this analysis lies in the fact that the ROC area can be interpreted as the performance of an ideal observer in making statements about the world given only the firing rate of a single neuron. A value of 0.5 indicates that even an ideal observer can only guess as to whether stimulus A or B was present (50% is chance performance for a choice between two possibilities A and B), whereas a value of 1 indicates that an ideal observer could make a correct choice on all trials.

Consider the experiment of Barlow and colleagues (1971). They assembled firing rate distributions for single ganglion cells under illuminations of: (1) zero quanta and (2) five quanta of light as shown in Fig. 1.1(b). Using ROC analysis, they were able to quantify how well a single ganglion cell communicated information about this small difference in illumination. The ROC analysis provides an estimate of how likely it is that illumination was actually present on that trial, *thus using the response of a single neuron to provide a probability estimate about some state of the external world.* By varying the amount of illumination (always compared to the no-illumination condition), one can assemble a sensitivity function for each ganglion cell under study. Different ganglion cells have different sensitivity profiles but, for a given illumination, a particular ganglion cell will have a maximal probability of detecting the stimulus. This led Barlow to formulate the lower envelope principle:

> sensory thresholds are set by the class of sensory neuron that has the lowest threshold for a particular stimulus, and they are little influenced by the presence or absence of responses in an enormous number of other neurons that are less sensitive to that stimulus.

The first part of this statement is quite intuitive, it simply states that discrimination performance is limited by how well we can perceive differences using our senses. It is the second part of the statement that is quite surprising and somewhat controversial, since it says that the performance of the organism is limited not by the average performance of

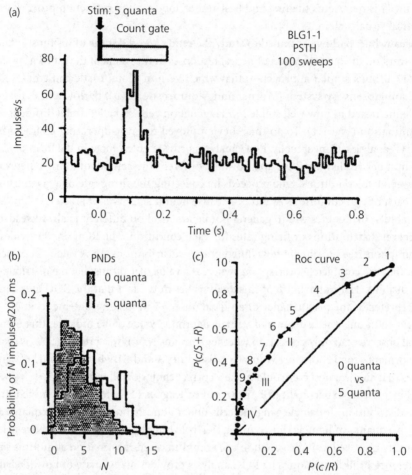

Fig. 1.1 *ROC analysis of neurons in the cat retina.* (a) Action potential (impulse) count histogram (peristimulus time histogram, PSTH) of a single neuron's response to brief illumination of light (5 quanta, stimulus duration 10 milliseconds). (b) Firing rate distributions (pulse number distributions, PNDs) for conditions of no stimulus present (0 quanta, shaded distribution), and for a weak flash of light (5 quanta, non-shaded distribution). Each curve represents the frequency (on the abscissa) of having observed a given number of action potentials in each of the two cases (on the ordinate). (c) Receiver-operating-characteristic (ROC) curve generated from the firing-rate distribution shown in (b). The ROC curve plots the probability of a correct detection (on the abscissa) against the probability of a false alarm (on the ordinate). Each point on the curve represents a different criterion impulse count (c), and thus relates the probability that the random background activity exceeded a criterion (c) spike count $P(c|c)$ to the probability that the activity elicited by the weak flash exceeded the same criterion (c). Each numbered point on the curve is generated by varying the criterion (c) from zero to the maximum number of spikes observed (17 in the present case). For example, neither distribution exceeds a criterion of 17, so this would generate a point on the ROC curve at the origin (0, 0). (Modified from Barlow *et al.* (1971).)

its relevant components but by the performance of the best components. According to this principle, badly performing neurons do not drag down the performance of the entire animal—it can always rely on the best neurons to support behaviour.

The work of Barlow in the retina was extended by David Tolhurst and co-workers (1983) in the *primary visual* cortex (V1) of the anaesthetized cat and monkey. Tolhurst and colleagues measured the contrast sensitivity of V1 neurons for sine-wave gratings of optimal spatial frequency, orientation, and drift-rate for the neuron under study. They generated ROC curves, and measured neural performance thresholds, which they then compared to measures of psychophysical performance of human and monkey observers. There was general agreement between the measures of behavioural and neural performance, although neural performance was somewhat worse than behavioural performance both in terms of threshold and slope. This prompted Tolhurst and colleagues to suggest that *to produce behaviour, the combination of a small number of selective units might be required such that, through a process of probability summation, these units together could perform better than any individual one.* The idea is that any individual neural response is noisy, so that it may or may not provide a reliable signal of stimulus presence on any given trial. However, the more neurons are considered together, the more likely it becomes that at least one of them has detected the stimulus resulting in correct behaviour for that particular trial. More recent results, however, suggest that the discrepancies between neural and behavioural performance may, in fact, have been due to the receptive field structure of V1 neurons (Hawken and Parker 1990). Using a more detailed model of receptive field structure, they found that there was, in fact, *quite good agreement between neural and behavioural performance*, suggesting that the lower envelope principle appears to hold in area V1. An important caveat in interpreting neural performance measures is that they are closely dependent on the length of time over which the firing rates of the neuron are computed. The longer this period is, the more accurate the rate estimates become as long as the process is stationary (i.e. does not change over time). Comparing neural performance between different conditions (i.e. different values of illumination or contrast) is unproblematic, but the absolute thresholds are somewhat arbitrary due to this dependence on integration time.

Soon after the discovery of orientation selectivity by Hubel and Wiesel (1959) in the anaesthetized preparation, they and others began to study neural activity in awake and behaving monkeys. The techniques for performing these recordings were pioneered by Edward Evarts (1966), who originally developed them to study motor cortex. A typical set-up is shown in Fig. 1.2, and consists of a device for fixing the head, a recording chamber for insertion of the electrodes, a scleral search coil for monitoring eye movements by means of electromagnetic induction, a screen or monitor for displaying visual stimuli, and a juice system for delivering a reward.

Many investigators began to study vision-related neural activity in various areas of the monkey brain and to relate it to different behaviours of interest. A detailed

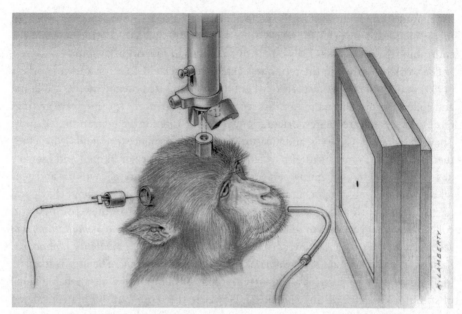

Fig. 1.2 *Single-unit recording in the behaving monkey.* Monkeys (most often macaques) are seated in primate chairs and often also have buttons or levers at their disposal for making manual responses (not shown). Stainless steel head-holders and recording chambers are implanted under general anaesthesia during sterile conditions with monkeys receiving postoperative antibiotics and analgesics. Eye position is monitored using a scleral search coil with metal contacts embedded in the head-holder. During recording sessions, the head is held in a steady position by a metal arm (shown above the monkey). Electrodes (usually made of platinum–iridium or tungsten) are inserted into the brain using manually or mechanically driven devices. Electrical signals are appropriately amplified and filtered (devices not shown). A reward is typically delivered in the form of apple juice or other varieties depending on the particular monkey's preferences.

account of these goes beyond the scope of this chapter, but further details on the historical developments can be found elsewhere (Gross 1998; Hubel 1995; Schiller 1986). We continue here by providing an overview of the cortical areas of the monkey that process visual information and discussing some of the relevant literature for each area.

Visual processing areas in the macaque brain

The macaque monkey brain contains more than 30 distinct visual areas (Fig. 1.3). These areas can be divided into a dorsal and a ventral processing stream (Ungerleider and Mishkin 1982), each of which includes primary visual cortex (V1) and adjacent occipital visual areas (V2, V3). Dorsal stream areas located mostly in parietal cortex are thought to be important for the visual guidance of movements towards objects and the coordinate transformations required to perform these movements (Andersen *et al.*

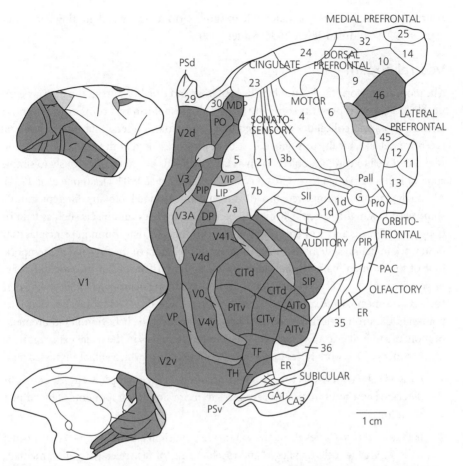

Fig. 1.3 *Map of the cortical areas of the macaque monkey*. Visual areas are shown shaded. Occipital visual areas include V1 (primary visual cortex), V2, V3, V3A, VP (ventral posterior), V4, V4t (transitional), and VOT (ventral occipitotemporal). Ventral stream areas include posterior (PIT), central (CIT), and anterior inferior temporal (AIT) cortex (both dorsal and ventral), posterior and anterior STP (superior temporal polysensory), TF, and TH. Dorsal stream areas include MT (middle temporal), dorsal and lateral MST (medial superior temporal), PO (parieto-occipital), 7a, DP (dorsal prelunate), MDP (medial dorsal prelunate), and several interparietal areas (lateral LIP, ventral VIP, and medial MIP). Finally the frontal eye fields (FEF) and area 46 of the frontal lobe are considered visual. (Modified from Felleman and Van Essen (1991).)

1997; Colby and Goldberg 1999; Milner and Goodale 1993; see also chapter 5, this volume). Areas of the ventral stream located in the temporal cortex are thought to be involved in object recognition and long-term memory storage (Gross 1992; Logothetis and Sheinberg 1996; Tanaka 1996; Miyashita 1993). The prefrontal cortex, which receives projections from both processing streams and contains many visually modulated neurons, is thought to play a major role in short-term memory and guiding behaviour (Fuster 1997; Goldman-Rakic 1996; Miller 2000).

Ventral stream

The pioneering work carried out by Charles Gross and collaborators in the inferior temporal (IT) cortex represents some of the first single-neuron recordings in the ventral stream. Gross and colleagues discovered that IT neurons tended to have large bilateral receptive fields, typically responded best to objects presented at the centre of gaze, and responded well to complex objects such as faces or hands but not as vigorously to simple spots of light or oriented bars (Gross *et al.* 1972; Perrett *et al.* 1982; Desimone *et al.* 1984). Although many IT neurons were broadly tuned and responded to many different stimuli, some fired in a highly specific fashion to behaviourally relevant objects such as fruit or body parts. The discovery of face-selective neurons suggests that common principles may be at work in neural systems as widely different as the retina of the frog and the temporal lobe of the monkey, namely, that neurons are tuned for features of the world that are important to the animal and is of interest for understanding neuropsychological disorders such as prosopagnosia (see Chapter 7, this volume). Indeed, as Desimone and colleagues point out, the strong selectivity for faces may in fact reflect the behavioural requirements of monkeys to make accurate judgements about differences in the facial expressions of other monkeys. This work raises important questions, two of which will be discussed here.

1. How is selectivity for complex stimuli such as faces implemented; can it be described as a combination of responses to more simple components of a complex stimulus?

2. Is face selectivity a result of the extensive experience primates have with other faces, or are face cells privileged and mechanisms for face selectivity fundamentally different from the selectivity for other objects?

Keiji Tanaka and co-workers (1991) conducted careful experiments to investigate complex feature selectivity. They employed a stimulus reduction technique, in which they initially isolated a neuron that was highly selective for a complex object and then simplified the object's features to find the minimal combination of features that still caused robust firing in that neuron. In a step-by-step procedure they were thus able to determine the minimal response features for many IT neurons. They concluded that, in general, moderately complex features such as filled circles with protrusions or combinations of hatched bars and ovals could elicit robust activity. Even neurons that appeared highly selective for real-world objects could be activated by much simpler features. These findings can be interpreted as evidence for a distributed code for complex objects, such that a given object would be represented by a unique firing pattern of a large ensemble of broadly tuned neurons, rather than very few highly selective neurons.

The question whether the highly specific face cells were fundamentally different from neurons selective for other objects was addressed by Nikos Logothetis and co-workers (1995). They reasoned that, if face cells were a result of extensive experience with faces, it should be possible to train monkeys to recognize arbitrary objects and then find neurons highly selective for these objects in IT cortex. Logothetis and colleagues employed three-dimensional stimuli that resembled amoebae and paperclips. After extensive training, monkeys were able to recognize these objects from different views. Recording from IT cortex in these trained monkeys, they found neurons with firing characteristics like those shown in Fig. 1.4.

Single IT neurons responded in a highly specific fashion to views of the trained paperclip objects, but showed little or no response to distractor paperclips even though these appeared very similar to the trained examples. In addition, the vast majority of selective IT neurons—like the ones in Fig. 1.4—were tuned to particular views of objects (view-tuned cells), and only very few responded in a view-invariant fashion. These studies have demonstrated that, as a result of experience, IT neurons can become tuned to arbitrary objects such as paperclips. Further evidence that experience can modify neural tuning properties in IT came from Yasushi Miyashita and co-workers. They employed a pair-association task, in which monkeys were trained to associate pairs of complex objects. They found that responses of IT neurons became correlated such that, after training, they tended to show similar responses to associated objects as compared to non-associated ones (Sakai and Miyashita 1991). Together, these and other studies suggest that IT cortex maintains representations of complex objects that are behaviourally important and that even the adult cortex shows plasticity—possibly accounting for improvement of performance after cortical damage (see Chapter 11, this volume). Further clues as to how this representation is formed and which processes may play a role in their formation come from examining activity in intermediate ventral stream areas such as area V4.

First described by Semir Zeki (1973) as the colour-processing area, V4 represents an intermediate processing stage between primary visual and inferior temporal cortex and is an area where neural activity is in fact modulated by both colour and form (Desimone and Schein 1987; Gallant et al. 1993; Pasupathy and Connor 1999). Landmark work concerning a possible function subserved by area V4 was performed by Jeffrey Moran and Robert Desimone (1985). They employed a paradigm in which two objects were simultaneously presented within the receptive field of a V4 neuron. Only one of these objects was relevant for the task; the other one was a distractor that could be ignored. They found that the relevant, attended object captured the response of the neuron and that the irrelevant distractor had little or no influence on the neural response. The importance of this work lies in the fact that *identical visual stimulation can result in very different neural activity patterns depending on where the monkey directs his attention.* Since then, effects of attention have been further studied in V4 (Connor et al. 1997; McAdams and Maunsell 1999) and also uncovered in other brain regions (Motter 1993). Different hypotheses have been proposed to account for attentional modulations. The strong effect that attention can have on neural responses highlights the fact that visual processing is not simply a passive 'bottom–up' process, but that sensory input is interpreted and modified in accordance with the internal state of the

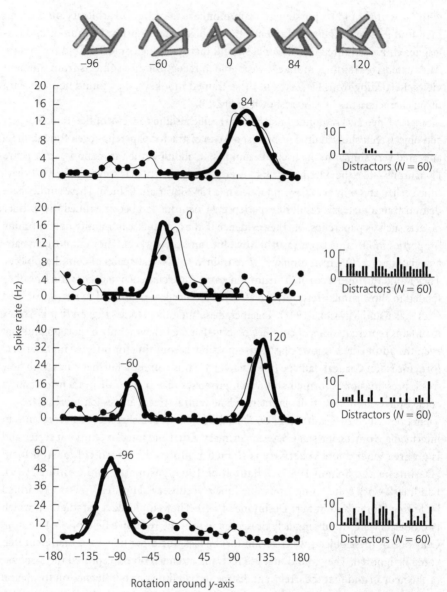

Fig. 1.4 *View-selective neurons in inferior temporal cortex.* Four examples of neurons recorded in the inferior temporal cortex of monkeys trained to recognize arbitrary three-dimensional objects resembling paperclips. Each of these neurons responded to a different view of the same object. The plots represent average firing rate during stimulus presentation (on the ordinate) as a function of rotation angle of the object (on the abscissa). The insets show the responses of each neuron to 60 distractor objects that appeared similar to the trained paperclip but which the monkey had not been trained to recognize. Neural responses to these distractors were low in all cases compared with the responses to the trained object. (Modified from Logothetis *et al.* (1995).)

brain at any given time, as is evident, e.g. in the neglect syndrome (see Chapter 7, this volume).

More evidence that neural activity does not simply reflect sensory inputs came from studies of binocular rivalry (Logothetis and Schall 1989; Leopold and Logothetis 1996; Sheinberg and Logothetis 1997). In these studies, a different visual stimulus is presented to each eye. Under these conditions, the viewer experiences perceptual alternations such that, typically, one or the other visual stimulus is dominant and 'seen', but rarely both together. Logothetis and co-workers found that activity in high-level ventral stream areas reflected the dominant percept, such that a neuron selective for the visual stimulus to the left eye would fire only when that visual stimulus was perceived, but not when the other stimulus was perceived even though sensory stimulation was constant. In early visual areas, on the other hand, only a small proportion of neurons changed activity when the perceptually dominant stimulus changed, with the majority of cells responding to the sensory characteristics of the stimuli.

Dorsal stream

The relation between neural and behavioural performance measures was further explored in awake monkeys by William Newsome and co-workers in the middle temporal (MT), the middle superior temporal (MST), and other cortical areas (Newsome *et al.* 1989; Britten *et al.* 1992). Of neurons in cortical area MT, 90% are motion-selective, responding optimally to stimulus motion in their preferred, but not in the opposite direction. Newsome and colleagues employed a random-dot stimulus that consisted of a large number of moving dots presented in the receptive field of the neuron under study. The coherence of the dots could be varied such that at 100% coherence all dots are moving in one direction (usually the preferred direction of the neuron under study), or else each dot moves in a random direction (0% coherence). Parametric variation of the coherence level allows simultaneous assessment of both neural and behavioural performance. The performance of a single neuron in this coherent motion task is depicted in Fig. 1.5.

Interestingly, Newsome and colleagues found that, under these conditions, *the sensitivity of most MT neurons was very similar to the psychophysical sensitivity of the monkeys.* In fact, there was often good quantitative agreement between parameters describing neuronal activity and behaviour as a function of stimulus coherence. This raised the possibility that psychophysical performance could be supported by relatively few statistically independent neurons, although larger ensembles would be required for partially intercorrelated neurons (Parker and Newsome 1998; Shadlen *et al.* 1996).

The parietal cortex contains several different areas that are thought to play a role in the coordinate transformations that are required to perform visually guided movements. The location where an object forms an image on the retina will depend on where the eyes happen to be looking at a given moment. To accurately reach for the object, eye position relative to the head as well as head position relative to the body have to be taken into account since a large variety of possible head and eye positions will require the same arm movement. Accordingly, parietal areas that are thought to be

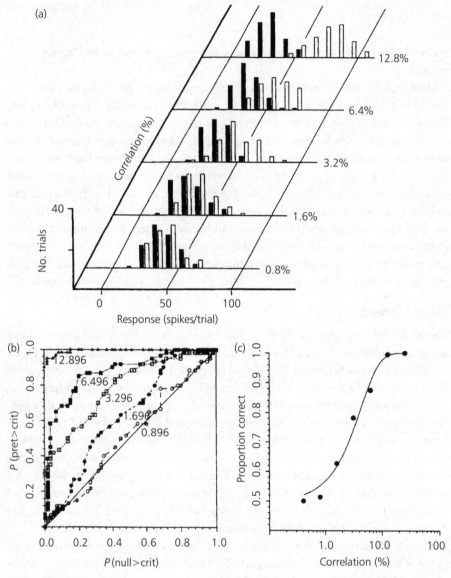

Fig. 1.5 *Processing of coherent motion in the middle temporal (MT) area.* (a) Response histograms for a single MT neuron as a function coherence of the moving dot pattern. The abscissa shows the neural firing rate obtained on a given trial, and the ordinate shows how often each value occurred. The dark bars represent the non-preferred or null direction, and the open bars represent the preferred direction. The depth axis represents different coherence levels. Each distribution is based on 60 trials (2 s duration each). (b) ROC curves comparing neural responses for the preferred to the null direction at different coherence levels. With increasing coherence level the separation between preferred and null direction increases and this leads to the ROC curve being further away from the diagonal, (c) This neurometric curve is generated by plotting the area under the ROC curve for each coherence level against stimulus coherence. It provides a measure of neural performance in motion discrimination that can be easily compared with behavioural performance. (Modified from Britten *et al.* (1992).)

involved in these transformations receive visual, somatosensory, and vestibular projections as well as efference copies of motor commands. One important concept for parietal cortex function is the gain field, which was described by Andersen and co-workers in parietal areas 7a and the lateral interparietal (LIP) cortex (Andersen and Mountcastle 1983; Andersen et al. 1985). Convergent eye position and visual signals produce visual neural responses in these areas that have retinocentric receptive fields and are modulated in a monotonic fashion by the orbital position of the eye. The term 'gain field' refers to the fact that eye position appeared to modify the gain of the visual responses. As Andersen and colleagues noted, *these gain fields represent a stage in the coordinate transformation required to perform accurate reaching movements.* Importantly, the activity of a single neuron does not unambiguously communicate information about stimulus and eye position—different combinations of retinocentric stimulus position and gain can lead to the same neural activity. *Only across a population of neurons will the ensemble activity be unique for each configuration.* Consistent with a general involvement in action, Michael Goldberg and co-workers have found evidence that *parietal cortex preferentially processes visual stimuli that appear relevant for behaviour, regardless of whether an eye movement is actually carried out or not.* For example, in a recent experiment conducted in the LIP (Gottlieb et al. 1998), monkeys were trained to make eye movements that brought a stimulus into the receptive field of the neuron under study. Gottlieb et al. found that the response of the neuron varied dramatically depending on whether the stimulus was salient for the monkey or not. If the stimulus had only recently appeared and was thus interesting or salient for the monkey, an LIP neuron gave a large response when the stimulus entered its receptive field after the saccade. These neurons showed little or no response when the same stimulus had been part of the display for a while and was thus nonsalient when it entered the neurons' receptive field. These two studies and a large body of additional work have begun to elucidate how visual information is processed and used to guide movements in parietal cortex.

Another area that plays a major role in sensorimotor transformations is the premotor cortex, where Giacomo Rizzolatti and collaborators have made important contributions. Premotor neurons show selective responses during tasks in which monkeys see and subsequently grasp objects (Murata et al. 1997). An example of such a neuron is shown in Fig. 1.6.

Because these responses occur both when monkeys are preparing to grasp known objects in complete darkness and also when they observe objects but never make subsequent grasping movements, they cannot be understood as exclusively visual or motor-related. Instead, *the premotor cortex represents objects in terms of their pragmatic or motor-related properties,* such as potential grasping movements that could be made towards them. This interpretation is consistent with mirror neurons, which Rizzolatti and colleagues (1996) have described in premotor cortex. These neurons are active both when a monkey performs a grasping movement himself, and also when the

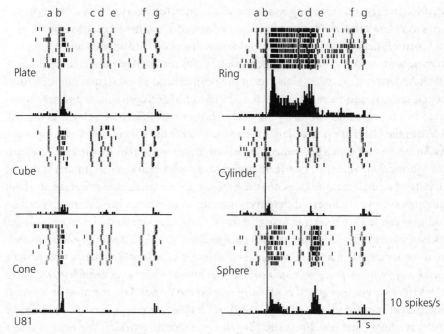

Fig. 1.6 *Grasping neuron in premotor cortex.* The response of a single neuron during the grasping of each of six objects is shown in raster format. Dark vertical bars represents action potentials, with subsequent trials shown in different rows. Activity histograms are shown for each object under the corresponding rasters. The trial began with the onset of a red light (a), which was the signal for the monkey to press a key (b). Upon pressing the key, an object was presented to the monkey for 1 second. Then, the onset of a green light (c) cued the monkey to release the key (d) and grasp the object, which occurred at time (e). The onset of a second green light (f) cued the monkey to release the object, which occurred at time (g). This premotor neuron thus showed robust activity during both observation and grasping of a ring. (After Murata *et al.* (1997).)

monkey observes a human while he makes a similar grasping movement. Further light on how premotor cortex represents visual attributes came from Michael Graziano and collaborators (1994). They demonstrated that *the premotor representation of visual space is in many cases anchored to the face or to the body parts.* That is, a neuron might represent the visual space right next to the monkey's arm, and would thus respond whenever a visual stimulus appeared near that arm, largely independent of the arm's actual position. Neurons of this kind were in general also selective for somatosensory stimulation, responding to touch of a body region near the visually modulated area. Such an arm-centred representation of space that combines both visual and somatosensory information could be very useful for goal-directed movement (Graziano and Gross 1998), which is thought to be a major function of the dorsal visual pathway.

Frontal cortex

Major progress was made in our understanding of the frontal cortex when Joaquin Fuster and Garrett Alexander (1971) discovered delay activity. They found that, during periods in which monkeys had to maintain the location of an item in short-term or working memory, neurons in the prefrontal cortex exhibited periods of sustained activity that could last for the entire duration of the delay. *This delay activity is thought to be the neural correlate of active maintenance of information in memory.* The working memory functions of the prefrontal cortex were further explored extensively by Patricia Goldman-Rakic and co-workers (Funahashi *et al.* 1989). They employed an oculomotor delayed-response task in which a monkey was briefly cued with a spot of light at a peripheral location. After a delay, the monkey had to execute an eye movement to the remembered location of the cue. Funahashi *et al.* found that delay activity of prefrontal neurons varied as a function of the location of the cue. An example is shown in Fig. 1.7.

Delay activity was found to be specific to the location of a particular cue, but does it reflect visual memory for the spot of light or movement preparation for the forthcoming saccade? In an experiment that allowed the dissociation between sensory- and motor-related activity, Funahashi and colleagues (1993) demonstrated that, in general, prefrontal neurons reflected both these processes but the majority coded the memory of the cue. However, prefrontal neurons not only support memory for spatial locations but also subserve working memory for objects (Rao *et al.* 1997; Rainer *et al.* 1998), hence lesions in these regions should interfere with spatial abilities. But does cue-specific memory actually reflect active maintenance or simply an automatic perseverance of sensory events? This question was addressed by Earl Miller and co-workers (1996), who employed a paradigm investigating working memory for objects. Miller and colleagues showed that delay activity for objects survived intervening stimuli in prefrontal, but not IT cortex. They employed a delayed-matching-to-sample task in which a cue object needed to be remembered and compared to up to five possible distractors presented sequentially and separated by delays. In the delays following the distractor objects, IT neurons tended to reflect the characteristics of these distractors, whereas neurons in prefrontal cortex maintained a memory of the initial cue object across the intervening stimuli, consistent with a role in the active short-term maintenance of information. This work demonstrates an important difference between prefrontal and IT object selectivity, and raises the question whether neurons in these areas exhibit other differences.

Recent work has addressed this question, and demonstrated that prefrontal object selectivity is tightly coupled to a monkey's behavioural performance (Rainer and Miller 2000). Using objects degraded with noise, Rainer and Miller showed that monkeys were better able to identify familiar objects in the presence of noise as compared to novel objects. This experience-dependent improvement was reflected in prefrontal neurons, in that their object selectivity was more robust to degradation for familiar than for novel objects. This suggests that prefrontal neurons have activity patterns consistent with

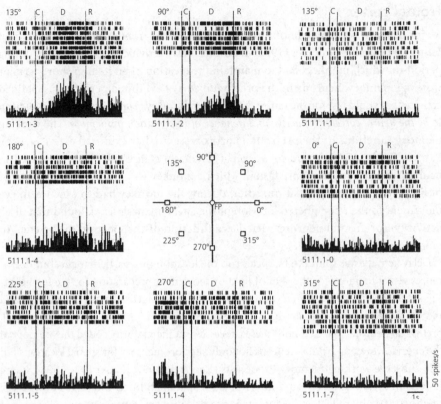

Fig. 1.7 *Working memory neuron in prefrontal cortex*. The response of a single neuron during the performance of an oculomotor delayed-response task is shown. A peripheral cue is briefly presented at one of eight locations located at 13° eccentricity (see centre panel), corresponding to the period marked (C) on each of the histograms. This is followed by a delay (D) and a response (R) period, in which the monkey had to maintain central fixation and make a saccadic eye movement to the remembered location of the cue, respectively. Above each histogram the action potentials for this neuron on several trials can be seen, with each vertical tick representing a single action potential. This single neuron showed robust activity whenever the monkey needed to remember a cue presented on the upper right (135°), with activity falling off rapidly towards the other locations. This delay activity is thought to be the neural correlate of working memory. (After Funahashi *et al.* (1989).)

a role in supporting behavioural performance, and that this selectivity can be strongly modulated by experience. Such changes are consistent with work by Jeff Schall and co-workers (Bichot *et al.* 1996) in the frontal eye field (FEF). Single neurons in the FEF are generally not object-selective but, after extensive training on a visual search task with coloured targets, Bichot and colleagues found that FEF neurons exhibited color selectivity. These and other studies *implicate the prefrontal cortex in short-term memory and, more generally, in the processing of currently relevant stimuli.*

Conclusions

The studies outlined in this chapter represent only a small sample of the wealth of information that has been accumulated by recording the activity of single neurons in monkeys. Yet it demonstrates that significant progress has been made, not only in our understanding of the representation of sensory stimuli, but also in uncovering neural correlates of cognitive operations such as attention, decision-making, or associative memory formation. Perhaps the most significant progress has been made by parametric studies, because they allow accurate quantification of effects and permit the most meaningful correlations with behavioural performance. Several new techniques for studying the brain have been developed recently. For example, functional magnetic resonance imaging (fMRI) allows the study of average activity levels across a large number of neurons (see Chapter 4, this volume), whereas two-photon microscopy permits the *in vivo* imaging of individual neurons and even synapses. In addition, *in vitro* physiology is continuing to provide a wealth of information about how activity can modulate synaptic efficacy by means of mechanisms such as long-term-potentiation (LTP) or depotentiation (LTD). The challenge for monkey electrophysiology will be to integrate knowledge from these and other techniques to uncover the mechanisms by which single neurons process information in a behaving cognitive organism, how neurons underlie our conscious experience, and how progress in understanding can be used to combat neurological disorder and disease.

References

Andersen, R.A. and Mountcastle, V.B. (1983). The influence of the angle of gaze upon the excitability of the light-sensitive neurons of the posterior parietal cortex. *J. Neurosci.* 3 (3), 532–48.

Andersen, R.A., Essick, G.K., and Siegel, R.M. (1985). Encoding of spatial location by posterior parietal neurons. *Science* 230 (4724), 456–8.

Andersen, R.A., Snyder, L.H., Bradley, D.C., and Xing, J. (1997). Multimodal representation of space in the posterior parietal cortex and its use in planning movements. *Ann. Rev. Neurosci.* 20, 303–30.

Barlow, H.B. (1953). Summation and inhibition in the frog's retina. *J. Physiol. (Lond.)* (119), 69–88.

Barlow, H.B., Levick, W.R., and Yoon, M. (1971). Responses to single quanta of light in retinal ganglion cells of the cat. *Vision Res. (suppl. 3)*, 87–101.

Bichot, N.P., Schall J.D., and Thompson, K.G. (1996). Visual feature selectivity in frontal eye fields induced by experience in mature macaques. *Nature* 381 (6584), 697–9.

Britten, K.H., Shadlen, M.N., Newsome, W.T., and Movshon, J.A. (1992). The analysis of visual motion: a comparison of neuronal and psychophysical performance. *J. Neurosci.* 12 (12), 4745–65.

Colby, C.L. and Goldberg, M.E. (1999). Space and attention in parietal cortex. *Ann. Rev. Neurosci.* 22, 319–49.

Connor, C.E., Preddie, D.G., Gallant, J.L., and Van Essen, D.C. (1997). Spatial attention effects in macaque area V4. *J. Neurosci.* 17 (9), 3201–14

Desimone, R. and Schein, S.J. (1987). Visual properties of neurons in area V4 of the macaque: sensitivity to stimulus form. *J. Neurophysiol.* 57 (3), 835–68.

Desimone, R., Albright, T.D., Gross, C.G., and Bruce, C. (1984). Stimulus-selective properties of inferior temporal neurons in the macaque. *J. Neurosci.* **4** (8), 2051–62.

Evarts, E.V. (1966). Methods for recording individual neurons in moving animals. In *Methods in medical Research* (ed. R.F. Rushman), pp. 241–50. Year book Medical Publishers, Chicago.

Felleman, D.J. and Van Essen, D.C. (1991). Distributed hierarchical processing in primate cerebral cortex. *Cereb. Cortex* **1** (1), 1–47.

Funahashi, S., Bruce, C.J., and Goldman-Rakic, P.S. (1989). Mnemonic coding of visual space in the monkey's dorsolateral prefrontal cortex. *J. Neurophysiol.* **61** (2), 331–49.

Funahashi, S., Chafee, M.V., and Goldman-Rakic, P.S. (1993). Prefrontal neuronal activity in rhesus monkeys performing a delayed antisaccade task. *Nature* **365** (6448), 753–6.

Fuster, J.M. (1997). *The prefrontal cortex: anatomy, physiology, and neuropsychology of the frontal lobe.* Lippincott–Raven, Philadelphia.

Fuster, J.M. and Alexander, G.E. (1971). Neuron activity related to short-term memory. *Science* **173** (997), 652–4.

Gallant, J.L., Braun, J., and Van Essen, D.C. (1993). Selectivity for polar, hyperbolic, and Cartesian gratings in macaque visual cortex. *Science* **259** (5091), 100–3.

Goldman-Rakic, R.S. (1996). The prefrontal landscape: implications of functional architecture for understanding human mentation and the central executive. *Phil. Trans. R. Soc. Lond. B, Biol. Sci.* **351** (1346), 1445–53.

Gottlieb, J.P., Kusunoki, M., and Goldberg, M.E. (1998). The representation of visual salience in monkey parietal cortex. *Nature* **391** (6666), 481–4.

Graziano, M.S. and Gross, C.G. (1998). Spatial maps for the control of movement. *Curr. Opin. Neurobiol.* **8** (2), 195–201.

Graziano, M.S., Yap, G.S., and Gross, C.G. (1994). Coding of visual space by premotor neurons. *Science* **266** (5187), 1054–7.

Gross, C.G. (1992). Representation of visual stimuli in inferior temporal cortex. *Phil. Trans. R. Soc. Lond. B Biol. Sci.* **335** (1273), 3–10.

Gross, C.G. (1998). *Brain, vision, memory.* MIT Press, Cambridge, Massachusetts.

Gross, C.G., Rocha-Miranda, C.E., and Bender, D.B. (1972). Visual properties of neurons in inferotemporal cortex of the macaque. *J. Neurophysiol.* **35** (1), 96–111.

Hartline, H.K. (1938). The response of single optic nerve fibers of the vertebrate eye to illumination of the retina. *Am. J. Physiol.* **121**, 400–15.

Hawken, M.J. and Parker, A.J. (1990). Detection and discrimination mechanisms in the striate cortex of Old-World monkey. In *Vision: coding and efficiency* (ed. C. Blakemore), pp. 103–16. Cambridge University Press, Cambridge.

Hubel, D.H. (1995). *Eye, brain, and vision,* Scientific American Library no. 22. W.H. Freeman, New York.

Hubel, D.H. and Wiesel, T.N. (1959). Receptive fields of single neurones in the cat's striate cortex. *J. Physiol. (Lond.)* **148**, 574–91.

Leopold, D.A. and Logothetis, N.K. (1996). Activity changes in early visual cortex reflect monkeys' percepts during binocular rivalry [see comments]. *Nature* **379** (6565), 549–53.

Lettvin, J.Y., Maturana, W.S., McCullogh, W.S., and Pitts, W.H. (1959). What the frog's eye tells the frog's brain. *Proc. Inst. Radio. Engr.* **47**, 1940–51.

Logothetis, N.K. and Schall, J.D. (1989). Neuronal correlates of subjective visual perception. *Science* **245** (4919), 761–3.

Logothetis, N.K. and Sheinberg, D.L. (1996). Visual object recognition. *Ann. Rev. Neurosci.* **19**, 577–621.

Logothetis, N.K., Pauls, J., and Poggio, T. (1995). Shape representation in the inferior temporal cortex of monkeys. *Curr. Biol.* **5** (5), 552–63.

McAdams, C.J. and Maunsell, J.H.R. (1999). Effects of attention on orientation-tuning functions of single neurons in macaque cortical area V4. *J. Neurosci.* **19** (1), 431–41.

Miller, E.K. (2000). The neural basis of top–down control of visual attention in the prefrontal cortex. In *Control of cognitive processes: attention and performance* (ed. S. Monsell and J. Driver), pp. 511–34. MIT Press, Cambridge, Massachusetts.

Miller, E.K., Erickson, C.A., and Desimone, R. (1996). Neural mechanisms of visual working memory in prefrontal cortex of the macaque. *J. Neurosci.* **16** (16), 5154–67.

Milner, A.D. and Goodale, M.A. (1993). Visual pathways to perception and action. *Prog. Brain Res.* **95**, 317–37.

Miyashita, Y. (1993). Inferior temporal cortex: where visual perception meets memory. *Ann. Rev. Neurosci.* **16**, 245–63.

Moran, J. and Desimone, R. (1985). Selective attention gates visual processing in the extrastriate cortex. *Science* **229** (4715), 782–4.

Motter, B.C. (1993). Focal attention produces spatially selective processing in visual cortical areas V1, V2, and V4 in the presence of competing stimuli. *J. Neurophysiol.* **70** (3), 909–19.

Murata, A., Fadiga, L., Fogassi, L., Gallese, V., Raos, V., and Rizzolatti, G. (1997). Object representation in the ventral premotor cortex (area F5) of the monkey. *J. Neurophysiol.* **78** (4), 2226–30.

Newsome, W.T., Britten, K.H., and Movshon, J.A. (1989). Neuronal correlates of a perceptual decision. *Nature* **341** (6237), 52–4.

Parker, A.J. and Newsome, W.T. (1998). Sense and the single neuron: probing the physiology of perception. *Ann. Rev. Neurosci.* **21**, 227–77.

Pasupathy, A. and Connor, C.E. (1999). Responses to contour features in macaque area V4. *J. Neurophysiol.* **82** (5), 2490–502.

Perrett, D.I., Rolls, E.T., and Caan, W. (1982). Visual neurones responsive to faces in the monkey temporal cortex. *Exp. Brain Res.* **47** (3), 329–42.

Rainer, G. and Miller, E.K. (2000). Effects of visual experience on the representation of objects in the prefrontal cortex [see comments]. *Neuron* **27** (1), 179–89.

Rainer, G., Asaad, W.F., and Miller, E.K. (1998). Memory fields of neurons in the primate prefrontal cortex. *Proc. Natl Acad. Sci., USA* **95** (25), 15008–13.

Rao, S.C., Rainer, G., and Miller, E.K. (1997). Integration of what and where in the primate prefrontal cortex. *Science* **276** (5313), 1821–4.

Rizzolatti, G., Fadiga, L., Gallese, V., and Fogassi, L. (1996). Premotor cortex and the recognition of motor actions. *Brain Res. Cogn. Brain Res.* **3** (2), 131–41.

Sakai, K. and Miyashita, Y. (1991). Neural organization for the long-term memory of paired associates [see comments]. *Nature* **354** (6349), 152–5.

Schiller, P.H. (1986). The central visual system. *Vision Res.* **26** (9), 1351–86.

Shadlen, M.N., Britten, K.H., Newsome, W.T., and Movshon, J.A. (1996). A computational analysis of the relationship between neuronal and behavioral responses to visual motion. *J. Neurosci.* **16** (4), 1486–510.

Sheinberg, D.L., and Logothetis, N.K. (1997). The role of temporal cortical areas in perceptual organization. *Proc. Natl Acad. Sci., USA* **94** (7), 3408–13.

Tanaka, K. (1996). Inferotemporal cortex and object vision. *Ann. Rev. Neurosci.* **19**, 109–39.

Tanaka, K., Saito, H., Fukada, Y., and Moriya, M. (1991). Coding visual images of objects in the inferotemporal cortex of the macaque monkey. *J. Neurophysiol.* **66** (1), 170–89.

Tolhurst, D.J., Movshon, J.A., and Dean, A.F. (1983). The statistical reliability of signals in single neurons in cat and monkey visual cortex. *Vision Res.* **23** (8), 775–85.

Ungerleider, L.G. and Mishkin, M. (1982). Two cortical visual systems. In *Analysis of visual behavior* (ed. D.J. Ingle, M.A. Goodale, and R.J.W. Mansfield), Vol. 18, pp. 549–86. MIT Press, Cambridge, Massachusetts.

Werner, G. and Mountcastle, V.B. (1963). The variability of central neural activity in a sensory system, and its implications for the central reflection of sensory events. *J. Neurophysiol.* **26**, 958–77.

Zeki, S.M. (1973). Colour coding in rhesus monkey prestriate cortex. *Brain Res.* **53** (2), 422–7.

Chapter 2

Cortical connections and functional interactions between visual cortical areas

Jean Bullier

Introduction

Since the late 1980s it has been usual to partition the cortical surface of vertebrates in a number of functional areas. These do not always correspond to the areas discovered by Brodmann and the cytoarchitectonic school of the beginning of the century. In the visual system, functional areas are usually smaller than cytoarchitectonic areas, with the exception of area 17, which corresponds exactly to area V1, and area 18, which, in some species such as the cat and the tree shrew (Kaas 1996), corresponds to area V2. The discovery of functional areas in the human brain is more recent but conforms to this general rule that functional areas are smaller than Brodmann's areas. The present chapter reviews what is known of the interconnections between visual areas in the two animals that have received the most attention, the macaque monkey and the cat. A simplified version of the visual cortical areas in these two animals is presented in Fig. 2.1.

Functional areas are interconnected by a very dense network of cortico-cortical connections, also called interarea or extrinsic connections. Connections exist between areas of the same cortical hemisphere (intrahemispheric connections), as well as between areas of opposite hemispheres (interhemispheric or callosal connections). Diagrams of the intrahemispheric connections between visual areas of the cat and monkey can be found in earlier reviews (Boussaoud *et al.* 1990; Bullier *et al.* 1996; Felleman and Van Essen 1991), and are summarized in later sections.

Interarea or extrinsic connections are made by pyramidal neurons, which also send collaterals to neighbouring neurons within a few millimetres. These connections, together with those of inhibitory γ-aminobutyric acid (GABA)ergic interneurons, are called intraarea, local, horizontal, or intrinsic connections. Although these connections are not the subject of the present review, they share several characteristics with interarea connections and much of the present line of research consists in distinguishing between influences mediated by intrinsic and by extrinsic cortico-cortical connections. All pyramidal neurons that send extrinsic cortico-cortical connections also send local

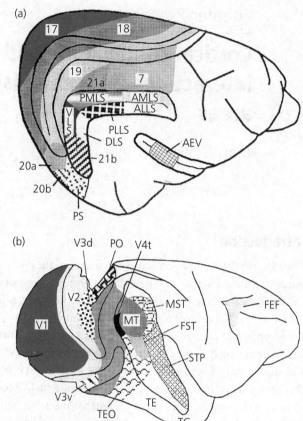

Fig. 2.1 Visual cortical areas in the cat and the monkey. (a) Lateral view of the cat visual cortex with the areas of the visual system. The lateral sulcus, the suprasylvian sulcus (containing PMLS, AMLS, VLS, PLLS, etc.), and the anterior ectosylvian sulcus (containing the anterior ectosylvian visual area (AEV)) have been opened for clarity. (b) Visual areas on a lateral view of the macaque monkey cortex. The lunate sulcus (containing V3d), the inferior occipital sulcus (containing V3v), and the superior temporal sulcus (containing MT) have been opened to reveal the areas inside.

arbors in their immediate vicinity, as illustrated in Fig. 2.2. Thus, extrinsic and intrinsic influences are inevitably related by the simple fact that whatever message is sent by a cortical neuron to neurons in other cortical areas through extrinsic connections is also transmitted by intrinsic connections to the immediate surroundings of the source neuron. The local connections of a neuron projecting to another cortical area appear to be almost exclusively targeted at pyramidal cells, some of them projecting to the same cortical area. It seems that neurons sending an axon to a given cortical area are also interconnected by local connections and that they receive reciprocal connections from their common projection targets (Johnson and Burkhalter 1997), thus defining a specific network across and within areas.

General characteristics of interarea cortico-cortical connections

Interarea connections are almost exclusively made by pyramidal neurons. A few exceptions have been noted—in the cat, some spiny stellate cells in area 17 send projections to area 18 (Meyer and Albus 1981). It has been reported that in the rat a small contingent

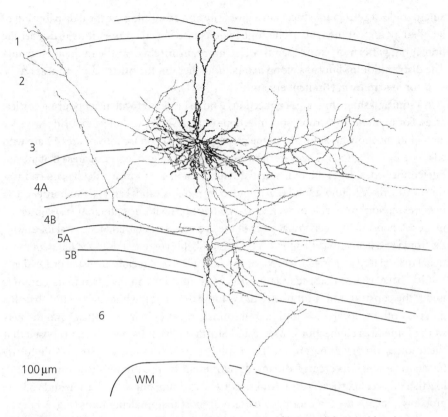

Fig. 2.2 Pyramidal neuron stained by intracellular injection of horseradish peroxidase in cat area 17. Note the dense arborization of the axon collaterals in area 17 and the axon leaving the cortex in the white matter. The local collaterals are the main source of the horizontal connections in the cortex (also called intrinsic connections). They carry the same messages as the axons of extrinsic connections that connect to other cortical areas. (Reproduced from Martin 1984.)

of GABAergic smooth stellate cells send connections between neighbouring cortical areas (McDonald and Burkhalter 1993). Interhemispheric connections have also been found to arise from a few presumably inhibitory interneurons in the rat (Hughes and Peters 1992a,b) and in the cat (Peters *et al.* 1990). Despite this evidence from anatomy, no monosynaptic inhibitory synaptic potential has ever been reported in electrophysiological studies of connections between cortical areas of the same or opposite hemisphere. It can therefore be concluded that interarea and interhemispheric cortico-cortical connections are excitatory. However, intra- and interhemispheric connections always contact excitatory pyramidal cells as well as inhibitory interneurons in the target area (see below for the proportions) and the net effect of cortico-cortical connections is therefore a mixture of excitatory and inhibitory influences.

It is known that, within the local intraarea network, the densest connections are with immediate neighbour neurons. This is demonstrated by placing small injections of anterograde or retrograde tracers in a given site and examining the local distribution of labelled axons and neurons. The higher density of local connections is due to the branching pattern of axons that arborize more profusely near the main axon trunk. The distribution of boutons along axonal branches, on the other hand, appears to be more or less uniform (Braitenberg and Schüz 1991).

In a similar fashion, interarea connections tend to be densest with neighbouring cortical areas. For example, the strongest connections of area V2 are with neighbouring areas V1 and V4 in the monkey. Similarly, in the cat, the strongest connections of area 17 are with adjacent areas 18 and 19. There are, however, a few examples of adjacent areas that are not interconnected, such as the retrosplenial visual area in the monkey that has no connections with area V1 although it is surrounded by it on its caudal and lateral borders. The major exception to the rule of preferential connections with neighbour areas is observed in the relationship between visual areas of the occipital, parietal, and temporal lobes with the frontal eye field area (FEF in Fig. 2.1). This probably corresponds to the different functional roles played by parietal, temporal, and frontal cortical regions in visual processing.

It has been argued that the organization of connectivity in the mammalian brain is under the constraint of minimizing the volume of cortical white matter and that this governs both the local organization of terminal arbors (patchy or diffuse) and the network of interarea connections (Murre and Sturdy 1995). It has also been proposed that the folding of cortex in gyri and deep sulci (Fig. 2.1) in most brains is due to the mechanical tensions created during development by the numerous axons that link together adjacent cortical areas (Van Essen 1997). Minimizing axon tension and volume probably explains the typical folded pattern of most mammalian brains (Fig. 2.1).

Feedforward, feedback, lateral connections

Definitions

Intrahemispheric cortico-cortical connections are often subdivided into three classes: feedforward; feedback; and lateral connections. The difference between feedforward and feedback originated in the distinction made by Rockland and Pandya (1979) who noted that some connections (forward-going) tended to originate in neurons located in supragranular layers (layers 2 and 3) and terminate around layer 4, whereas reciprocal connections (backward-directed) were predominantly made by neurons in infragranular layers (layers 5 and 6) and project outside layer 4. This was later formalized by Maunsell and Van Essen (1983) and Felleman and Van Essen (1991) who defined feedforward, feedback, and lateral connections and used this classification to construct the hierarchy of cortical areas (see the section 'Hierarchical organization of cortical areas'). Lateral connections do not fit into either feedforward or feedback classes. Their neurons of origin belong to infra- and supragranular layers and their terminals arborize in all layers (Fig. 2.3).

These three groups of cortico-cortical connections are not as homogeneous as implied by the synthetic presentation of Van Essen and his colleagues. Quantitative estimates of the proportions of source neurons in infragranular (layers 5 and 6) versus

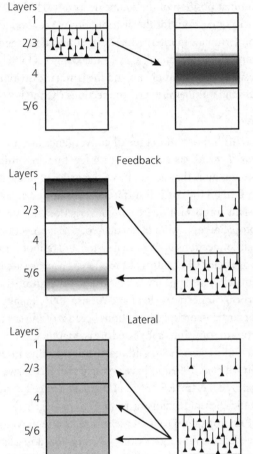

Fig. 2.3 Schematic representation of the distribution of source neurons (little black triangles) and axonal terminal arborization (shading density corresponds to bouton density) of axons of the three major types of extrinsic cortico-cortical connections (feedforward, feedback, and lateral). Numbers refer to cortical layers.

supragranular layers (layers 2 and 3) reveal that there is a continuum in the organization of feedback and feedforward connections instead of two homogeneous populations (Barone *et al.* 2000). Although this has not been quantified, it appears that a similar continuum is found when the depth level of axonal arborization is considered. As argued earlier (Salin and Bullier 1995), the archetypal organization of feedback connection (neurons in infragranular layers providing input into layers 1 and 2) is only found for connections between areas that are distant on the cortical surface and in the hierarchy of cortical areas. In contrast, feedback connections between neighbouring areas, which are extremely numerous, do not follow the archetypal model and originate from neurons in supra- as well as infragranular layers and terminate in all layers except the lower portion of layer 4. Such is the case for the very dense feedback connections from area V2 to V1 in the monkey (Kennedy and Bullier 1985; Kennedy *et al.* 1989).

Interhemispheric connections have morphological characteristics that class them in the feedforward group for the laminar position of the source neurons (in layers 2 and 3) and in the feedforward or feedback connections for the distributions of the axon terminals. In fact, the organization of axon terminals in interhemispheric connections tends to follow that of intrahemispheric connections. In general, a given area connects to the same areas in the same and in the opposite cortical hemipheres and the laminar distributions of the terminals are similar for inter- and intrahemispheric connections (Kennedy *et al.* 1991).

Retinotopic organization

All anatomical studies show an important degree of convergence and divergence in cortico-cortical connections. Typically, a cortical zone a few hundred microns wide projects to and receives from a region that is usually of the order of a few millimetres wide, but can cover up to 15 mm on the cortical surface of a connected area (see review in Salin and Bullier 1995). This important degree of convergence and divergence has consequences for the retinotopic organization of cortico-cortical connections.

It is usually assumed that all connections in the visual system are retinotopically organized, meaning that the receptive field (RF) centres of the afferent neurons are included in the RF centre of the recipient cell. This appears to be the case for a number of connections such as the thalamocortical connections (Reid and Alonso 1995; Tanaka 1983), but cannot be true for all types of cortico-cortical connections because of the large difference in RF sizes between the neurons in some interconnected areas. Mapping studies in the cat (Price *et al.* 1994; Sherk and Ombrellaro 1988) and inactivation studies in the monkey (Girard and Bullier 1989; Girard *et al.* 1991*a,b*) have revealed that feedforward connections are retinotopically organized, i.e. the RF centre of the recipient cell corresponds to the sum of the RF centres of the afferent feedforward connections (Fig. 2.4).

Because the RF centres of neurons tend to increase in size as one moves away from area V1, it is clear that the feedback connections cannot be organized in a similar fashion. Earlier mapping studies showed that the organization of feedback connections is compatible with the rule that neurons tend to interconnect if their RF centres overlap at least partially (Salin *et al.* 1992). As a consequence, the extent of visual field represented by the feedback connections corresponds to the sum of twice the average diameter of the RF centre in the source area and the average RF centre in the recipient area (Fig. 2.4). Given that some projections to area V1 in the macaque come from inferotemporal cortex neurons (Kennedy and Bullier 1985; Rockland *et al.* 1994), which have very large receptive fields, it is evident that such connections enable V1 neurons to be influenced by information coming from the highest stages of processing and concerning very large portions of the visual field.

In a similar way, but to a much smaller scale, the horizontal connections link together neurons with neighbouring and partially overlapping receptive fields. The region of the visual field covered by the horizontal connection array approximately corresponds to the point image (the average scatter of RF centres plus the average RF

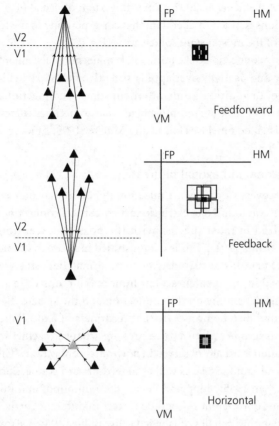

Fig. 2.4 Retinotopic organization of feedforward, feedback, and horizontal connections. The left part of the figure represents schematically areas V1 and V2 seen from above. Triangles correspond to neuron cell bodies. The direction of the connection is indicated by the arrows on the simplified axons. On the right is represented the right lower visual field of the animal (FP, fixation point; HM, horizontal meridian; VM, vertical meridian). For the feedforward connections, the large square represents the receptive field (RF) centre of the V2 neuron receiving convergent information from the V1 neurons that have the small black squares as RF centres. The combination of RF centres of the afferent V1 neurons make up the RF centre of the target V2 neuron: feedforward connections are visuotopically organized. For the feedback connections, the small black square represents the RF centre of the V1 neuron receiving convergent information from V2 neurons with the large open squares as RF centres. The RF centres of V2 neurons cover a larger region of visual field than that covered by the RF centre of their target neuron in area V1. The feedback connections are only loosely retinotopic and can be used to mix information from distant regions of the visual field. For the horizontal connection, the grey square represents the RF centre of the V1 neuron receiving convergent horizontal connections from neighbouring neurons with RF centres indicated by the black square. The combination of the horizontal afferents covers a larger part of the visual field than the RF centre of the target neuron. Horizontal connections are loosely retinotopic.

centre diameter; Angeluci *et al.* 2002). Thus, the extent of visual field concerned with the local connections is much smaller than that corresponding to the feedback connections from some of the most distant source areas (Fig. 2.4).

Interhemispheric connections, like horizontal connections, also interconnect neurons with overlapping and partially overlapping receptive fields, particularly around the vertical meridian. In addition, some interhemispheric connections appear to link together neurons with separate receptive fields that sometimes correspond to mirror images in both visual hemifields (Houzel and Milleret 1999; Innocenti 1986; Kennedy *et al.* 1991).

Patchy organization and axonal bifurcation

Following the discovery of patchy organization in horizontal connections (Rockland and Lund 1982), it was found that extrinsic cortico-cortical connections also tend to be similarly organized in most species, with the possible exception of the mouse (Braitenberg and Schüz 1991). This is demonstrated in neuroanatomical tracing studies that show that neurons retrogradely filled by a small deposit of retrograde tracer tend to be grouped in small patches a few hundred microns wide and separated by 500–1000 microns depending on the connection and the species. Results of anterograde tracer studies also demonstrate that terminals of axons labelled by a small amount of tracer placed in a given cortical area are grouped together in small patches.

Patchy arborization is usually observed in horizontal connections (Gilbert and Wiesel 1983; Rockland and Lund 1982), as well as in feedforward connections (Bullier 1984; DeYoe and Van Essen 1985; Shipp and Zeki 1985; Symmonds and Rosenquist 1984). Coupled injections of different retrograde tracers in different cortical areas produce mostly non-overlapping patches of labelled cells (Bullier 1984; DeYoe and Van Essen 1985; Shipp and Zeki 1985), with very few double labelled cells in the regions of overlap. This suggests that a given cortical area sends feedforward connections to several other areas through a system of interdigitating neuronal patches that probably share common functional properties and are interconnected by patchy horizontal connections. Although less frequently demonstrated because of the small number of studies using coupled anterograde tracers, patches of terminal axons also appear to segregate at least partially in the target area for feedforward and interhemispheric connections (Goldman-Rakic and Schwartz 1982; Morel and Bullier 1990).

It is likely that the patchy organization and lack of axonal bifurcation in feedforward connections is the mark of the functional specificity of such connections. This is suggested by the results of Movshon and Newsome (1996) who demonstrated that the V1 neurons projecting to area MT (middle temporal) belong to a specific type with homogeneous properties. This result is comparable to that of an earlier work by Henry and his collaborators (1978) that also demonstrated the specific functional properties of neurons projecting from area 17 to the posterior mediolateral suprasylvian sulcus (PMLS) in the cat. The patchy distribution of feedforward terminals presumably results from the convergence of axon terminals coming from neurons with some common functional properties. This is suggested by the elegant experiments of Sherk in the lateral suprasylvian sulcus (LS) area (slightly larger area than area PMLS in Fig. 2.1; Sherk 1990). Using a neurotoxin, she killed the neurons in a small region of that area and recorded from what presumably corresponds to the terminals of afferent axons. She found that axons tend to group together according to the direction selectivity, thus suggesting that neurons with the same optimal direction tend to terminate in common patches. The neurons innervated by this axon group presumably inherit the property of direction selectivity transmitted by the converging feedforward axons.

The prevalence of patchy organization is more variable for feedback connections. In general, when relatively extensive injections of retrograde tracers are placed in a given area, neurons in extrastriate areas do not group themselves in well-defined patches as in the case of feedforward connections (Kennedy and Bullier 1985; Perkel et al. 1986). On the other hand, more localized injections in the supragranular layers produce patchy distributions of retrogradely labelled cells in supragranular layers (Salin et al. 1994; Shipp and Grant 1991). Similarly, injections of anterograde tracers produce patchy distributions of terminals, particularly in the supragranular layers (Henry et al. 1991; Salin et al. 1994; Wong-Riley 1979b), whereas a continuous distribution of anterograde labelling has been reported on other occasions (Maunsell and Van Essen 1983; Ungerleider and Desimone 1986).

The major reason for the larger variability of the results concerning the patchy distribution of feedback compared to feedforward connections may be that there is more variability in the laminar distribution of axon terminals in feedback than in feedforward connections. Indeed, direct comparisons of labelled cells or axon terminals distributions in different layers for feedback connections show that patchy distributions exist in the connections between supragranular layers, whereas connections from infragranular layers appear to be less segregated, and afferent terminals in the lamina 1 always arborize in a diffuse manner (Henry et al. 1991; Salin et al. 1992; Shipp and Grant 1991). Similar differences between the topographic organizations of terminals in different laminae are also observed when individual axonal arbors are traced in the target area, as demonstrated by the work of Rockland and colleagues (Rockland and Drash 1996; Rockland et al. 1994).

It is interesting that the laminar differences observed for the patchy character of feedback connections are echoed by similar differences in the pattern of axonal bifurcation. Thus, in feedback connections, the proportion of neurons sending bifurcating axons to two cortical areas is higher in infragranular than in the supragranular layers (Bullier and Kennedy 1987). Also, the results of Rockland and her associates (1994) demonstrate that some feedback axons have long axonal collaterals in layer 1 that arborize extensively over at least two cortical areas, whereas terminals in supragranular layers are restricted to one cortical area.

This difference in organization across layers suggests that, for a given set of feedback connections between two areas, different roles are played by different subsets of connections corresponding to different laminar distributions in the source and target areas. Thus, the variability of laminar distribution among feedback connections between areas at different distances on the cortical surface (see the section 'Definitions') may correspond to different functional roles played by distant feedback connections (for example TE to V1) compared to those between adjacent areas (like V2 to V1).

Assuming that the patchy and unbranched nature of feedforward connections reflects the necessity to organize inputs according to specific properties, the more diffuse character of the feedback connections to layer 1 suggests that it plays a more general role such as controlling the contrast gain or membrane potential of target neurons. Such a general role cannot be extended to all feedback connections because feedback connections to layers 2 and 3, with their patchy organization, probably play a very specific role in the processing of visual information (see below).

What differentiates neurons with axonal bifurcation to several cortical areas from neurons that project to only one cortical area? This question is particularly interesting for the feedback connections from the infragranular layers that contain a sizeable proportion of axonal bifurcation (Bullier and Kennedy 1987). It is possible that such bifurcation concerns preferentially axons with fast conduction velocity. As shown by modelling studies (Murre and Sturdy 1995), axon size is under strong constraints in the brain of large mammals. Projection of thick axons to several areas by way of bifurcation is one way of limiting their number. Indeed, there are many examples of thick axons that bifurcate. Y cells in the cat lateral geniculate nucleus (LGN) that have the largest axons send bifurcation to areas 17 and 18 (Bullier and Kennedy 1987) and Meynert cells in layer 6 of area V1 send bifurcating axons to at least area MT and the superior colliculus (Fries *et al.* 1985). In functional terms, the bifurcation of thick axons to several cortical areas is an efficient way to rapidly and simultaneously coactivate several cortical areas.

Synaptic transmission

Reports of electron microscopy (EM) studies on cortico-cortical connections all agree that such connections make excitatory synapses on their target neurons (Anderson *et al.* 1998; Gonchar and Burkhalter 1999; Johnson and Burkhalter 1996; Lowenstein and Somogyi 1991). Given the laminar and morphological differences between feedforward and feedback connections reviewed above, it is expected that the synaptic organization of these different sets of connections will also show differences. The morphology of feedforward connections from V1 to V5 was recently investigated by Anderson and his collaborators (1998). Terminal boutons formed asymmetric (presumably excitatory) synapses and tended to contact preferentially spiny neurons (excitatory, mostly pyramidal), but also terminated on smooth, presumably inhibitory, cells in 20% of the cases. Very similar proportions were reported by Lowenstein and Somogyi (1991) in their study of the feedforward projection from area 17 to PMLS in the cat, an area that has been considered homologous to area MT of primates (Payne 1993). In a study of feedforward connections between visual cortical areas in the rat, Johnson and Burkhalter (1996) reported a smaller proportion of contacts on to synaptic shafts (10%).

Less is known concerning the synaptic organization of feedback connections. The early results of Johnson and Burkhalter (1996) suggested that feedback connections contact more specifically spines of pyramidal cells (98% of the cases) and rarely terminate on dendritic shafts. However, a more recent report by the same group found similar proportions of terminals on parvalbumin-rich GABAergic interneurons (10%) in feedforward and in feedback connections in the rat visual system (Gonchar and Burkhalter 1999). Differences were found in the site of termination, with feedback connections terminating on distal parts of the dendrites of GABAergic parvalbumin-rich interneurons whereas feedforward connections contact dendritic regions closer to the cell body (Gonchar and Burkhalter 1999). This is in keeping with functional data from the same group showing that feedback connections have mostly an excitatory influence, whereas electrical stimulation of intrinsic and feedforward connections tend to recruit inhibitory circuits at higher stimulus intensities (Shao and Burkhalter 1996). The latter results, however, should be treated with caution since electrical stimulation acts exclusively on axonal branches (Nowak and Bullier 1998a,b) and therefore stimulating in one area stimulates orthodromically the efferent axons as well as the afferent axons antidromically. It is impossible to differentiate the synaptic potentials evoked by direct orthodromic activation from those evoked by recurrent collaterals of antidromically activated axons. This confusion probably explains why the laminar pattern of electrical activation elicited in a given cortical area by electrical stimulation in another does not always fit with that predicted from the laminar distribution of axon terminals (Domenici et al. 1995; Nowak et al. 1997).

The low proportion of terminals on dendritic shafts reported for feedback connections by Burkhalter and his colleagues contrasts with the results of an earlier EM study of the feedback connections between areas 18 and 17 in the cat (Fisken et al. 1975). In that study the authors concluded that more than 30% of the terminals of feedback connections were located on dendritic shafts. Whether this discrepancy is related to a species difference or whether there is indeed a strong feedback projection to dendritic shafts remains to be determined by further studies.

Hierarchical organization of cortical areas

The classification of cortico-cortical connections in feedforward, feedback, and lateral connections led Maunsell and Van Essen (1983) to define a hierarchy of cortical areas on the basis of a simple rule: the areas are arranged in a series of levels defined by their connections with each other. At the lowest level is found the area that receives only feedback connections and sends only feedforward connections to other areas (area V1 in the monkey, area 17 in the cat). At the next level is found V2 which receives feedforward connections from V1 but receives only feedback connections from other areas. Above V2 is found V3 which receives feedforward connections from V1 and V2 and feedback connections from other areas. In addition, it is possible for two areas to belong to the same level if they exchange lateral connections.

It is remarkable that this simple set of rules is in most cases internally consistent. If area A sends feedforward connections to area B, then area B sends feedback connections to area A; if area A sends lateral connections to B, B sends lateral connections to A. A small number of exceptions have been noted (Felleman and Van Essen 1991). Applying these rules to the areas of the macaque monkey initially generated the pattern shown in Fig. 2.5(a). More recent versions (Fig. 2.5(b)) have a similar organization but become more complicated as more connections have been discovered (DeYoe *et al.* 1994; Felleman and Van Essen 1991).

This method helps in organizing the large number of cortical areas of the monkey visual system in a small number of distinct levels but it has two disadvantages: (1) it is an anatomical classification that says little about the functional interactions between the areas (we will come back to this question below); (2) it is largely underdetermined as pointed out by Malcolm Young and his associates (Hilgetag *et al.* 1996). This means that the set of rules used to construct the hierarchy leads to many different ways of classifying cortical areas in different levels. Optimal solutions lead to smaller numbers of rule violations, but it is impossible to claim that one configuration is optimal because of the lack of knowledge concerning many connections. As shown in Fig. 2.5(c), the consequence of the underdetermined character of the hierarchical scheme is that a given cortical area such as area MT can occupy levels 5–10. As a consequence, for most pairs of cortical areas beyond V1, V2, and V3, it is difficult to determine whether one area is at a lower or at a higher level, or whether they belong to the same level in the hierarchy.

An attempt has been made recently to reduce this underdetermined character by quantifying the proportions of source neurons in supragranular versus infragranular layers (Barone *et al.* 2000). When this is done, a reasonably good match to the original hierarchy of Felleman and Van Essen is obtained and, provided a few adjustments are made, the proportion of labelled neurons in supragranular layers is a good predictor of the hierarchical level (Fig. 2.6). However, when Figs 2.5 and 2.6 are compared, there are discrepancies between the levels at which a given area belongs. Note, for example, how the FEF belongs to the highest level in the original map (Fig. 2.5(a)), to the eighth level in the 1991 version (Fig. 2.5(b)), and is brought down to the fourth level when attention is paid to the proportions of supragranular layer neurons (Fig. 2.6).

The underdetermined character and the variability of classification of different schemes shown in Figs 2.5 and 2.6 suggest that caution should be applied when attempts are made at deriving functional interpretations from the hierarchical classification. Furthermore, as mentioned below (see section on timing), the latencies of neurons in different cortical areas cannot be predicted from the hierarchy of cortical areas, as would be expected if the hierarchical organization corresponded to a functional model with a succession of processing stages along the hierarchy.

Another interpretation of the laminar organization of neurons and axon terminals of different cortico-cortical connections has been proposed by Barbas (Barbas 1986; Barbas and Rempel-Clower 1997) for the connections in the monkey frontal cortex.

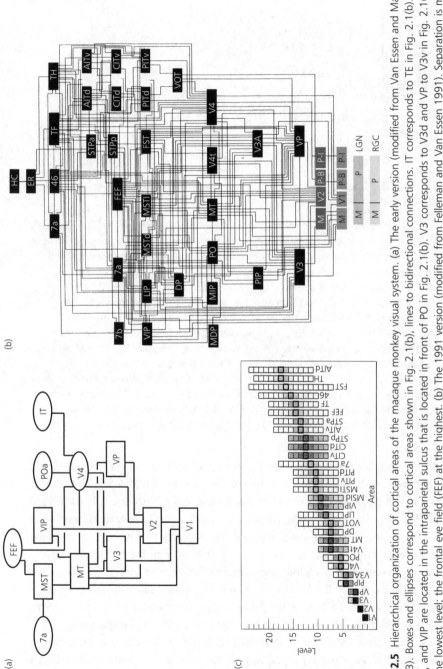

Fig. 2.5 Hierarchical organization of cortical areas of the macaque monkey visual system. (a) The early version (modified from Van Essen and Maunsell 1983). Boxes and ellipses correspond to cortical areas shown in Fig. 2.1(b), lines to bidirectional connections. IT corresponds to TE in Fig. 2.1(b). 7a, POa, and VIP are located in the intraparietal sulcus that is located in front of PO in Fig. 2.1(b). V3 corresponds to V3d and VP to V3v in Fig. 2.1(b). V1 is at the lowest level; the frontal eye field (FEF) at the highest. (b) The 1991 version (modified from Felleman and Van Essen 1991). Separation is made between magno- and parvocellular layers in the LGN (M and P) and in the retinal ganglion cells (RGC). In V1 the magno stream (M) is separated from the parvo-blob (P-B) and the parvo-interblob (P-I) streams (see Fig. 2.8 for a more up-to-date version of the streams in areas V1 and V2). At the highest level are found the hippocampal formation (HC) and the entorhinal cortex (ER). The frontal eye field (FEF) is at 7 levels above V1. (c) Underdetermined character of the hierarchical levels for different cortical areas. Each area (except V1 and V2) can occupy several different levels. This uncertainty reflects the poor knowledge of the type (feedforward, feedback, lateral) of many connections in the visual system. (Modified from Hilgetag et al. 1996.)

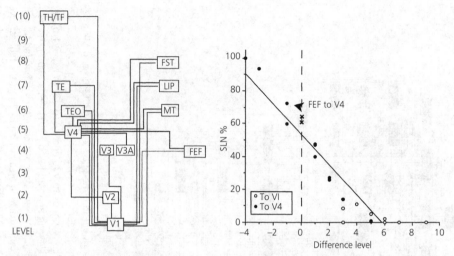

Fig. 2.6 Correlation between hierarchical levels and the proportion of neurons in supragranular layers (layers 2 and 3) participating in different types of connections. The scattergram on the right illustrates the proportion of supragranular layer neurons (SLN) for connections linking different levels of the modified hierarchy shown on the left (negative difference levels correspond to feedforward and positive values to feedback connections). Connections with negative difference levels contain high proportions of supragranular layer neurons, which corresponds to the fact that feedforward connections are mostly made by these neurons (Fig. 2.3). Horizontal connections (crosses) contain about 60% supragranular neurons. Feedback connections from distant sources (high positive difference levels) are made almost exclusively by infragranular layer neurons (as indicated by the low proportions of supragranular layer neurons). On the left is shown the hierarchical organization modified to fit the linear relationship between proportion of supragranular layer neurons and difference level. The main difference with the original hierarchy (Fig. 2.5(b)) is in the low level of FEF and the higher level of MT compared to V4. (Modified from Barone *et al.* 2000; left side modified from Felleman and Van Essen 1991.)

This author claims that the laminar organization of a given connection can be predicted from the structure of the source and target areas. Most sensory areas have a classic organization with six layers and a well identified layer 4 (or granular layer). In the frontal cortex, there are also 'agranular' areas, lacking the characteristic layer 4, and several areas belonging to the limbic type of cortex with a dense population of neurons in the deep layers. It has been argued that evolutionary steps can be identified by the structural character of different cortical regions, from ancient limbic-type cortex to more recent granular cortex (Sanides 1970). Barbas shows that the laminar distributions of neurons of origin and the terminal arbors in the projection area are related to the difference in structure between the source and target area. Thus, areas of the granular type project from the supragranular layers and send terminals mostly in the middle and deep layers of less laminated areas, whereas the return projections originate from the deep layers and preferentially target the upper layers (Barbas and Rempel-Clower 1997). Thus the differences between feedforward and feedback connections in occipital, parietal, and temporal cortex may simply reflect differences in organization between sensory cortices of the occipital cortex with well differentiated structures (areas V1 and V2) and areas with less differentiated structures in the parietal and temporal cortices. One advantage of this model is that it predicts the observed progressive shift toward projections from infragranular layers terminating at higher levels in the target area with increasing distance (in terms of levels of organization that reflect distance on the cortical surface). The interpretation of laminar organization of cortico-cortical connections in terms of the phylogenetic evolution of cortex is supported by the results from development studies that show major reorganizations of this organization during pre- and postnatal development (see the section 'Development of cortico-cortical connections').

Functional streams and channels in feedforward cortico-cortical connections

The extensive array of connections between cortical areas shown in Fig. 2.5(b) contains a number of streams or channels that group some connections together. The idea of functional streams goes back to the classification of retinal ganglion cells and thalamocortical neurons. In the 1970s, the population of cat retinal ganglion cells was subdivided into X and Y and W cells. Each of these classes was found to be connected to different neuronal subgroups in the LGN and cortex (Stone 1983). Subsequently, a similar division was found in the retinogeniculostriate system of monkeys with the characterization of magnocellular, parvocellular, and koniocellular streams in the retinogeniculate system (Hendry and Reid 2000; Hendry and Yoshioka 1994; Merigan and Maunsell 1991).

Another functional subdivision of the visual system was proposed at the same period— that between structures subserving form and space vision. The separation between space and form vision was already present in the early models of the visual system based on the study of non-primate species, with the superior colliculus involved in space vision and the visual cortex dealing with form vision (Schneider 1969). A similar distinction was made between structures dealing with focal and ambient vision (Trevarthen 1968). Since the beginning of the twentieth century, it was known that, in humans, lesions in the parietal and temporal cortex lead to deficits in space and form vision, respectively. All these ideas were synthesized in the concept of two functional streams in the primate visual cortex, with the ventral occipitotemporal stream dealing with form vision and the dorsal occipitoparietal stream involved in space vision. The success of this subdivision was established by the demonstration in the monkey of a double dissociation of the effects of lesions in the parietal and inferotemporal cortex (Pohl 1973) that mirrored the clinical observations in humans, and by the tracing of anatomical connections between striate cortex and parietal and inferotemporal cortex (Ungerleider and Mishkin 1982). The segregation of cortical connections into dorsal and ventral streams was confirmed by the results of mathematical models grouping together the densest connections between different cortical areas of the monkey (Jouve et al. 1998; Young 1992).

Since then, questions have been raised concerning the roles of the two cortical streams. The initial idea was that the dorsal stream is involved in processing *where* an object is located in the visual field, whereas the ventral stream is engaged in the recognition of objects (the 'where/what' of Ungerleider and Mishkin 1982). More recently, the emphasis has shifted to the visuomotor aspects of processing in the dorsal stream. In addition to dealing with where an object is located, the dorsal stream is important for grasping and manipulating an object (Goodale and Milner 1992; Jeannerod *et al.* 1995). Despite these evolutions, the basic idea that parietal and inferotemporal cortices deal with different aspects of vision has stood the test of time. More recent work showed that the two streams remain partially separate in the frontal cortex and that there are regions of convergence in frontal cortex and in the depths of the superior temporal sulcus (Baizer *et al.* 1991; Bullier *et al.* 1996; Morel and Bullier 1990). Various diagrams of the two visual streams are presented in Fig. 2.7.

The two visual streams have been integrated in the hierarchical organization of cortical areas: in the diagrams of Van Essen and his colleagues, the ventral stream is to the right and the dorsal stream to the left (Fig. 2.5(b)), whereas they are located above each other in the Ungerleider and Desimone's version of the hierarchy (Fig. 2.7(b)).

In 1984, in a sweeping synthesis, Livingstone and Hubel attempted to combine together the magno/parvo subdivision in retino-thalamo-cortical pathways and the two cortical visual streams in primates. The impetus behind this new synthesis was the discovery of the subdivisions in V1 and V2 revealed by reacting the tissue for cytochrome oxidase, a metabolic enzyme sensitive to neural activity (Wong-Riley 1979*a*). This showed the presence of cytochrome oxidase-rich blobs in V1 (Horton and Hubel 1981) and the thin, thick, and pale cytochrome oxidase bands in V2 (Livingstone and Hubel 1984, 1987*a*). Cytochrome oxidase bands in V2 became particularly important when it was demonstrated that they mark the territories providing inputs to the dorsal and ventral streams (Fig. 2.8). The thick cytochrome oxidase bands in V2 were found to project to area MT and from there to the dorsal stream. The thin and pale bands project to V4 (DeYoe and Van Essen 1985; Shipp and Zeki 1985) that constitutes the entry to the ventral stream (Fig. 2.8). The interconnections between these different territories were thought to be minimal, suggesting the presence of two (or three) parallel and independent cortical channels beginning in V2. The story became even more interesting when Hubel and Livingstone showed that the blobs in V1 project to the thin bands in V2, whereas the interblob regions in layers 2–3 of V1 project to the pale bands of V2. Finally, layer 4B in V1 projects to the thick bands in V2 that relay information to area MT (Fig. 2.8). Although connections between them have since been demonstrated (Levitt *et al.* 1994; Yoshioka *et al.* 1994), these channels are usually considered as transferring information in parallel from V1 to areas V4 and MT, in a manner similar to that of the parallel channels through the LGN.

Because it was thought at the time that blobs and interblobs receive exclusively parvocellular inputs, Livingstone and Hubel proposed that the parvo/magno division in the LGN continues in the cortex, with the parvocellular neurons driving the ventral

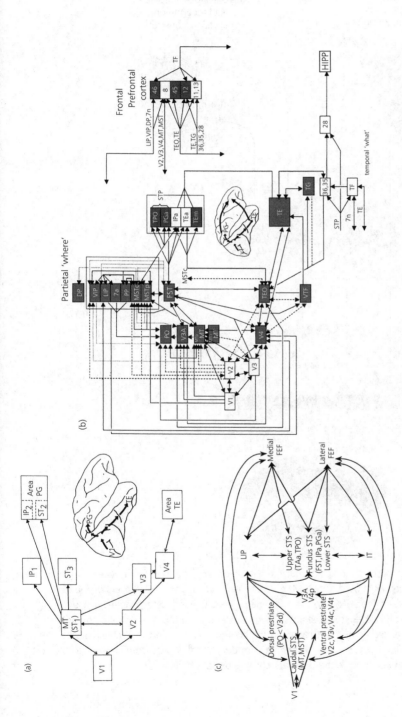

Fig. 2.7 The two visual streams story. (a) The original version (modified from (Ungerleider 1985). (b) The more recent version (modified from http://lbc.nimh.nih.gov/people/ungerleider/ungerlei.html). The ventral stream is below; the dorsal stream above. Successive levels in the hierarchy are found as one progresses from left to right. To the right are illustrated the connections with the frontal cortex. (c) A simplified version of the two-streams story, emphasizing the links between the two streams and the connections with the frontal eye field (FEF; modified from Bullier *et al.* 1996). STS, superior temporal sulcus; LIP, lateral intraparietal area (also called POa by some authors); IT, inferotemporal cortex (corresponds to TE). IPa, PGa, TPO, TAa are found in the depths of the superior temporal sulcus; V4c and V4p correspond to the regions of V4 coding central and peripheral visual fields; same convention for V2c. This diagram shows that the two streams communicate mostly through the depths of the superior temporal sulcus and areas V3A and V4. Note also that the ventral stream connects to the lateral FEF, whereas the dorsal stream projects to the medial and lateral FEF.

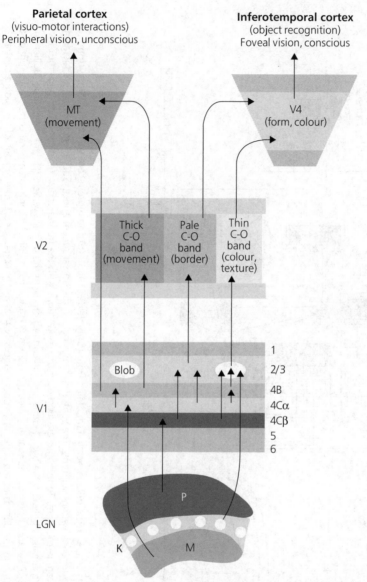

Fig. 2.8 The magno-, parvo-, and koniocellular streams. For simplicity, only feedforward connections have been illustrated. P and M, parvocellular and magnocellular layers of the LGN. K, koniocellular layers of the LGN, also called interlaminar. C-O band, cytochrome-oxidase band. Note that beyond the first stages in V1 (layer 4Cα and β), the magno, parvo, and konio streams are no longer segregated as they are in the LGN. Note also that the parietal cortex is mostly under the influence of the magno stream with direct connections from layer 4B to MT and indirect connections through the thick cytochrome oxidase bands.

stream with a blob–thin band–area V4 channel devoted to colour and an interblob–pale band–area V4 channel devoted to form, whereas the dorsal stream is activated by the magnocellular system and processes movement and depth in the visual field (Livingstone and Hubel 1987*b*).

As shown in Fig. 2.8, the presently accepted scheme of connections is slightly more complicated: the cytochrome oxidase blobs in V1 are driven by magno, parvo, and konio layers of the LGN and the magno stream also drives cells in the interblob regions (Callaway 1998; Nealey and Maunsell 1994). Furthermore, it was shown that cells in V4 are activated by magno as well as parvocellular cells of the LGN (Ferrera *et al.* 1994). Thus, it is clear that the ventral stream receives input from all three LGN channels. On the other hand, it appears that the dorsal stream is mainly under the influence of the magno stream, as shown by the anatomy (Fig. 2.8) and by functional experiments (Maunsell *et al.* 1990).

The idea of separate channels for colour and form across V1, V2, and V4 has not been confirmed by subsequent studies. Although some specific types of colour-selective cell are probably restricted to the thin cytochrome oxidase bands in V2, selectivity for the colour of the stimulus is found in all subdivisions in V1 and V2. In fact, the published accounts of quantitative measurements of different receptive field properties (colour, orientation, depth selectivity) have concluded that these different selectivities are distributed among the different channels with little evidence for specificity (Peterhans 1997; Salin and Bullier 1995). The functional significance of these well defined anatomical structures remains therefore a mystery. It has been proposed recently that the pale cytochrome oxidase bands may be involved in form vision (Heider 2000; Zeki 1993). The support for this hypothesis comes from clinical observations of the deficits of patients with carbon monoxide poisoning. These patients appear to suffer from a selective deficit of form vision that could be due to a selective lesion in the pale bands that would be less protected from the effects of hypoxia than the cytochrome-oxidase-rich thin and thick bands. The role of pale bands in form vision is further supported by the observation that they contain numerous neurons selective for occlusion cues (Peterhans and Heydt 1993). The involvement in form vision of the interblob–pale bands–V4 channel is in keeping with the role of boundary contour system attributed to it by Grossberg (1994) who suggested that the blob–thin band–V4 system would be involved in surface filling-in and that the thick band–MT system deals with detection of motion boundaries. The shorter latencies to visual stimulation observed in the pale and thick cytochrome oxidase bands compared to thin bands (Munk 1995*a*) would be consistent with the necessity to determine the boundaries of objects before surface filling-in takes place.

Functional roles of feedforward and feedback connections

Feedforward connections

A number of functional studies have attempted to discover the role of feedforward connections by reversible inactivation. In the cat, the early work was intended to test to what extent the organization of the cat visual system differs from that of primates. In cats, as in other non-primate mammalian species, inactivating or lesioning area 17 does not lead to a complete cessation of visual responses in other visual cortical areas (see Bullier et al. 1994 and Salin and Bullier 1995 for review) in contrast to the results reported in monkeys (see later in this section).

The specific role of the feedforward connections from area 17 to area 18 cells in the cat was assessed by methods comparing visual responses before and during reversible inactivation of area 17. Inactivation of a large region of area 17 produced a general decrease of visual responses in numerous BA18 neurons, with a few specific effects (Sherk 1978). In particular, it was noted that the effects of area 17 inactivation were more pronounced for low stimulus velocities, in keeping with the finding of Dreher and Cottee (1975) that cells in area 18 are tuned to higher velocities after lesion of area 17. These results suggest that area 17, which contains cells tuned to lower velocities than area 18 (Orban et al. 1981), potentiates the responses of A18 neurons to low-velocity stimuli.

Similar methods were used to investigate the role of feedforward connections from area 17 to area 21a in the cat (Wimborne and Henry 1992). Inactivation of a large region of area 17 led to a strong decrease of response of many area 21a neurons and a complete silencing of others. It is quite remarkable that the orientation selectivities of the neurons in area 21a were retained even when the inactivation of area 17 led to an almost total cessation of the responses. This suggests that area 17 neurons providing feedforward connections to area 21 are very homogeneous in their orientation selectivity, a likely possibility in view of the results obtained in the monkey (Movshon and Newsome 1996). There is also the possibility that specific mechanisms strengthen orientation selectivity within area 21a.

Some of the recent studies have used more localized inactivation techniques and their conclusions point to a specific role for feedforward connections. Molotchnikoff and his colleagues presented evidence for changes in direction selectivity in many 'simple' cells in area 18 during inactivation of a small zone of area 17 a few hundred microns wide. In most cases, this effect was due to a selective decrease of the response to the optimal direction and in a few cases to an increase in the non-preferred direction (Casanova et al. 1992). They also demonstrated that local inactivation of area 17 produced changes in orientation tuning curves in A18 neurons and that the effects were specific for the cell type ('simple' or 'complex' cells) (Chabli et al. 1998). Such results confirm that feedforward connections can have a very strong driving input into cortical neurons and that they are organized in a precise column-to-column fashion. It is, however, difficult to deduce from these studies that specific properties such as direction or orientation selectivity are set up by feedforward inputs from 17 to 18. Indeed, the reported changes with localized inactivation of A17 could be due to a loss of balance between the excitatory inputs coming from different columns in area 17 converging on the recorded neuron in area 18.

The driving role of feedforward connections in the cat is confirmed by the work of Vanduffel and collaborators (1997). In awake cats, they used radioactive 2-deoxyglucose to assess the residual neural activity in visual areas during reversible inactivation by cooling of cortical areas in the suprasylvian sulcus. The results show strong decreases of activity in areas that receive feedforward connections from areas of the suprasylvian sulcus, in contrast to areas receiving feedback connections that show a smaller decrease of activity.

In the monkey, our knowledge of the role of feedforward connections is mostly derived from the results of reversible inactivation or lesions in area V1 and their effects on responses in other cortical areas. In contrast to the results obtained in the cat, inactivation or lesion of V1 leads to a complete cessation of activity in a number of cortical areas, such as area V2, V3, V4, and the inferotemporal cortex (see review by Bullier *et al.* 1994). These areas belong mostly to the ventral or occipitotemporal stream that channels information from V1 to the inferotemporal cortex. In contrast, areas of the dorsal occipitoparietal stream remain visually responsive in the absence of input from area 17. At least in the case of area MT, the residual input is channelled through the superior colliculus (see review in Bullier *et al.* 1994).

The present consensus is that feedforward connections carry the drive of lower-order areas and that the selectivities of neurons in higher-order areas result mostly from the converging feedforward inputs of neurons in lower-order areas. This is well illustrated by the study of Movshon and Newsome (1996) who found that the neurons in V1 that project to area MT have receptive fields exactly superimposed on those of the recipient neurons. A similar result had also been found earlier for cortico-cortical connections in the cat (Bullier *et al.* 1988; Henry *et al.* 1978). Such electrical stimulation studies also produced interesting results concerning the cell types that project to a given area. Both in the cat (Henry *et al.* 1978) and in the monkey (Movshon and Newsome 1996), the neurons that send feedforward connections away from area V1 appear to belong to a relatively homogeneous population of neurons in terms of functional properties. The results of Sherk (1990) on the patchy organization of area 17 inputs to PMLS described above are also consistent with such a role of convergent feedforward inputs.

This suggests that feedforward connections are important for carrying the visual drive from one neuronal population to the next and that their arrangement is important for shaping the selectivities of neurons in higher-order areas. Thus, feedforward connections belong to the 'driver' category of the classification of connections by Sherman and Guillery (1998) and Crick and Koch (1998).

It should be noted, however, that the selective properties of cortical neurons are not entirely explained by the properly arranged convergence of feedforward connections. This question has been central to the controversy concerning the mechanisms underlying orientation and direction selectivity of area 17 neurons. Do they result mostly from the arrangement of their thalamic inputs as predicted by Hubel and Wiesel (1962), or are they mainly shaped by the local network of horizontal connections? Until recently, the presence of inhibitory inputs to cortical neurons proved to be elusive and it was thought that the orientation selectivity in area 17 neurons results mainly from the convergence of excitatory thalamic inputs (Douglas *et al.* 1991; Ferster *et al.* 1996; Hubel 1996). This has changed with the discovery of strong shunting inhibitory inputs into cortical cells (Borg-Graham *et al.* 1998) and the demonstration that local cortical inactivation has strong and specific effects on the orientation tuning curves of cortical cells (Crook *et al.* 1997). The results of Grinvald's group with optical imaging techniques are also consistent with a major role for local horizontal connections. They showed that a cortical neuron gives spikes when the network of interconnected cortical patches in area 17 is activated. Most remarkably, this was observed for visually driven as well as for spontaneous activity (Tsodyks *et al.* 1999). This suggests that local horizontal connections have a major impact on the excitability of cortical neurons and that the response of a neuron in area 17 cannot simply be explained by the simultaneous firing of afferent thalamic neurons. Instead, it appears that the cortical network governs the excitability of the cell and that the thalamic input plays the role of a trigger. It remains to be seen if similar mechanisms are at play between feedforward, horizontal, and feedback cortico-cortical connections.

Feedback connections

Effects on responses to RF centre stimulation

Fewer experiments have been devoted to feedback connections. Several groups have inactivated large portions of a higher-order cortical area to assess the role of feedback connections in anaesthetized animals. All concluded that feedback connections mostly tend to facilitate the responses of neurons in lower-order areas. Sandell and Schiller (1982) inactivated by cooling a region of area V2 in the squirrel monkey and reported effects on a third of the neurons in area V1. Most effects were decreases of responses to visual stimulation and were strongest in the infragranular layers. These results are in keeping with those of Mignard and Malpeli (1991) who concluded that feedback connections from area 18 predominantly exert a facilitatory effect upon neurons in area 17 in the cat. Similar conclusions were reached by Dreher and his collaborators for the feedback connections from area 21a to area 17 in the cat (Wang *et al.* 2000) and our group for the feedback connections from area MT to areas VI, V2, and V3 in the monkey (Hupé *et al.* 1998). In general, effects were observed for a fraction of the population of recorded neurons (10–40%). In addition, no clear effects have been reported on orientation tuning curves during inactivation of higher-order areas (Wang *et al.* 2000).

Overall, inactivating feedback connections produces smaller effects than for feedforward connections: a smaller proportion of neurons are affected and the response changes are less dramatic. In no case does inactivation of a cortical area lead to a complete cessation of responses in an area receiving feedback connections, as was the case for feedforward connections to the ventral stream in the monkey. As mentioned above, a direct comparison between the effect of inactivating area PMLS on cortical areas receiving feedforward and feedback connections from that area has been made recently (Vanduffel *et al.* 1997). The results show that both feedforward and feedback connections have a net excitatory role on their target areas but the effects are stronger for areas receiving feedforward than for those receiving feedback connections.

Not only do feedback connections have a weaker effect on their target neurons than feedforward connections, they also do not appear to be able to drive neurons in the absence of a feedforward drive. Several lines of evidence support this conclusion. There is a complete lack of responses of neurons in V2 to visual stimulation when V1 is inactivated in the monkey (Girard and Bullier 1989; Schiller and Malpeli 1977). Although there are strong feedback projections from area MT to V2 (Kennedy and Bullier 1985), and numerous MT neurons, remain visually responsive when V1 is inactivated (Girard *et al.* 1992; Rodman *et al.* 1989), these feedback connections appear unable to drive V2 neurons when they are deprived of their feedforward drive from V1. Another line of evidence comes from the observation that the potentiating effect of feedback connections is present only for the excitatory centre of the receptive field (Hupé *et al.* 2001*b*), which presumably reflects the converging feedforward inputs, despite the wide spatial convergence of feedback connections (Fig. 2.4).

Such a nonlinear interaction between feedforward and feedback connections is also suggested by the results of Mignard and Malpeli (1991) in the cat. They compared the effects of inactivating the A layers of the LGN on the responses of neurons in upper layers of area 17 when area 18 is intact or lesioned. When area 18 is intact, most neurons in the upper layers of area 17 retain a strong level of visual responses when the A layers are inactivated (Malpeli 1983). This contrasts with the strong decrease in visual responses of these neurons during inactivation of the A layers when area 18 had been lesioned (Mignard and Malpeli 1991). Without LGN blocking, direct inactivation of area 18 produces a mild response decrease in BA17cells (Sherk 1978). Thus, the feedforward input from the A layers of the LGN and the feedback input from area 18 each have a relatively weak influence on upper layer neurons of area 17 but their combination has a dramatic effect on the visual responses.

This suggests that feedback connections act by nonlinear mechanisms to potentiate the responses of neurons in lower-order areas. This effect is particularly evident for weak responses, as seen in intracellular recordings (Fig. 7 in Shao and Burkhalter 1999), as well as in extracellular recordings (Bullier *et al.* 2001). An interesting possibility is that this nonlinear mechanism is used to gate the flow of different circuits in lower-order areas, thus allowing higher-order areas to rapidly reorganize processing in lower-order areas.

More specific effects of feedback inactivation were demonstrated by Alonso and his collaborators (1993*a,b*) who blocked a small region of layer 5 of area 18 while recording in layer 5 of area 17 in the cat. The effects were strong and frequent when the authors inactivated area 18 neurons with overlapping receptive fields and the same properties as the recorded neurons in area 17. Effects were observed on the orientation tuning curves and on the speed selectivity of the neurons. Some were compatible with a facilitatory action of the feedback and other effects suggested an inhibitory effect. The specificity of the demonstrated effect was particularly striking in the case of speed selectivity. Alonso and co-workers (1993*a*) demonstrated that 40% of the neurons in layer 5 of area 17 increased their responses to high velocities when the corresponding region of layer 5 of area 18 was blocked. This result suggests that the selectivity for low-stimulus velocities of neurons in layer 5 of area 17 is due, at least in part, to an inhibitory input from area 18 neurons, which are known to respond to high velocities. Thus, at least in that particular case, feedback connections appear to play a role in sharpening the selectivity of neurons in another cortical area.

The results of Alonso and his colleagues make the important point that feedback connections can have very specific effects and are not limited to the diffuse and unselective role that is often attributed to them. Similar experiments conducted on the interactions between the upper layers of BA18 and the upper layers of area 17 produced more variable results (Martinez-Conde *et al.* 1999) on orientation tuning curves of area 17 neurons. As argued above for the work of Casanova *et al.* (1992) on feedforward connections, such results could be due to the fact that only a small region of area 18 was inactivated, thus possibly producing a loss of balance between different converging inputs.

Feedback influences on centre-surround interactions

So far, we have examined the contribution of feedback connections to the response of the RF centre. However, the important degree of spatial divergence and convergence of these connections (Fig. 2.4) suggests that they might regulate the strength of the centre-surround interactions. This is indeed what was found in our recent study on the role of feedback connections from area MT to areas V1, V2, and V3. Feedback connections appear to potentiate the strength of the inhibitory influence of the RF surround on the response generated by stimulating the RF centre (Bullier *et al.* 2001; Hupé *et al.* 1998). However, this effect was found to be specific for stimuli of low salience (a low-contrast bar moving on a noisy background). When the stimulus is of high salience (a high-contrast bar moving on a low-contrast noisy background), the contribution of the MT feedback to the centre-surround inhibitory interactions is small (Bullier *et al.* 2001; Hupé *et al.* 1998). This is in keeping with the lack of effect of feedback connections from V2 to V1 on centre-surround interactions in V1 neurons (Hupé *et al.* 2001*a*).

The relative roles of horizontal and feedback connections in shaping the modulatory regions of the receptive field surround of a cortical neuron is a subject of debate (Angeluci *et al.* 2002; Bullier *et al.* 2001). It appears that the spatial extent of horizontal connections is too small to carry information from more than a few millimetres away on the cortical surface. Because of the high magnification factor in the central visual field, a few millimeters on the surface of area 17 represents only a few tenths of a degree of visual angle. This is much smaller than the size of the RF surround of most V1 neurons (Levitt and Lund 1997). This distance in visual field is also far too small to explain the large extent of the interaction field beyond the RF centre demonstrated by using collinear lines in a noisy background (Ito and Gilbert 1999; Kapadia 1995). Thus, it is impossible that monosynaptic horizontal connections can subserve by themselves alone the far-reaching contextual effects demonstrated in area 17. One possibility is offered by multisynaptic information transfer through horizontal connections. However, horizontal connections are much too slow (Girard *et al.* 2001) to account for the rapid contextual effects seen in responses of neurons in area 17 (Ito and Gilbert 1999). Because of the high conduction velocity of feedforward and feedback axons (Girard *et al.* 2001) and the large spatial convergence and divergence of feedback connections (Fig. 2.4), it is likely that the latter play a major role in shaping the long-range centre-surround interactions in the receptive fields of cortical neurons. Experiments are needed to test directly this prediction on behaving animals performing a visual task requiring attention to long-range interactions across the visual field, such as that used by Gilbert and his colleagues (2000).

Feedback influences on the synchrony of neurons in lower-order areas

A number of studies have shown that cortical neurons tend to synchronize the time of emission of their action potentials (see review by Nowak and Bullier 2000). As mentioned above, neurons in a given cortical column send projections to several columns in other cortical areas. The exact cell-to-cell connectivity within this column-to-column network is not known but it is likely that it is similar to that found for intrinsic connections. Each axon gives only a few contacts to some neurons in a column and each neuron in a target column receives convergent input from several neurons. In that case, a powerful way to modulate transfer from one column to another is to synchronize the spike discharges of the neurons belonging to the source column or to change the firing pattern from regular to bursty. It has been proposed that feedback corticogeniculate connections switch the firing mode from bursting to tonic in lateral geniculate neurons through activation of metabotropic receptors (Godwin *et al.* 1996). The results of Sillito and his group (1994) further indicated that feedback corticothalamic connections synchronize the firing of LGN neurons. However, recent results suggest that there may be an important effect of feedback connections on slow modulation of rate changes instead of a direct effect on spike-to-spike synchronization (Brody 1998).

Lesion studies showed that, when higher-order areas are lesioned in the cat, certain types of synchronization between neurons located in lower-order cortical areas in opposite hemispheres disappear (Munk *et al.* 1995*b*). This suggests that feedback connections are involved in the synchronization of activity in neurons of lower-order cortical areas. We tested this hypothesis directly by measuring changes in synchronization of spike firing induced by inactivating higher-order areas. Indeed, we found changes in the cross-correlograms and the auto-correlograms of neighbouring neurons showing changes in response strength (Hupé, Girard, and Bullier, unpublished observations). However, we never observed a change in the strength of the cross-correlograms when there was no change in firing rate in at least one of the neurons. Therefore, despite its attractiveness, the idea that feedback connections control specifically the synchronization of lower-order neurons independently of their firing rate does not seem tenable at the moment. On the other hand, it would be interesting to determine whether inactivation or activation of a higher-order area leads to a change in the firing pattern of neurons in lower-order area, as suggested by the conclusions reached by Sherman and his collaborators for the corticogeniculate feedback connections (see above).

Figure–ground segregation, attention, top–down activation by internal images

A role for feedback connections in attention has been postulated in many studies but has not been directly tested yet. Attending to a visual stimulus increases the gain of neuronal responses in most visual cortical areas (Reynolds *et al.* 2000; Treue and Maunsell 1999). It has been shown that attention strongly potentiates responses to low-contrast stimuli and has little effect on high-contrast stimuli (Reynolds *et al.* 2000). This is reminiscent of the effects of inactivating area MT on the responses of neurons in areas VI, V2, and V3 which were strongest for low-salience stimuli, as reviewed above (Bullier *et al.* 2001; Hupé *et al.* 1998). It is therefore possible that the mechanisms revealed by inactivation of feedback connections may be at play during the modulation of sensitivity of lower-order areas by spatially directed attention.

It has been claimed that feedback connections play a role in the modulation of responses of neurons in VI when their receptive field is inside a square object that pops out from the background because of its difference in orientation of the lines composing the pattern or movement direction of random dots (Lamme *et al.* 1998; Lamme 1995). The argument rests on the observation that such modulatory effects are delayed by 40–100 ms with respect to the beginning of the response and that these effects disappear during anaesthesia. However, given that higher-order area neurons can have very short latencies (Nowak and Bullier 1997) and that feedback effects appear to be extremely rapid (Hupé *et al.* 2001*b*), it is not clear that delayed-response modulations are necessarily due to feedback influences. The disappearance of the effect during anaesthesia does not speak to the source of the effects since it was shown by several studies reviewed above that clear influences of feedback connections can be revealed during anaesthesia. It remains to be tested by directly influencing the responses of neurons in higher-order areas whether the modulatory effects corresponding to pop-out are transferred from higher-order areas by feedback connections.

A recent study of Miyashita and his group demonstrated a role that has been long suspected for feedback connections, that of activating lower-order area neurons with top–down signals conveying information about categorization of visual images (Tomita *et al.* 1999). By using a split-brain preparation, they were able, in inferotemporal cortex neurons, to distinguish activation by feedforward connections from the drive of feedback connections from the frontal cortex. This is the first direct evidence that feedback connections carry signals corresponding to internal images to lower-order areas of the visual system.

Temporal aspects of cortical interactions

Until recently, little attention has been paid to the temporal aspects of interactions between cortical areas (Nowak and Bullier 1997). The hierarchical model of visual cortical areas suggests that information is processed through a succession of stages corresponding to the different levels of the hierarchy. This leads to the prediction that successive levels should contain neurons responding with increasingly longer latencies to visual stimulation, the increase of latency reflecting processing occurring at the different levels. Direct tests of this hypothesis, however, have not confirmed such a model of a cascade of processors. Latencies of neurons in different areas are only loosely correlated to their location in the hierarchy of cortical areas (Fig. 2.9(a)). For example, neurons in the FEF area have latencies that are longer by only a few milliseconds than those of area 17 (Nowak and Bullier 1997; Schmolesky et al. 1998), despite the five levels difference between the two areas (Fig. 2.5). Similarly, latencies of neurons in MT and V2 are comparable ((Raiguel et al. 1989), Fig. 2.9(a)), even though area MT is placed at three levels above V2 in the cortical hierarchy (Fig. 2.5(b)).

It was also found that areas of the dorsal stream tend to have short latencies to visual stimulation (Nowak and Bullier 1997; Schmolesky et al. 1998). This is apparent in Fig. 2.9(a) with short latencies for areas V1, V2, MT, MST, and FEF and longer latencies for areas of the inferotemporal cortex (TEm, TEa, IT, Tpo, PGa, IPa, TE2, TE1, TAa, TS). That neurons of the dorsal pathway respond rapidly to visual stimuli is in keeping with their role in visuomotor interactions. To correct a hand movement in time to catch a ball on a windy day it is necessary to rapidly process visual information across the different cortical areas involved in the parietal and frontal cortex. In contrast, areas of the ventral stream tend to contain neurons with longer latencies to visual stimulation, in keeping with the role of this pathway in object recognition, for which speed is presumably less essential than for visuomotor interactions.

There is an interesting correlation between the short latencies of neurons in the dorsal stream and the rapidity of axons in this pathway. Staining for myelin reveals that the density of myelin is much higher in the grey matter of areas of the dorsal stream than that of those of the ventral stream, indicating a higher incidence of myelin sheaths, which are known to increase conduction velocity (Nowak and Bullier 1997). Indeed, the hallmark of area MT is the presence of a high density of myelin that has been observed in all primate species so far investigated. Also, it has been found that connections to the dorsal stream involve much higher densities of neurofilament protein than those to the ventral stream (Hof et al. 1996), indicating a much higher proportion of large myelinated axons that conduct faster than small axons (Nowak and Bullier 1997). In particular, all V1 neurons projecting to area MT contain neurofilament protein (Hof et al. 1996), in keeping with the very fast conduction velocities of these axons (Movshon and Newsome 1996).

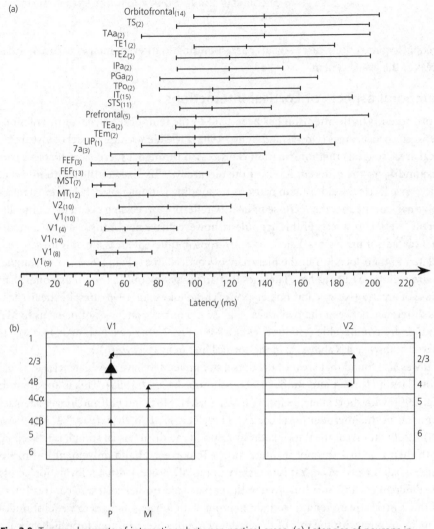

Fig. 2.9 Temporal aspects of interactions between cortical areas. (a) Latencies of neurons in different cortical areas of the macaque monkey. Behaving monkeys in all cases except (10). Small flashed stimuli in all cases except (7) and (12) for which motion onset was used. No difference was found between latencies to motion onset and to small flashed stimuli (Raiguel *et al.* 1999). For each published study, the central bar represents the median and the extremities of the line represent the 10 and 90 percentiles. (1) Barash *et al.* 1991; (2) Baylis *et al.* 1987; (3) Bushnell *et al.* 1991; (4) Celebrini *et al.* 1993; (5) Funahashi *et al.* 1990; (6) Goldberg and Bushnell 1991; (7) Kawano *et al.* 1994; (8) Knierim and Van Essen 1992; (9) Maunsell and Gibson 1992; (10) Nowak *et al.* 1995; (11) Perrett *et al.* 1982; (12) Raiguel *et al.* 1999; (13) Thompson *et al.* 1996; (14) Thorpe *et al.* 1983; (15) Vogels and Orban 1994. Note that the FEF latencies are similar to those in VI despite the large distance of these two areas in the cortical hierarchy (Fig. 2.5); the same remark holds for V2 and MT. Thus, the cortical hierarchy is a poor predictor of the timing of activation of neurons in different cortical areas, (b) A model combining the fast input from magnocellular LGN cells and the rapid effect of feedback connections. A first-pass analysis is made by the M input that is rapidly sent to higher-order areas. This first-pass analysis reorganizes the processing at lower levels through feedback connections in time for the arrival of the parvocellular stream that is delayed by 20 milliseconds compared to the magno input.

The elevated level of neurofilament protein in callosal connections afferent to the border between areas V1 and V2 suggests that these connections are very rapid, a necessary condition given the long distance covered by callosal axons (Hof *et al.* 1997) and the necessity of rapidly integrating information across the two visual hemifields (Kennedy *et al.* 1991). The high proportion of neurofilament protein in the feedback connections from all cortical areas (Hof *et al.* 1996) is strongly suggestive that these connections are fast. Indeed, we found that, in the rat as well as the monkey, feedback connections are matched in conduction speed to feedforward connections (Girard *et al.* 2001; Nowak *et al.* 1997). This means that information is transferred as rapidly in the forward as in the feedback direction.

This finding together with the rapid effect of the feedback connections led us to propose a functional model for the visual system that differs from that suggested by the hierarchical organization of cortical areas (Bullier 2001). According to this model (Fig. 2.9(b)), after a stimulus is flashed in the visual field (or after the eyes land on a visual target), the first wave of activity that reaches area 17 is carried by the axons of magnocellular LGN cells into layer 4Cα. After a relay in the adjacent layer 4B, this information is sent to areas V2, V3, and MT, the three main targets of feedforward axons from area V1. Because of the early activation of layer 4B neurons (Nowak *et al.* 1995) and their fast conducting axons, activity is very rapidly transferred to these areas from where they can be relayed to other higher-order areas. This early wave of activity enables a first step of computation to be achieved in higher-order areas. Results of these first computations are sent back through fast feedback connections to neurons in lower-order areas in order to optimize the subsequent processing. Such optimization could be achieved by potentiating the responses of some neuronal populations and increasing their centre-surround interactions, as shown above for the role of feedback connections, while possibly inhibiting the responses of other neuronal populations. Presumably, this early first-pass processing and signal routing can be done in time for the arrival of the input from the LGN parvocellular neurons that arrive some 20 milliseconds later. Although this model fits with a number of observations made concerning the rapid effects of feedback connections and the rapid axons of feedforward and feedback axons, much remains to be tested before it is established.

Development of cortico-cortical connections

During the 1970s and 1980s, the consensus among students of cortical development was that the precise pattern of cortico-cortical connectivity emerges from a totally undifferentiated set of diffuse connectivity. This was largely based on the results of connectivity studies done in the interhemispheric pathway in the cat. When retrograde tracers are placed in the visual cortex of the kitten, a very wide distribution of labelled neurons is observed with a large number of labelled neurons in the region of area 17 that codes for the peripheral visual field. This contrasts with the situation in the adult cat where labelled neurons are concentrated near the area 17–18 border, a region coding for central visual field (Innocenti *et al.* 1977). This has been the impetus for a large number of studies that have stressed the importance of the supernumerary aspect of callosal connectivity at the earliest stages of development followed by selective pruning during prenatal and postnatal development. A popular idea at the time was that information contained in the genome was not sufficient to code for the details of adult brain connectivity and that experience was needed to specify the adult pattern of connections (Changeux and Danchin 1976; Innocenti 1988).

Experimental results in the 1990s have led to a revision of this model of development of cortical connectivity. There was first the discovery that, in the monkey, the adult pattern of callosal connectivity characteristic of area 17 (with practically no callosal neurons within area 17) is already present at the earliest stages of prenatal development (Dehay *et al.* 1988). This raised questions concerning the generality of the principle of pruning of cortical connections during development. Not all of the precise connection patterns are the result of a period of exuberance followed by a period of selective elimination. As argued by Chalupa and Dreher (1991), this may be related to the necessity of a more precise 'blueprint' at the initial stages of development of highly interconnected brains like those of primates. Quantitative studies of the distribution of callosal neurons in the neonatal rat revealed that the adult pattern is already present at birth with higher neuron densities (Hernit *et al.* 1996). Thus, as argued elsewhere (Kennedy and Dehay 1997), the adult pattern of callosal connections in area 17 of cats and rats, instead of being sculpted out of a uniform distribution across the surface of area 17, may be the result of a more or less uniform reduction in cell density and axonal branches. Similar conclusions have been reached for studies of the development of corticospinal neurons in the ferret (Meissirel *et al.* 1993) and the development of intrahemispheric cortico-cortical connections in the cat (Kennedy *et al.* 1994). One could therefore conclude that the adult connectivity pattern of cortical connections simply results from a massive uniform reduction of connections during development, if there was not a specific reduction of neurons with exuberant connections. For example, in cat visual cortex, especially after injections involving the white matter, labelled neurons are found at great distances of the main concentration of labelled neurons in visual areas (Kennedy *et al.* 1994; Luhmann *et al.* 1990). Labelled neurons are also observed in nonvisual areas after postnatal injections in areas 17 and 18 of the cat (Dehay *et al.* 1984; Innocenti 1988). It is likely that these early exuberant connections are eliminated by selective pruning.

Thus, bulk injections of retrograde tracers during development reveal limited adjustments of the initial pattern of cortico-cortical connectivity with elimination of a small proportion of exuberant connections and a general reduction of the density of connections. There is also evidence for local reorganization of cortical connections. Small injections of retrograde tracers placed early in development produce a non-patchy distribution of neurons in afferent areas in the ipsilateral and contralateral hemisphere (Innocenti 1981; Price 1985), suggesting that the patchy organization of feedforward and interhemispheric connections is achieved also by selective pruning. Repeated injections of different fluorescent dyes showed that a number of neurons providing early connections to the other hemisphere do not die during development but reorganize their connectivity pattern. This is consistent with the demonstration that axonal branching is much more frequent during the early stages of development than in the adult (Bullier *et al.* 1990) and that single axons change their targets during development. The specificity of adult connectivity is therefore achieved by a combination of selective removal of axonal branches and regrowth of other branches. In addition, cell death in cortex has been shown to be important in the early stages of cortical organization (Blaschke *et al.* 1996), and it is therefore likely that it also plays a role in the reorganization of cortico-cortical connectivity during development.

The results of 30 years of investigation on the development of cortical connections therefore lead to a more balanced view of the mechanisms involved. There is an early specification of the connectivity pattern that involves regional and areal specification. During a period of reorganization, some neurons die, a number of axonal branches are retracted, others are extended, and the adult pattern emerges. Since this reorganization begins early, long before birth and eye opening in some species (Chalupa and Dreher 1991; Kennedy and Dehay 1993), there is little control of the visual responses of neurons on the early stages of this process. Effects of postnatal manipulation on the development of cortical connections have been studied mostly for the interhemispheric connections. The initial conclusion that artificially induced strabismus tends to preserve the diffuse immature pattern of callosal neurons on the cortical surface of area 17 (Lund *et al.* 1978) has not been confirmed by quantitative measurements of neuron density (Bourdet *et al.* 1996), although it has been shown that convergent strabismus does affect the functional interhemispheric connectivity (Milleret and Houzel 2001). Effects of early monocular and binocular eyelid sutures on the distribution pattern of callosal neurons in areas 17 and 19 of the cat have been demonstrated (see review by Innocenti 1986).

That the axonal pattern of cortico-cortical connections can be modified by such massive insults to the normal system as monocular or binocular deprivation tells us little about the changes in functional interactions between cortical areas that occur during normal development. Although it is likely that the postnatal modifications in the cortico-cortical connectivity are somewhat related to the learning phase during which young mammals learn to use their cortex to interact with the world, little direct evidence for this has been provided. A set of observations by Kennedy and Barone is particularly interesting in this respect. They showed that, at birth, feedforward connections from V2 to V4 in the monkey are already as patchy as in the adult (Barone *et al.* 1996). This contrasts with the situation for feedback connections that are not adult-like before 1 month of age (Barone *et al.* 1995). Since much of the acquisition of visually driven behaviour occurs during the first months of life in the monkey, it is likely that this progressive reorganization of feedback connections during postnatal life is related to processes of learning. Such a hypothesis is consistent with recent results in the study of the plasticity of the thalamocortical connections showing that the upper layers of area 17 are the first stage affected by peripheral manipulation such as eye closure or strabismus and that reorganization of layer 4 follows that of upper layers (Rathjen and Löwel 2000; Trachtenberg *et al.* 2000). This suggests that plasticity of ocular dominance columns in layer 4 of area 17 is not explained by a competitive interaction between the incoming feedforward thalamocortical inputs from the two eyes, but results from a top–down influence from upper layers. This represents an important paradigm shift, after many years of models of neural plasticity based on Hebbian mechanisms of competition between feedforward inputs. Transposed to the level of the cortico-cortical network, this would mean that feedback connections could be heavily involved in the reorganization of the cortical network during the early stages of postnatal life, in connection with plasticity and learning.

Acknowledgements

I thank Frédéric Sarrato for his expert help with the iconography.

References

Alonso, J.M., Cudeiro, J., Perez, R., Gonzalez, F., and Acuna, C. (1993*a*). Influence of layer V of area 18 of the cat visual cortex on responses of cells in layer V of area 17 to stimuli of high velocity. *Exp. Brain Res.* **93** (2), 363–6.

Alonso, J.M., Cudeiro, J., Perez, R., Gonzalez, F., and Acuna, C. (1993*b*). Orientational influences of layer V of visual area 18 upon cells in layer V of area 17 in the cat cortex. *Exp. Brain. Res.* **96** (2), 212–20.

Anderson, J.C., Binzegger, T., Martin, K.A., and Rockland, K.S. (1998). The connection from cortical area V1 to V5: a light and electron microscopic study. *J. Neurosci.* **18** (24), 10525–40.

Angeluci, A., Levitt, J.B., and Lund, J.S. (2002). Anatomical origins of the classical receptive field and modulatory surround field of single neurons in macaque visual cortical area V1. *Prog. Brain Res.* in press.

Baizer, J.S., Ungerleider, L.G., and Desimone, R. (1991). Organization of visual inputs to the inferior temporal and posterior parietal cortex in macaques. *J. Neurosci.* **11**, 168–90.

Barash, S., Bracewell, R.M., Fogassi, L., Gnadt, J.W., and Andersen, R.A. (1991). Saccade-related activity in the lateral intraparietal area. I. Temporal properties; comparison with area 7a. *J. Neurophysiol.* **66**, 1095–108.

Barbas, H. (1986). Pattern in the laminar origin of corticocortical connections. *J. Comp. Neurol.* **252** (3), 415–22.

Barbas, H. and Rempel-Clower, N. (1997). Cortical structure predicts the pattern of corticocortical connections. *Cereb. Cortex* **7** (7), 653–46.

Barone, P., Batardiere, A., Knoblauch, K., and Kennedy, H. (2000). Laminar distribution of neurons in extrastriate areas projecting to V1 and V4 correlates with the hierarchical rank and indicates the operation of a distance rule. *J. Neurosci.* **20**, 3263–81.

Barone, P., Dehay, C., Berland, M., Bullier, J., and Kennedy, H. (1995). Developmental remodeling of primate visual cortical pathways. *Cereb. Cortex* **5**, 22–38.

Barone, P., Dehay, C., Berland, M., and Kennedy, H. (1996). Role of directed growth and target selection in the formation of cortical pathways: prenatal development of the projection of area V2 to area V4 in the monkey. *J. Comp. Neurol.* **374**, 1–20.

Baylis, G.C., Rolls, E.T., and Leonard, C.M. (1987). Functional subdivisions of the temporal lobe neocortex. *J. Neurosci.* **7**, 330–42.

Blaschke, A.J., Staley, K., and Chun, J. (1996). Widespread programmed cell death in proliferative and postmitotic regions of the fetal cerebral cortex. *Development* **122**, 1165–74.

Borg-Graham, L., Monier, C., and Frégnac, Y. (1998). Visual input evokes transient and strong shunting inhibition in visual cortical neurons. *Nature* **393**, 369–73.

Bourdet, C., Olavarria, J.F., and Van Sluyters, R.C. (1996). Distribution of visual callosal neurons in normal and strabismic cats. *J. Comp. Neurol.* **366** (2), 259–69.

Boussaoud, D., Ungerleider, L.G., and Desimone, R. (1990). Pathways for motion analysis: cortical connexions of the MST and fundus of the superior temporal sulcus visual areas in the macaque. *J. Comp. Neurol.* **296**, 462–95.

Braitenberg, V. and Schüz, A. (1991). *Anatomy of the cortex. Statistics and geometry.* Springer-Verlag, Berlin.

Brody, C.D. (1998). Slow covariations in neuronal resting potentials can lead to artefactually fast cross-correlations in their spike trains. *J. Neurophysiol.* **80** (6), 3345–51.

Bullier, J. (2001). An integrated model of the visual system. *Brain Res. Rev.* **36**, 96–107.

Bullier, J. and Kennedy, H. (1987). Axonal bifurcation in the visual system. *Trends Neurosci.* **10**, 205–10.

Bullier, J., Kennedy, H., and Salinger, W. (1984). Branching and laminar origin of projections between visual cortical areas in the cat. *J. Comp. Neurol.* **228**, 329–41.

Bullier, J., McCourt, M.E., and Henry, G.H. (1988). Physiological studies on the feedback connection to the striate cortex from cortical areas 18 and 19 of the cat. *Exp. Brain Res.* **70**, 90–8.

Bullier, J., Dehay, C., and Dreher, B. (1990). Bihemispheric axonal bifurcation of the afferents to the visual cortical areas during postnatal development in the rat. *Eur. J. Neurosci.* **2**, 332–43.

Bullier, J., Girard, P., and Salin, P.A. (1994). The role of area 17 in the transfer of information to extrastriate visual cortex. In *Primary visual cortex in primates* (ed. A. Peters and K.S. Rockland), Vol. 10, pp. 301–30. Plenum, New York.

Bullier, J., Schall, J.D., and Morel, A. (1996). Functional streams in occipito-frontal connections in the monkey. *Behav. Brain Res.* **76**, 89–97.

Bullier, J., Hupé, J.-M., James, A., and Girard, P. (2001). The role of feedback connections in shaping the responses of visual cortical neurons. *Prog. Brain Res.* **134**, 193–204.

Bushnell, M.C., Goldberg, M.E., and Robinson, D.L. (1991). Behavioral enhancement of visual responses in monkey cerebral cortex. I. Modulation in posterior parietal cortex related to selective visual attention. *J. Neurophysiol.* **46**, 755–72.

Callaway, E.M. (1998). Local circuits in primary visual cortex of the macaque monkey. *Ann. Rev. Neurosci.* **21**, 47–74.

Casanova, C., Michaud, Y., Morin, C., McKinley, P.A., and Molotchnikoff, S. (1992). Visual responsiveness and direction selectivity of cells in area 18 during local reversible inactivation of area 17 in cats. *Vis. Neurosci.* **9** (6), 581–93.

Celebrini, S., Thorpe, S., Trotter, Y., and Imbert, M. (1993). Dynamics of orientation coding in area V1 of the awake primate. *Vis. Neurosci.* **10**, 811–25.

Chabli, A., Ruan, D.Y., and Molotchnikoff, S. (1998). Influences of area 17 on neuronal activity of simple and complex cells of area 18 in cats. *Neuroscience* **84** (3), 685–98.

Chalupa, L.M. and Dreher, B. (1991). High precision systems require high precision blueprints: a new view regarding the formation of connections in the mammalian visual system. *J. Cogn. Neurosci.* **3**, 209–18.

Changeux, J.-P. and Danchin, A. (1976). Selective stabilisation of developing synapses as a mechanism for the specification of neural networks. *Nature* 264, 705–12.

Crick, F. and Koch, C. (1998). Constraints on cortical and thalamic projections: the no-strong-loops hypothesis. *Nature* 391, 245–50.

Crook, J.M., Kisvarday, Z.F., and Eysel, U.T. (1997). GABA-induced inactivation of functionally characterized sites in cat striate cortex: effects on orientation tuning and direction selectivity. *Vis. Neurosci.* 14 (1), 141–58.

Dehay, C., Bullier, J., and Kennedy, H. (1984). Transient projections from the fronto-parietal and temporal cortex to areas 17, 18, and 19 in the kitten. *Exp. Brain Res.* 57, 208–12.

Dehay, C., Kennedy, H., Bullier, J., and Berland, M. (1988). Absence of interhemispheric connections of area 17 during development in the monkey. *Nature* 331, 348–50.

DeYoe, E.A. and Van Essen, D.C. (1985). Segregation of efferent connections and receptive field properties in visual area V2 of the macaque. *Nature* 317, 58–61.

DeYoe, E.A., Felleman, D.J., Van Essen, D.C., and McClendon, E. (1994). Multiple processing streams in occipitotemporal visual cortex. *Nature* 371 (6493), 151–4.

Domenici, L., Harding, G.W., and Burkhalter, A. (1995). Patterns of synaptic activity in forward and feedback pathways within rat visual cortex. *J. Neurophysiol.* 74 (6), 2649–64.

Douglas, R.J., Martin, K.A.C., and Whitteridge, D. (1991). An intracellular analysis of the visual responses of neurones in cat visual cortex. *J. Physiol.* 440, 659–96.

Dreher, B. and Cottee, L.J. (1975). Visual receptive-field properties of cells in area 18 of cat's cerebral cortex before and after lesions in area 17. *J. Neurophysiol.* 38, 735–50.

Felleman, D.J. and Van Essen, D.C. (1991). Distributed hierarchical processing in the primate cerebral cortex. *Cereb. Cortex* 1, 1–47.

Ferrara, V.P., Nealey, T.A., and Maunsell, J.H. (1994). Responses in macaque visual area V4 following inactivation of the parvocellular and magnocellular LGN pathways. *J. Neurosci.* 14(4), 2080–8.

Ferster, D., Chung, S., and Wheat, H. (1996). Orientation selectivity of thalamic input to simple cells of cat visual cortex. *Nature* 380 (6571), 249–52.

Fisken, R.A., Garey, L.J., and Powell, T.P.S. (1975). The intrinsic, association and commissural connections of area 17 of the visual cortex. *Phil. Trans. R. Soc., Lond.* 272, 487–536.

Fries, W., Keizer, K., and Kuypers, H.G. (1985). Large layer VI cells in macaque striate cortex (Meynert cells) project to both superior colliculus and prestriate visual area V5. *Exp. Brain Res.* 58 (3), 613–16.

Funahashi, S., Bruce, C.J., and Godman-Rakic, P.S. (1990). Visuospatial coding in primate prefrontal neurons revealed by oculomotor paradigms. *J. Neurophysiol.* 63, 814–31.

Gilbert, C.D. and Wiesel, T.N. (1983). Clustered intrinsic connections in cat visual cortex. *J. Neurosci.* 3, 1116–33.

Gilbert, C., Ito, M., Kapadia, M., and Westheimer, G. (2000). Interactions between attention, context and learning in primary visual cortex. *Vision Res.* 40(10–12), 1217–26.

Girard, P. and Bullier, J. (1989). Visual activity in area V2 during reversible inactivation of area 17 in the macaque monkey. *J. Neurophysiol.* 62, 1287–302.

Girard, P., Salin, P.A., and Bullier, J. (1991a). Visual activity in areas V3A and V3 during reversible inactivation of area V1 in the macaque monkey. *J. Neurophysiol.* 66, 1493–503.

Girard, P., Salin, P.A., and Bullier, J. (1991b). Visual activity in macaque area V4 depends on area 17 input. *Neuroreport* 2, 81–4.

Girard, P., Salin, P.A., and Bullier, J. (1992). Response selectivity of neurons in area MT of the macaque monkey during reversible inactivation of area V1. *J. Neurophysiol.* 67, 1–10.

Girard, P., Hupé J.M., and Bullier, J. (2001). Feedforward and feedback connections between areas V1 and V2 of the monkey have similar rapid conduction velocities. *J. Neurophysiol.* **85**, 1328–31.

Godwin, D.W., Vaughan, J.W., and Sherman, S.M. (1996). Metabotropic glutamate receptors switch visual response mode of lateral geniculate nucleus cells from burse to tonic. *J. Neurophysiol.* **76** (3), 1800–16.

Goldberg, M.E. and Bushnell, M.C. (1991). Behavioral enhancement of visual responses in monkey cerebral cortex. II. Modulation in frontal eye fields related to saccades. *J. Neurophysiol.* **46**, 773–87.

Goldman-Rakic, P.S., and Schwartx, M.L. (1982). Interdigitation of contralateral and ipsilateral projections of frontal association cortex in primates. *Science* **216**, 755–7.

Gonchar, Y. and Burkhalter, A. (1999). Differential subcellular localization of forward and feedback interareal inputs to parvalbumin expressing GABAergic neurons in rat visual cortex. *J. Comp. Neuro.* **406** (3), 346–60.

Goodale, M.A. and Milner, A.D. (1992). Separate visual pathways for perception and action. *Trends Neurosci.* **15**, 20–5.

Grossberg, S. (1994). 3-D vision and figure–ground separation by visual cortex. *Perception Psychophys.* **55**, 48–120.

Heider, B. (2000). Visual form agnosia: neural mechanisms and anatomical foundations. *Neurocase* **6**, 1–12.

Hendry, S.H. and Reid, R.C. (2000). The koniocellular pathway in primate vision. *Ann. Rev. Neurosci.* **23**, 127–53.

Hendry, S.H.C. and Yoshioka, T.Y. (1994). A neurochemically distinct third channel in the macaque dorsal lateal geniculate nucleus. *Science* **264**, 575–7.

Henry, G.H., Lund, J.S., and Harvey, A.R. (1978). Cells of the striate cortex projecting to the Clare–Bishop area of the cat. *Brain Res.* **151**, 154–8.

Henry, G.H., Salin, P.A., and Bullier, J. (1991). Projections from area 18 and 19 to cat striate cortex: divergence and laminar specificity. *Eur. J. Neurosci.* **3**, 186–200.

Hernit, C.S., Murphy, K.M., and Van Sluyters, R.C. (1996). Development of the visual callosal cell distribution in the rat: mature features are present at birth. *Vis. Neurosci.* **13**, 923–43.

Hilgetag, C.C., O'Neill, M.A., and Young, M.P. (1996). Indeterminate organization of the visual system [see comments]. *Science* **271** (5250), 776–7.

Hof, P.R., Ungerleider, L.G., Webster, M.J., Gattass, R., Adams, M.M., Sailstad, C.A., and Morrison, J.H. (1996). Neurofilament protein is differentially distributed in subpopulations of corticocortical projection neurons in the macaque monkey visual pathways. *J. Comp. Neurol.* **376**(1), 112–27.

Hof, P.R., Ungerleider, L.G., Adams, M.M., Webster, M.J., Gattass, R., Blumberg, D.M. and Morrison, J.H. (1997). Callosally projecting neurons in the macaque monkey V1/V2 border are enriched in nonphosphorylated neurofilament protein. *Vis. Neurosci.* **14**(5), 981–7.

Horton, J.C. and Hubel, D.H. (1981). Regular patchy distribution of cytochrome oxidase staining in primary visual cortex of macaque monkey. *Nature* **209**, 762–4.

Houzel, J.C. and Milleret, C. (1999). Visual inter-hemispheric processing: constraints and potentialities set by axonal morphology. *J. Physiol. Paris* **93** (4), 271–84.

Hubel, D. (1996). A big step along the visual pathway. *Nature*, **380** (6571), 197–8.

Hubel, D.H. and Wiesel, T.N. (1962). Receptive fields, binocular interaction and functional architecture in the cat visual cortex. *J. Physiol. Lond.* **160**, 106–54.

Hughes, C.M. and Peters., A. (1992a). Symmetric synapses formed by callosal afferents in rat visual cortex. *Brain Res.* **583**, 271–8.

Hughes, C.M. and Peters, A. (1992b). Types of callosally projecting nonpyramidal neurons in rat visual cortex identified by lysosomal HRP retrograde labeling. *Anat. Embryol. (Berl.)* **186**, 183–93.

Hupé, J.M., James, A.C., Payne, B.R., Lomber, S.G., Girard, P., and Bullier, J. (1998). Cortical feedback improves discrimination between figure and background by V1, V2 and V3 neurons. *Nature* 394, 784–7.

Hupé, J.M., James, A.C., Girard, P., and Bullier, J. (2001a). Response modulations by static texture surround in area V1 of the macaque monkey do not depend on feedback connections from V2. *J. Neurophysiol.* 85, 146–63.

Hupé, J.M., James, A.C., Girard, P.S.L., Payne, B., and Bullier, J. (2001b). Feedback connections act on the early part of the responses in monkey visual cortex. *J. Neurophysiol.* 85, 134–45.

Innocenti, G.M. (1981). Growth and reshaping of axons in the establishment of visual callosal connections. *Science* 212 (4496), 824–7.

Innocenti, G.M. (1986). General organization of callosal connections in the cerebral cortex. In *Cerebral cortex* (ed. E.G. Jones and A. Peters), Vol. 5. Plenum Press, New York.

Innocenti, G.M. (1988). Loss of axonal projections in the development of the mammalian brain. In *The making of the nervous system* (ed. J.G. Parnavelas, C.D. Stern, and R.V. Stirling), pp. 319–39. Oxford University Press, Oxford.

Innocenti, G.M., Fiore, L., and Caminiti, R. (1977). Exuberant projection into the corpus callosum from the visual cortex of newborn cats. *Neurosci. Lett.* 4, 237–42.

Innocenti G.M., Berbel, P., and Clarke, S. (1988). Development of projections from auditory to visual areas in the cat. *J. Comp. Neurol.* 272, 242–59.

Ito, M. and Gilbert, C.D. (1999). Attention modulates contextual influences in the primary visual cortex of alert monkeys. *Neuron* 22 (3), 593–604.

Jeannerod, M., Arbib, M.A., Rizzolatti, G., and Sakata, H. (1995). Grasping objects: the cortical mechanisms of visuomotor transformation. *Trends Neurosci.* 18 (7), 314–20.

Johnson, R.R. and Burkhalter, A. (1996). Microcircuitry of forward and feedback connections within rat visual cortex. *J. Comp. Neurol.* 368, 383–98.

Johnson, R.R. and Burkhalter, A. (1997). A polysynaptic feedback circuit in rat visual cortex. *J. Neurosci.* 17 (18), 7129–40.

Jouve, B., Rosenstiehl, P., and Imbert, M. (1998). A mathematical approach to the connectivity between the cortical visual areas of the macaque monkey. *Cereb. Cortex* 8, 28–39.

Kaas, J.H. (1996). Theories of visual cortex organization in primates: areas of the third level. *Prog. Brain Res.* 112, 213–21.

Kapadia, M.K., Ito, M., Gilbert, C.D., and Westheimer, G. (1995). Improvement in visual sensitivity by changes in local context: parallel studies in human observers and in V1 of alert monkeys. *Neuron* 15 (4), 843–56.

Kawano, K., Shidara, M., Watanabe, Y., and Yamane, S. (1994). Neural activity in cortical area MST of alert monkey during occular following responses. *J. Neurophysiol.* 71, 2305–24.

Kennedy, H. and Bullier, J. (1985). A double-labelling investigation of the afferent connectivity to cortical areas V1 and V2 of the macaque monkey. *J. Neurosci.* 5, 2815–30.

Kennedy, H. and Dehay, C. (1993). Cortical specification of mice and men. *Cereb. Cortex* 3 (3), 27–35.

Kennedy, H. and Dehay, C. (1997). The nature and nurture of cortical development. In *Normal and abnormal development of cortex* (ed. A.M. Galaburda and Y. Christen), pp. 25–56. Springer-Verlag, Berlin.

Kennedy, H., Bullier, J., and Dehay, C. (1989). Transient projection from the superior temporal sulcus to area 17 in the newborn macaque monkey. *Proc. Natl Acad. Sci., USA* 86, 8093–7.

Kennedy, H., Meissirel, C., and Dehay, C. (1991). Callosal pathways in primates and their compliancy to general rules governing the organization of cortico-cortical connectivity. In (ed. C. Dillon)

Vision and visual dysfunction, Vol. 3, Neuroanotomy of the visual pathways and their development. Macmillan Press.

Kennedy, H., Salin, P.-A., Bullier, J., and Horsburgh, G. (1994). The topography of developing thalamic and cortical pathways in the visual system of the cat. *J. Comp. Neurol.* **348**, 298–319.

Knierim, J.J. and Van Essen, D.C. (1992). Neuronal responses to static texture patterns in area V1 of the alert macaque monkey. *J. Neurophysiol.* **67**, 961–80.

Lamme, V.A.F. (1995). The Neurophysiology of figure ground segregation in primary visual-cortex. *J. Neurosci.* **15** (2), 1605–15.

Lamme, V.A., Super, H., and Spekreijse, H. (1998). Feedforward, horizontal, and feedback processing in the visual cortex. *Curr. Opin. Neurobiol.* **8** (4), 529–35.

Levitt, J.B. and Lund, J.S. (1997). Spatial summation properties of macaque striate neurons. *Soc. Neurosci. Abstr.* **23**, 455.

Levitt, J.B., Yoshioka, T., and Lund, J.S. (1994). Intrinsic cortical connections in macaque visual area V2: evidence for interaction between different functional streams. *J. Comp. Neurol.* **342**, 551–70.

Livingstone, M.S. and Hubel, D.H. (1984). Anatomy and physiology of a color system in the primate visual cortex. *J. Neurosci.* **4**, 309–56.

Livingstone, M.S. and Hubel, D.H. (1987a). Connections between layer 4b of area 17 and the thick cytochrome oxidase stripes of area 18 in the squirrel monkey. *J. Neurosci.* **7**, 3371–7.

Livingstone, M.S. and Hubel, D.H. (1987b). Psychophysical evidence for separate channels for the perception of form, color, movement and depth. *J. Neurosci.* **7**, 3416–68.

Lowenstein, P.R. and Somogyi, P. (1991). Synaptic organization of cortico-cortical connections from the primary visual cortex to the posteromedial lateral suprasylvian visual area in the cat. *J. Comp. Neurol.* **310** (2), 253–66.

Luhmann, H.J., Singer, W.,and Martínez-Millán, L. (1990). Horizontal interactions in cat striate cortex: 1. Anatomical substrate and postnatal development. *Eur. J. Neurosci.* **2**, 344–57.

Lund, R.D., Mitchell, D.E., and Henry, G.H. (1978). Squint-induced modification of callosal connections in cats. *Brain Res.* **144**, 169–72.

Malpeli, J.G. (1983). Activity of cells in area 17 of the cat in absence of input from layer A of lateral geniculate nucleus. *J. Neurophysiol.* **49**, 595–610.

Martin, K.A.C. (1984). Neuronal circuits in cat striate cortex. In *Cerebral cortex*, Vol. 2 (ed. E.G. Jones and A. Peters), pp. 241–84. Plenum, New york.

Martinez-Conde, S., Cudeiro, J., Grieve, K.L., Rodriguez, R., Rivadulla, C., and Acuna, C. (1999). Effects of feedback projections from area 18 layers 2/3 to area 17 layers 2/3 in the cat visual cortex. *J. Neurophysiol.* **82** (5), 2667–75.

Maunsell, J.H.R. and Gibson, J.R. (1992). Visual response latencies in striate cortex of the macaque monkey. *J. Neurophysiol.* **4**, 1332–4.

Maunsell, J.H.R. and Van Essen, D.C. (1983). The connections of the middle temporal visual area (MT) and their relationship to a cortical hierarchy in the macaque monkey. *J. Neurosci.* **3**, 2563–86.

Maunsell, J.H., Nealey, T.A., and DePriest, D.D. (1990). Magnocellular and parvocellular contributions to responses in the middle temporal visual area (MT) of the macaque monkey. *J. Neurosci.* **10** (10), 3323–34.

McDonald, C.T. and Burkhalter, A. (1993). Organization of long-range inhibitory connections with rat visual cortex. *J. Neurosci.* **13** (2), 768–81.

Meissirel, C., Dehay, C., and Kennedy, H. (1993). Transient cortical pathways in the pyramidal tract of the neonatal ferret. *J. Comp. Neurol.* **338**, 193–213.

Merigan, W.H. and Maunsell, J.H.R. (1991). How parallel are the primate visual pathways? *Ann. Rev. Neurosci.* **16**, 369–402.

Meyer, G. and Albus., K. (1981). Spiny stellates as cells of origin of association fibres from area 17 to area 18 in the cat's neocortex. *Brain Res.* **210**, 335–41.

Mignard, M. and Malpeli, J.G. (1991). Paths of information flow through visual cortex. *Science* **251** (4998), 1249–51.

Milleret, C. and Houzel, J.-C. (2001). Visual interhemispheric transfer to areas 17 and 18 in convergent strabismic cats. *Euro. J. Neurosci.* **13**, 137–52.

Morel, A. and Bullier, J. (1990). Anatomical segregation of two cortical visual pathways in the macaque monkey. *Visual Neurosci.* **4**, 555–78.

Movshon, J.A. and Newsome, W.T. (1996). Visual response properties of striate cortical neurons projecting to area MT in macaque monkeys. *J Neurosci.* **16** (23), 7733–41.

Munk, M.H.J., Nowak, L.G., Girard, P., Chounlamountri, N., and Bullier, J. (1995*a*). Visual latencies in cytochrome oxidase bands of macaque area V2. *Proc. Natl Acad. Sci., UAS*, 988–92.

Munk, M.H.J., Nowak, L.G., Nelson, J.I., and Bullier, J. (1995*b*). The structural basis of cortical synchronization. II. Effects of cortical lesions. *J. Neurophysiol.* **74**, 2401–14.

Murre, J.M.J. and Sturdy, D.P.F. (1995). The connectivity of the brain: multi-level quantitative analysis. *Biol. Cybern.* **73**, 529–45.

Nealey, T.A. and Maunsell, J.H. (1994). Magnocellular and parvocellular contributions to the responses of neurons in macaque striate cortex. *J. Neurosci.* **14** (4), 2069–79.

Nowak, L.G. and Bullier, J. (1997). The timing of information transfer in the visual system. In *Cerebral cortex.* Vol. 12: *Extrastriate visual cortex in primates* (ed. K.S. Rockland, J.H. Kaas, and A. Peters), pp. 205–41. Plenum Press, New York.

Nowak, L.G. and Bullier, J. (1998*a*). Axons, but not cell bodies are activated by electrical stimulation in cortical gray matter. I. Evidence from chronaxie measurements. *Exp. Brain Res.* **118**, 477–88.

Nowak, L.G. and Bullier, J. (1998*b*). Axons, but not cell bodies, are activated by electrical stimulation in cortical grey matter. II. Evidence from selective inactivation of cell bodies and axon initial segments. *Exp. Brain Res.* **118**, 489–500.

Nowak, L.G. and Bullier, J. (2000). Cross correlograms for neuronal spike trains. Different types of temporal correlation in neocortex, their origin and significance. In *Time and the brain, conceptual advances in brain research* (ed. R. Miller), pp. 53–96. Harwood Academic Publishers, Amsterdam.

Nowak, L.G., Munk, M.H.J., Girard, P., and Bullier, J. (1995). Visual latencies in areas V1 and V2 of the macaque monkey. *Vis. Neurosci.* **12** (2), 371–84.

Nowak, L.G., James, A.C., and Bullier, J. (1997). Corticocortical connections between visual areas 17 and 18a of the rat studied *in vitro*: spatial and temporal organisation of functional synaptic responses. *Exp. Brain Res.* **117**, 283–305.

Orban, G.A., Kennedy, H., and Maes, H. (1981). Response to movement of neurons in areas 17 and 18 of the cat: velocit sensitivity. *J. Neurophysiol.* **45**, 1059–73.

Payne, B.R. (1993). Evidence for visual cortical area homologs in cat and macaque monkey. *Cereb. Cortex* **3**, 1–25.

Perkel, D.J., Bullier, J., and Kennedy, H. (1986). Topography of the afferent connectivity of area 17 of the macaque monkey: a double-labelling study. *J. Comp. Neurol.* **253**, 374–402.

Perrett, D.L., Rolls, E.T., and Caan, W. (1982). Visual neurons responsive to faces in the monkey temporal cortex. *Exp. Brain Res.* **47**, 329–42.

Peterhans, E. (1997). Functional organization of area V2 in the awake monkey. In *Cerbral cortex.* Vol. 12: *Extrastriate cortex in primates* (ed. K.S. Rockland, J.H. Kaas, and A. Peters), Plenum Press, New York.

Peterhans, E. and Heydt, R.V.D. (1993). Functional organization of area V2 in the alert macaque. *Eur. J. Neurosci.* 5, 509–24.

Peters, A., Payne, B., and Josephson, K. (1990). Transcallosal non-pyramidal cell projections from visual cortex in the cat. *J. Comp. Neurol.* 302, 124–42.

Pohl, W. (1973). Dissociation of spatial discrimination deficits following frontal and parietal lesions in monkeys. *J. Comp. Physiol. Psychol.* 82, 227–39.

Price, D.J. (1985). Patterns of cytochrome oxidase activity in areas 17, 18 and 19 of the visual cortex of cats and kittens. *Exp. Brain Res.* 58, 125–33.

Price, D.J., Ferrer, J.M.R., Blakemore, C., and Kato, N. (1994). Functional organization of corticocortical projections from area 17 to area 18 in the cat's visual cortex. *J. Neurosci.* 14, 2732–46.

Raiguel, S.E., Lagae, L., Gulyas, B., and Orban, G.A. (1989). Response latencies of visual cells in macaque areas V1, V2 and V5. *Brain Res.* 493, 155–9.

Raiguel, S.E., Xiao, D.K., Marcar, V.L., and Orban, G.A. (1999). Response latency of macaque area MT/V5 neurons and its relationship to stimulus parameters. *J. Neurophysiol.* 82 (4), 1944–56.

Rathjen, S. and Löwel, S. (2000). Early postnatal development of functional ocular dominance columns in cat primary visual cortex. *Neuroreport* 11, 2363–7.

Reid, C.R., and Alonso, J.-M. (1995). Specificity of monosynaptic connections from thalamus to visual cortex. *Nature* 378, 281–4.

Reynolds, J.H., Pasternak, T., and Desimone, R. (2000). Attention increases sensitivity of V4 neurons. *Neuron* 26 (3), 703–14.

Rockland, K.S. and Drash, G.W. (1996). Collateralized divergent feedback connections that target multiple cortical areas. *J. Comp. Neurol.* 373, 529–48.

Rockland, K.S. and Lund, J.S. (1982). Widespread periodic intrinsic connections in the tree shrew visual cortex. *Science* 215, 1532–4.

Rockland, K.S and Pandya, D.N. (1979). Laminar origin and terminations of cortical connections of the occipital lobe in the rhesus monkey. *Brain Res.* 179, 3–20.

Rockland, K.S., Saleem, K.S., and Tanaka, K. (1994). Divergent feedback connections from areas V4 and TEO. *Vis. Neurosci.* 11, 579–600.

Rodman, H.R., Gross, C.G., and Albright, T.D. (1989). Afferent basis of visual response properties in area MT of the macaque: I. Effects of striate cortex removal. *J. Neurosci.* 9, 2033–50.

Salin, P.-A. and Bullier, J. (1995). Corticocortical connections in the visual system: Structure and function. *Physiol. Rev.* 75, 107–54.

Salin, P.A., Girard, P., Kennedy, H., and Bullier, J. (1992). The visuotopic organization of corticocortical connections in the visual system of the cat. *J. Comp. Neurol.* 320, 415–34.

Salin, P.-A., Kennedy, H., and Bullier, J. (1994). Spatial reciprocity of connections between areas 17 and 18 of the cat. *Can. J. Physiol. Pharmacol.*

Sandell, J.H. and Schiller, P.H. (1982). Effect of cooling area 18 on striate cortex cells in the squirrel monkey. *J. Neurophysiol.* 48 (1), 38–48.

Sanides, F. (1970). Functional architecture of motor and sensory cortices in primates in the light of a new concept of neocortex evolution. In *The primate brain: advances in primatology* (ed. C.R. Noback and W. Montagna), pp. 137–208. Appleton-Century-Crofts, New York.

Schiller, P.H. and Malpeli, J.G. (1977). The effect of striate cortex cooling on area 18 cells in the monkey. *Brain Res.* 126, 366–9.

Schmolesky, M.T., Wang, Y., Hanes, D.P., Thompson, K.G., Leutgeb, S., Schall, J.D., and Leventhal, A.G. (1998). Signal timing across the macaque visual system. *J. Neurophysiol.* 79 (6), 3272–8.

Schneider, G.E. (1969). Two visual systems. *Science* 163, 895–902.

Shao, Z. and Burkhalter, A. (1999). Role of GABAB receptor-mediated inhibition in reciprocal interareal pathways of rat visual cortex. *J. Neurophysiol.* **81** (3), 1014–24.

Shao, Z.W. and Burkhalter, A. (1996). Different balance of excitation and inhibition in forward and feedback circuits of rat visual cortex. *J. Neurosci.* **16**, 7353–65.

Sherk, H. (1978). Area 18 cell responses in cat during reversible inactivation of area 17. *J. Neurophysiol.* **41** (1), 204–15.

Sherk, H. (1990). Functional organization of input from areas 17 and 18 to an extrastriate area in the cat. *J. Neurosci.* **10**, 2780–90.

Sherk, H. and Ombrellaro, M. (1988). The retinotopic match between area 17 and its targets in visual suprasylvian cortex. *Exp. Brain Res.* **72**, 225–36.

Sherman, S.M. and Guillery, R.W. (1998). On the actions that one nerve cell can have on another: distinguishing 'drivers' from 'modulators'. *Proc. Natl Acad. Sci., USA* **95** (12), 7121–6.

Shipp, S. and Grant, S. (1991). Organization of reciprocal connections between area 17 and the lateral suprasylvian area of cat visual cortex. *Vis. Neurosci.* **6**, 339–55.

Shipp, S. and Zeki, S.M. (1985). Segregation of pathways leading from area V2 to areas V4 and V5 of macaque monkey visual cortex. *Nature* **315**, 322–5.

Sillito, A.M., Jones, H., Gerstein, G.L. and West, D.C. (1994). Feature-linked synchronization of thalamic relay cell firing induced by feedback from the visual cortex. *Nature* **369**, 479–82.

Stone, J. (1983). *Parallel processing in the visual system. The classification of retinal ganglion cells and its impact on the neurobiology of vision.* Plenum Press, New York.

Symmonds, L.L. and Rosenquist, A.C. (1984). Corticocortical connections among visual areas in the cat. *J. Comp. Neurol.* **229**, 1–38.

Tanaka, K. (1983). Cross-correlation analysis of geniculostriate neuronal relationships in cats. *J. Neurophysiol.* **49**, 1303–18.

Thompson, K.G., Hanes, D.P., Bichot, N.P., and Schall, J.D. (1996). Perceptual and motor processing stages identified in the activity of macaque frontal eye field neurons during visual search. *J. Neurophysiol.* **76**, 4040–55.

Thorpe, S.J., Rolls, E.T., and Maddison, S. (1983). The orbitofrontal cortex: neuronal activity in the behaving monkey. *Exp. Brain Res.* **49**, 93–115.

Tomita, H., Ohbayashi, M., Nakahara, K., Hasegawa, I., and Miyashita, Y. (1999). Top-down signal from prefrontal cortex in executive control of memory retrieval. *Nature* **401** (6754), 699–703.

Trachtenberg, J.T., Trepel, C., and Stryker, M.P. (2000). Rapid extragranular plasticity in the absence of thalamocortical plasticity in the developing primary visual cortex. *Science* **287** (5460), 2029–32.

Treue, S. and Maunsell, J.H. (1999). Effects of attention on the processing of motion in macaque middle temporal and medial superior temporal visual cortical areas. *J. Neurosci.* **19** (17), 7591–602.

Trevarthen, C.B. (1968). Two mechanisms of vision in primates. *Psychol. Forsch.* **31**, 299–337.

Tsodyks, M., Kenet, T., Grinvald, A., and Arieli, A. (1999). Linking spontaneous activity of single cortical neurons and the underlying functional architecture. *Science* **286** (5446), 1943–6.

Ungerleider, L.G. (1985). The corticocortical pathways for object recognition and spatial perception. In *Pattern recognition mechanisms* (ed. C. Chagas, R. Gattass, and C. Gross), pp. 21–37. Pontifical Academy of Sciences, Vatican City.

Ungerleider, L.G. and Desimone, R. (1986). Cortical connections of visual area MT in the macaque. *J. Comp. Neurol.* **248**, 190–222.

Ungerleider, L.G. and Mishkin, M. (1982). Two cortical visual systems. In *Analysis of visual behavior* (ed. D.J. Ingle, M.A. Goodale, and R.J.W. Mansfield), pp. 549–86. MIT Press, Cambridge, Massachusetts.

Vanduffel, W., Payne, B.R., Lomber, S.G., and Orban, G.A. (1997). Functional impact of cerebral connections. *Proc. Natl Acad. Sci. USA* **94**, 7617–20.

Van Essen, D.C. (1997). A tension-based theory of morphogenesis and compact wiring in the central nervous system. *Nature* **385** (6614), 313–18.

Van Essen, D.C. and Maunsell, J.H.R. (1983). Hierarchical organization and functional streams in the visual cortex. *Trends in Neurosci.* **6**, 370–5.

Vogels, R. and Orban, G.A. (1994). Activity of inferior temporal neurons during orientation discrimination with successively presented gratings. *J. Neurophysiol.* **71**, 1428–51.

Wang, C., Waleszczyk, W.J., Burke, W., and Dreher, B. (2000). Modulatory influence of feedback projections from area 21a on neuronal activities in striate cortex of the cat. *Cereb. Cortex* **10** (12), 1217–32.

Wimborne, B.M. and Henry, G.H. (1992). Response characteristics of the cells of cortical area 21a of the cat with special reference to orientation specificity. *J. Physiol.* **449**, 457–78.

Wong-Riley, M.T.T. (1979a). Changes in the visual system of monoculary sutured or enucleated cats demonstrable with cytochrome oxidase histochemistry. *Brain Res.* **171**, 11–28.

Wong-Riley, M.T.T. (1979b). Columnar cortico-cortical interconnections within the visual system of the squirrel and macaque, monkeys. *Brain Res.* **162**, 201–17.

Yoshioka, T., Levitt, J.B., and Lund, J.S. (1994). Independence and merger of thalamocortical channels within macaque monkey primary visual cortex: anatomy of interlaminar projections. *Vis. Neurosci.* **11**, 467–89.

Young, M.P. (1992). Objective analysis of the topological organization of the primate cortical visual system. *Nature* **358**, 152–5.

Zeki, S. (1993). *A vision of the brain.* Blackwell Scientific, London.

Part 2

Sum potentials in humans: electroencephalography and magnetoencephalography

Chapter 3

Electro- and magneto-encephalographic and event-related potential studies of visual processing in normals and neurological patients

Thomas F. Münte and Hans-Jochen Heinze

Owing to its relatively easy accessibility and the availability of suitable animal models, the visual system is one of the best studied areas of the human brain. Electrophysiological and behavioural investigations of non-human primates have shown dozens of anatomically and functionally distinct areas active in the processing of visual input (Van Essen 1995; Van Essen *et al.* 1992). In the monkey it is possible to delineate, at the single-cell and ensemble levels, the timing and location of electrical activity related to the processing of spatial location, orientation, colour, and motion of a stimulus (Ferrera and Lisberger 1997; Chelazzi 1995; Watanabe and Iwai 1996; see also Chapter 5 this volume). Moreover, cells have been found that appear to respond specifically to faces and even to the gaze direction of these faces (Hietanen *et al.* 1992; Milders and Perrett 1993; Oram *et al.* 1992; see also Chapter 1, this volume). In addition, functional imaging studies using positron emission tomography (PET) and functional magnetic resonance imaging (fMRI) methodologies have yielded insights into the anatomical organization of visual processing in humans at an ever increasing pace. These exciting developments are reviewed in Chapters 4 and 7, this volume.

In this chapter, we will give an overview of non-invasive electrophysiological studies of the human visual system. We will first examine the effects of passive visual stimulation using different stimuli, followed by a review of the effects of attention to location and other visual features on event-related brain potentials. Finally, we will address recent findings related to complex visual stimuli such as hierarchically structured objects and faces.

Electroencephalograms and event-related potentials: some basic facts

In the late 1920s, Hans Berger, a German psychiatrist, was the first to record the electroencephalogram (EEG) of the human from the intact scalp. The spontaneous EEG generally contains potentials with amplitudes of up to 50 μV. Such potentials are usually generated by neurons in the neocortex. However, cells in structures located deeper in the brain, e.g. some brainstem structures, can also generate electrical fields that can be measured at the scalp. These are much smaller though, with amplitudes of 1 μV or less, and are buried in the ongoing EEG. Cells in the neocortex are arranged in an orderly fashion, which allows some speculation as to which cells and structures are responsible for the surface potentials. Top candidates are pyramidal cells of the cortex that are oriented perpendicular to the cortical layers and parallel to each other. These pyramidal cells often are activated simultaneously by input into the cortical columns. The geometry of the neurons suggests that it is likely that the excitatory postsynaptic potentials (EPSPs) that are responsible for triggering the action potentials sum up to produce the field potentials detectable at the scalp.

In this chapter, we will mostly discuss event-related brain potentials (ERPs). These are small voltage fluctuations that occur in response to external or internal events in a time-locked fashion. ERPs (i.e. the signal of interest) are generally too small to be seen in the spontaneous EEG and must therefore be extracted from the background activity. The most common technique for improving the ERP signal-to-noise ratio is signal-averaging in the time-domain. In this simple procedure, data points from each of the trials of one experimental condition are aligned with respect to the onset of the event of interest. Then, for each time point preceding or following this event, the arithmetic mean of the recorded samples is computed. This averaging procedure offers an increase in the signal-to-noise ratio of $1/\sqrt{n}$ (where n is the number of averaged trials). Consequently, the number of stimuli needed for the computation of 'clean' ERPs depends on the size of the effect. As a general rule of thumb, the studies discussed in this chapter deal with small ERP effects and, therefore, a large number of repetitions is required, usually several hundred trials. In other domains, e.g. language, ERP effects are much larger and allow experiments with 50 or even fewer trials per condition.

The resulting ERP is characterized by a series of peaks and troughs. In a plethora of papers it has been shown that the characteristics of these peaks, such as amplitude, latency, and topography, vary with the perceptual, attentional, or cognitive aspects entailed in the processing of the stimulus. Therefore, the ERPs can be used in addition to traditional behavioural measures, e.g. reaction times, to characterize the cognitive architecture and timing of human information processing and its disturbances in neuropsychological patients. Moreover, for many ERP components it has been possible to pinpoint their anatomical origins using source modelling techniques. Thus, ERP results can be linked to data from animal research and functional neuroimaging and neuropsychological evidence from patients with brain lesions. A fuller account of the physiological, technical, and psychological aspects of ERPs can be found in Münte *et al.* (2000).

Electrophysiological effects due to passive stimulation

Potentials evoked in response to stimuli passively viewed by the patient have been used by neurologists to assess the integrity of the visual system for many years. We will not be concerned with the many clinical applications of visual evoked potentials here (see Bodis-Wollner, 1992 for a review).

Passive viewing situations, i.e. situations in which subjects do not have a task, have been used to some extent in conjunction with ERPs and magnetoencephalography (MEG) to assess basic properties of the visual system. One of the goals of these studies is to provide a cortical cartography similar to the one elaborated for the monkey brain by using stimuli that specifically involve certain visual areas.

For example, in an effort to record electrophysiological activity from the human analogue of area V4, 'Mondrian' stimuli made up from coloured or grey patches were presented (Buchner *et al.* 1994; Plendl *et al.* 1993). Three active brain regions were identified by spatiotemporal dipole modelling that were interpreted to correspond to areas V1, V2, and V4. When difference potentials 'colour minus grey' were subjected to source analysis, colour-related activity could be modelled in isolation and located to area V4. Source activity in V4 was observed from approximately 100 to 150 ms after stimulus onset.

Allison *et al.* (1993) recorded brain activity from 13 candidates for epilepsy surgery that were implanted with intracranial electrodes. They used different stimuli designed to elicit colour-related activity and found that a region of inferior occipital cortex, primarily the posterior portion of the fusiform gyrus, is involved in colour perception (see also chapter 8, this volume). They therefore reasoned that this area might be homologous with area V4 in monkeys. Further regions with colour-related activity were situated in the dorsolateral surface cortex, which was speculated to be involved in selective attention to colour.

In a similar vein, several groups have employed MEG and ERPs to identify the human homologue of area MT/V5 that is involved in the processing of motion. For example, Anderson *et al.* (1996) found motion-related activity near the occipitotemporal border in a minor sulcus immediately below the superior temporal sulcus. In another MEG study, Uusitalo *et al.* (1997) could differentiate between transient and sustained activity to moving stimuli at the parietooccipitotemporal border. The former was attributed to the detection of changes in the environment, while the latter was interpreted as the possible substrate of conscious perception of the moving stimulus.

Attention to location and to other features: active stimulation

Beginning with early studies by Harter (reviewed in White and White 1995), the sensitivity of ERP components to attentional manipulations has been shown many times. These seminal investigations have opened the door to a cognitive neuroscience of the visual system (Harter and Aine 1986; Hillyard and Mangun 1986).

In one typical task, stimuli are presented rapidly in at least two 'channels' defined by, say, their location. Paying attention to one location in order to detect slightly altered target stimuli among similar frequent standard stimuli increases the amplitude of several ERP components when compared with the same stimuli when unattended. The earliest component that is enhanced by spatial attention is the occipitotemporal P1

Fig. 3.1 Typical ERPs obtained in a sustained visual attention task. In these tasks, subjects are required to covertly focus attention to one side of a stimulus display, while they fixate a fixation aid in the centre of the display. ERPs to stimuli from the attended location elicit larger temporo-occipital P1 and N1 components. In addition, a frontal negativity is observed that is similarly enhanced. Components emanating from primary visual cortex (C1) are not changed by spatial attention (after data from Hillyard and Anllo–Vento 1998).

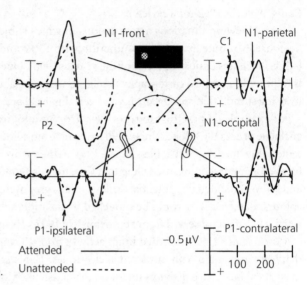

(latency about 120 ms) component emanating from the extrastriate cortex (Gomez *et al.* 1994) followed by a similarly enhanced negative component (N1) with a peak latency of approximately 170 ms. These attention effects are more pronounced over the scalp contralateral to the stimulus. Depending on the nature of the stimuli, they are sometimes followed by additional enhanced components. Over anterior scalp regions an earlier N1 negativity (around 150 ms) has been shown to be sensitive to spatial attention (Fig. 3.1).

A novel approach to spatial attention, using steady-state evoked responses, has been reported recently by Morgan *et al.* (1996) and Müller *et al.* (1998*a,b*). In these studies rapidly flickering light-emitting diodes (LEDs) were presented at the attended and unattended location 5 degrees to the left and to the right of a fixation point (Fig. 3.2). The flicker frequency at the two locations differed (e.g. 20.8 versus 27.8 Hz). For any given trial, subjects were instructed to attend to one of the locations. In random order and with an interstimulus interval (ISI) of 400–700 ms, some of the LEDs at the attended and unattended side changed colour. Subjects had to respond to a particular combination of colour-changed LEDs (target stimuli). Frequency domain analysis showed that the flickering stimulus at the attended side yielded an increased power at its frequency. Moreover, as illustrated by Fig. 3.2(b), the increase in power for the attended flicker stimulus appeared to be highly correlated with a steep increase in target detection rate. These steady-state evoked potentials can therefore serve as a continuous measure of the time course of attentional switching. Müller *et al.* (1998*a,b*) interpreted these effects as supportive of a sensory gain control mechanism enhancing the signal-to-noise ratio and, consequently, the discriminability of the attended stimuli. The scalp

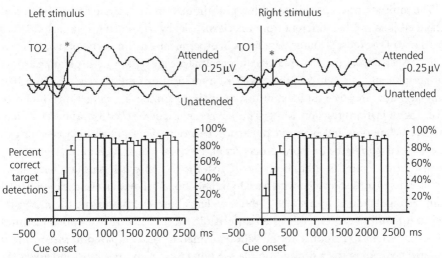

Fig. 3.2 Attention-related amplitude change of a steady state evoked potential driven by an LED at an attended spatial location. The figure illustrates that the attention-related gain in amplitude occurs about 300 ms after an attention-directing cue. The corresponding changes in behavioural accuracy suggest that identification of target stimuli is aided by the attention mechanisms indexed by the steady-state response (after data from Müller et al. 1998a).

distribution of this attention-driven steady-state evoked potential was narrowly focused over the posterior scalp contralateral to the side of stimulation (Müller et al. 1998a,b).

Attention to features other than location gives rise to different ERP components. Harter and Guido (1980) and Hillyard and Münte (1984) showed that attentional selection according to colour gives rise to a 'selection negativity' in the 150–350 ms range maximal over parietotemporal areas. The selection for colour was hierarchically dependent on the prior selection for location, when multidimensional stimuli were presented. Thus, the selection negativity for stimuli of the attended colour was only present if the stimuli also fulfilled the relevant location attribute. The selection negativity has been replicated in many studies (e.g. Smid et al. 1999) and is present for other features as well. For example, in recent studies comparing attention to colour and motion, Anllo-Vento and Hillyard (1996; Anllo-Vento et al. 1998) could show that attention to both features is accompanied by a selection negativity. Surprisingly, this negativity had a very similar timing and morphology regardless of the attended feature, in spite of the fact that colour is presumably processed by the so-called ventral stream, while motion is a feature analysed by the dorsal visual pathway (see Chapters 2 and 5, this volume). It remains to be shown whether subtle differences in scalp distribution of this selection negativity can be traced back to separate cortical origins compatible with dorsal and ventral stream locations.

The tonic attention paradigm with rapid stimulation from two or several different channels is somewhat different from the classic trial by trial-cueing approach that has been one of the most favoured paradigms in experimental neuropsychology. In this task (the 'Posner' task), a cue is presented either centrally (e.g. a left- or right-pointing arrow) or peripherally (e.g. a box at the possible target location) followed several hundred milliseconds later by a target stimulus requiring a simple (i.e. detection) or choice (i.e. discrimination) reaction. Most of the targets appear at the cued, or primed, location. Thus, reaction time and error rate differences between validly and invalidly cued targets can be used to infer the temporal properties of the visual spatial attention system.

In a series of studies, it has been shown that the ERP-effects in this task have many similarities to those obtained with fixed tonic attentional set over an entire experimental run (Mangun and Hillyard 1990, 1991). A central pre-cue indicating the likely site of an upcoming target leads to an amplitude increase for the temporooccipital P1-component in response to the validly primed target compared to the invalidly primed target in both choice and simple reaction tasks. In contrast, the subsequent N1 component was enhanced by validly cued stimuli in the choice reaction task condition only. These findings support models proposing that the behavioural effects of precueing expected target locations can be traced back to changes in sensoriperceptual processing within secondary modality-specific cortex. These areas have been shown to be under control of parietal supervisory systems (Gitelman *et al.* 1999; Mesulam 1990). As expected, in an ERP study using the Posner task in patients with parietal damage, Verleger *et al.* (1996) found a selective reduction of the attention effect for the left cue/right target combination.

Cross-modal interactions and visual attention

It is quite obvious in everyday life that an integration of information from several modalities is to the organism's advantage: we might be able to identify the image of the tiger faster if we know where the roar comes from. That our supramodal integration can be fooled is attested by the ventriloquist illusion, where the voice of the ventriloquist is erroneously attributed to his puppet, and the McGurk effect (Campbell *et al.* 1990*a*). In a series of elegant studies Driver and Spence (Driver and Spence 1998*a,b*; Spence and Driver 1996, 1997) have shown that divided attention to concurrent events in different modalities is generally more effective when stimuli have come from the same location. These multiple interactions of visual and auditory modalities at the behavioural level indicate that attention is at least partly dependent on spatial representations that have multimodal properties.

From a cognitive neuroscience perspective the question arises, at what stage of the information-processing cascade do cross-modal interactions take place? Can effects of cross-modal interaction be found in modality-specific cortex or are they confined to supramodal tertiary association cortex? Animal anatomy and physiology indicate that neurons at several levels in the nervous system (midbrain/superior colliculus, polysensory areas of the parietal, superior temporal, and frontal lobes) are responsive to stimuli from multiple modalities (Stein *et al.* 1993).

Event-related brain potentials are ideally suited to tackle this question in the human. In an early study, Hillyard and colleagues (1984) rapidly presented visual (flashes) and auditory (tones) stimuli at locations left and right of a fixation point. One group of subjects attended only to visual stimuli, directing their attention to one of the two locations in turn to detect slightly altered target stimuli; a second group of subjects attended only to auditory stimuli and was instructed to ignore the visual stimuli. In spite of the limited electrode array, typical visual and auditory spatial attention effects could be observed when these modalities were attended. Moreover, modulations of ERPs in the unattended modality depended on the direction of spatial attention in the attended modality. This is illustrated in Fig. 3.3 by data from a follow-up study using

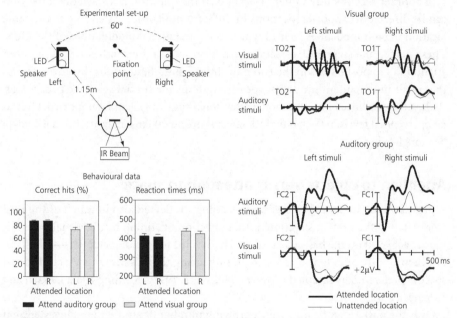

Fig. 3.3 Cross-modal spatial attention experiment; The upper left part of the figure illustrates the experimental set-up. Subjects either attended to rapid sequences of auditory stimuli presented over two speakers to the left and right of a fixation aid, or they attended to visual stimuli coming from the same locations. Each subject only attended one modality and attended location (left/right) was changed from run to run. In the subject group that attended to visual stimuli only (upper right part of figure) the typical temporo-occipital spatial attention effects were observed. The auditory stimuli that had no task relevance for this group showed an attention carry-over effect: auditory stimuli coming from the same location as the attended visual stimuli showed an enhanced negativity (Nd wave). Likewise, in the subject group that always attended to auditory stimuli, a typical auditory attention effect was present (lower right). Again, a carry-over effect to the unattended (visual) modality was observed. The visual stimuli coming from the same location as the attended auditory stimuli showed a frontocentral positive shift in addition to a modulation of the posterior N1 component (after data from Teder-Sälejärvi *et al.* 1999).

an extended electrode array (Teder-Sälejärvi *et al.* l999; see also Eimer and Schröger 1998). Again, two groups attended exclusively to either visual or auditory stimuli. In the attend-visual group, ERPs to auditory stimuli showed a typical modulation resembling the effect of spatial attention directed to auditory stimuli albeit with a smaller amplitude. The visual ERPs in the attend-auditory group showed a small but significant enhancement of the posterior and anterior N1 effects as a sign of cross-talk between the modalities. The effects were much smaller than the effects of visual spatial attention proper, though.

Because of the close similarity of attention effects and cross-modal attentional carry-over effects, these studies can be taken to suggest that intermodal attention operates by a selective modulation of modality-specific areas. These modulations have to be carried out by a supramodal attentional system.

In another recent study Eimer (1999) asked the question as to whether attention can be directed to opposite locations in different modalities. Attending to the same location in both modalities yielded typical early attentional modulations of the ERPs. These perceptual stage ERP effects were not present in the condition that required attention to opposite sides in the two modalities. Thus, these results disprove theories that posit independent modality-specific systems for spatial selective processing. Rather, the existence of a supramodal attentional control system is supported. Only at postperceptual levels, reflected by ERP effects beyond 200 ms, may attentional control be more flexible.

Attention to objects versus attention to space

A prevailing theme in experimental psychology, reflected also in much of the ERP work cited in the previous section, is that selection of stimuli by the visual system is mostly achieved on the basis of location. This has led to several metaphors—spotlight, gradients, and zoom lens—all of them indicating that a selected subset of visual space is preferentially sampled (Posner 1980; Yantis 1992; Downing 1988; Eriksen and St James 1986).

Over the past 15 years, however, a growing number of studies has suggested that more elaborate levels of representation, such as objects themselves, rather than their spatial location can serve as the basis for attentional selection of information (Duncan 1984; Vecera and Farah 1994, 1997; Kramer *et al.* 1997). So far, only a few recent ERP studies have tackled this fundamental issue. Clearly, showing a modulation of exogenous components in situations that require an object-based selection of information would place these mechanisms at the front end of the information-processing cascade. On the other hand, late effects would rather indicate that object-based selection is taking place at later postperceptual stages.

One elegant set of studies by Valdes-Sosa *et al.* (1998) used spatially interspersed dots of different colours as stimuli. Two conditions were used. In one condition, the dots did not move during the baseline stimulation. This led to the perception of *one object* composed of many dots. In the other condition, the dots of one colour were rotating in one direction, whereas the dots of the second colour moved in the opposite direction during baseline stimulation. They were thus perceived as two different objects. Critically, the two objects shared the same location. Stimuli were defined as brief displacements of the dots of one colour in several directions, one of which was designated the target direction. Subjects were instructed to attend to displacements of the dots of one (attended) colour and to ignore the displacements or the dots in the other colour. When these displacements were presented in the condition with stationary dots, the stimuli were perceived as displacements of one part of a single object. In the rotating baseline condition, the stimuli can be thought of as displacements of one of two objects. Since the dots of the two colours were interspersed, spatial selection could not be used by the subjects. The results for standard stimuli are shown in Fig. 3.4. Dramatic differences

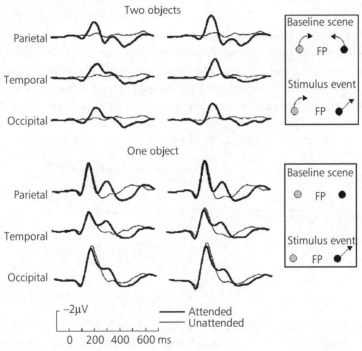

Fig. 3.4 Experiment addressing the role of objects in visual attention. In condition 'Two objects' (upper part), stimuli are created by dots of two colours rotating in opposite directions. This creates the perception of two separate objects at the same location. Target stimuli are created by dislocation of one set of dots. Attended colour stimuli are characterized by an enhanced P1 and N1 component, thus indicating very early attentional selection mechanisms. In the control condition 'One object' (lower part), stationary dots were used leading to the perception of just one object. The ERPs to the attended stimuli are characterized by a later selection negativity in this condition (after data from Valdes-Sosa *et al.* 1998).

emerged between the two-object (rotating baseline) and one-object (stationary baseline) conditions. A modulation of the P1 and N1 components was found in the two-object condition, indicating that very early perceptual processes located in extrastriate cortex are involved in object-based attention. On the other hand, when the baseline compelled the subjects into viewing one object, movement of one set of dots led to a typical selection negativity with an onset of about 150 ms as described previously for colour and motion selection (Anllo-Vento and Hillyard 1996; Hillyard *et al.* 1984). These results indicate that perceptual organization (into objects) acts as a supplementary attentional selection process at very early levels. Further studies suggest that there might be an interaction between selection based on location and selection based on objects. More work comparing space-based and object-based attention and employing methods of source localization is needed to specify more precisely the time-course and anatomical basis of object-based selection and its independence from spatial attention.

Visual search

Screening a complex visual scene for some relevant item or feature is a prerequisite for the survival of the individuum. Experimental psychologists have shown that, in essence, there are two different search modes. In parallel search, illustrated in Fig. 3.5(a), subjects have to search for a distinguishing feature that is present only for the target item, in this case an extra line extending from the base of one triangle.

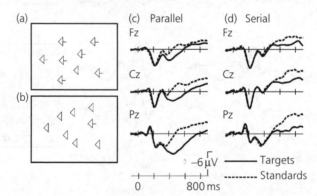

Fig. 3.5 Illustration of typical ERP findings in parallel and serial search modes. (a) In the serial search mode subjects are required to detect a target item characterized by the *missing* of a stimulus feature (in this case an additional horizontal line) shared by all other items. Only half of the stimuli in the experiment contained a target item. (b) In the parallel search mode the task is to detect target items characterized by an additional feature. This latter task can be accomplished much faster, as all items can be screened for the additional feature at the same time (in parallel). (c) ERPS in the parallel search task show a peaked P3 component for the target stimuli. Target and standard stimuli diverge at about 350 ms. (d) This separation occurs much later in the serial search task. Moreover, the serial nature of the task tends to smear out the P3 peak (unpublished data from Münte).

All items of a complex array can be searched for this distinguishing feature in parallel and reaction time does not increase with increased numbers of items in an array. In one type of serial search mode (Fig. 3.5(b)), on the other hand, all items, except for the target item, possess a feature, in this case the additional line. In this condition, an observer has to scan each item serially in order to detect the missing line, leading to a massive increase in reaction time as a function of the number of items within an array.

These tasks have been translated into the electrophysiological domain by Luck and Hillyard (1990, 1994 a,b). They found that the latency and the amplitude of the P3 component differed radically for the two search modes. In the parallel search mode, a high-amplitude P3 with a circumscribed peak occurred for target stimuli, whereas in the serial task the divergence between standard and target stimuli was much later (see Fig. 3.5(c),(d) for similar data). Furthermore, the latency of the P3 varied with the number of distractor items within an array.

Some clinical applications, e.g. on patients with Huntington's disease (Münte et al. 1997) or brain injury (Heinze et al. 1992), have been reported. In general, it was found that the simple, parallel search mode was more or less preserved in patients with neuro-logical disorders, while the more complex serial search task showed differences between patients with various pathologies and normal controls.

In more recent investigations, Luck and colleagues have concentrated on the so-called N2pc component (Luck and Hillyard 1995; Luck et al. 1996; Luck and Ford 1998). This component is a negative deflection in the 200–300 ms time range that is typically observed at posterior scalp sites contralateral to the location of a target item in a search task. The N2pc reflects the focusing of attention on to the target item to filter out irrelevant information from adjacent distractor items within an array. The functional parallels between the N2pc component and the attentional suppression effects present in single-unit recordings from area V4 in the macaque brain have been discussed by Luck and colleagues (1997).

In one recent series of experiments (see Fig. 3.6), Luck and Ford (1998) compared feature extraction and conjunction tasks. In the feature extraction task (Fig. 3.6(a)), subjects viewed an array containing 10 grey and 2 coloured items and were required to report whether a particular colour was present within an array. This task was per-formed either alone or in conjunction with a second task that required the subjects to indicate whether a centrally presented letter was a vowel or a consonant. Only a small N2pc component was present for the feature task that was completely abolished when the subjects had to perform the letter classification task in parallel. This was taken to suggest that the feature task does not require the perceptual level attentional mecha-nism that is indexed by the N2pc component.

In a second, more complex search task subjects had to search for rectangles that had a particular colour and orientation. Again, this task was either executed alone or in conjunction with a central letter discrimination. Only for the conjunction task (colour and orientation) did a sizeable N2pc emerge, which persisted in the dual-task situation

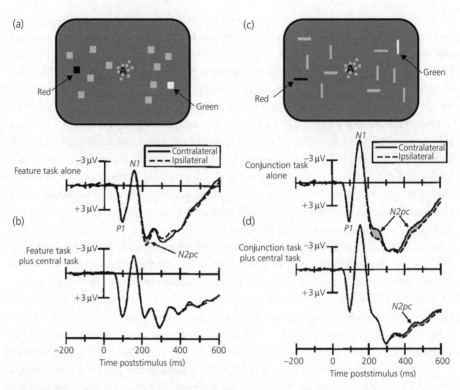

Fig. 3.6 Two different varieties of a visual search task. (a) A feature detection task is illustrated. In this task, a target item is characterized by a distinguishing feature, i.e. its colour, that is not shared by any of the distractor items. (b) ERPs from two different versions of the feature detection task. When the feature task is the only task of the subjects, waveforms show a so-called N2pc (for posterior contralateral) component (middle left), which is abolished when subjects have to simultaneously execute a letter discrimination task presented in the centre of the video screen. This suggests that, although the observers were able to accurately detect the feature target while performing the concurrent letter discrimination task, attention was not necessary for feature detection. (c) A similarly constructed conjunction search experiment is illustrated. In this task, target items are characterized by features (in this case horizontal orientation and red colour) that are shared by the distractor items, necessitating an exhaustive serial search strategy. (d) A large N2pc wave is seen for the conjunction task when it was performed alone (middle right). When the central letter discrimination task was added, an N2pc was still observed but was considerably delayed and smeared out in time (after data from Luck and Ford 1998).

but was shifted towards a later latency. Because of the nature of the discrimination task, requiring the subjects to combine colour and orientation features of target items, attention was necessary to execute the task as reflected in the higher-amplitude N2pc in the conjunction task alone condition. During the second attention-demanding task, the N2pc was smeared out and shifted in time. Luck and Ford's interpretation of this latency shift was that subjects accessed the iconic image of the search array after they finished the central task.

Hierarchical visual stimuli

A sizeable literature within neuropsychology has addressed the brain's processing of hierarchically structured visual objects (Kimchi 1992; Lamb *et al.* 1990). While in the real world global (e.g. a forest) and local levels (e.g. the trees) are quite different, research has concentrated on objects that have similar elements on global and local levels, e.g. a large H made up of small Hs (Fig. 3.7). Patients with lesions at the temporoparietal junction but not in frontal areas exhibit marked problems with the analysis of global (right lesions) and local (left lesions) aspects of such hierarchical stimuli (Robertson *et al.* 1988, 1991).

Recent neuroimaging data (Fink *et al.* 1999; Heinze *et al.* 1998) have shown that, in addition to the temporoparietal areas, secondary visual areas in the extrastriate cortex might be involved in global/local processing. Neuroimaging studies, however, have the disadvantage that they have to direct the attention of the subject to one level of the stimuli. Electrophysiological studies, on the other hand, can assess processing of global and local levels of stimuli in more natural, divided-attention tasks, in which subjects have to identify target items on global and local levels of the stimuli simultaneously.

Heinze and Münte (1993), in a study of young adults having to detect target letters at both global and local levels, have shown that a negativity in the 150–300 ms range with a maximum at temporoparietal sites indicated the detection of target letters. Moreover, this selection negativity showed a differential hemispheric distribution for local (left preponderant) and global (right preponderant) targets, with an interaction between the two levels. Using the same task, Heinze *et al.* (1997) investigated patients with malignant brain tumours including the temporoparietal junction. A clear dissociation of left- and right-hemisphere patients could be shown, in that right-hemisphere patients had a grossly attenuated selection negativity for targets at the global level, while the reverse was true for left-hemisphere patients (Fig. 3.8).

In another study, selective and divided attention between local and global levels of hierarchical letter stimuli was directly compared (Heinze *et al.* 1998). When attention was divided between global and local levels, the N2 component elicited by the target stimuli showed asymmetries in amplitude over the two hemispheres as in earlier studies. During selective attention to either global or local targets, asymmetries of the N2

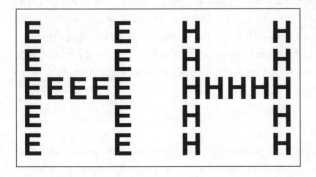

Fig. 3.7 Illustration of typical hierarchical stimuli used in experiments addressing global and local stimulus perception.

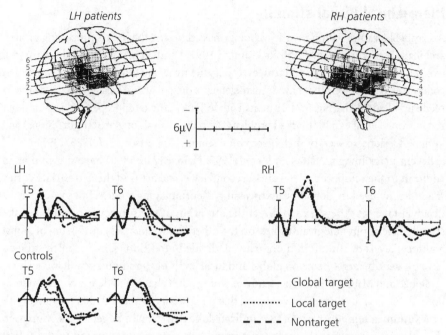

Fig. 3.8 Data from a task assessing global and local target detection. Stimuli comprised large letters (global level, e.g. the letter H) made up from smaller letters (local level, e.g. letter S). In any given run, one letter was designated as a target letter in response to which subjects had to press a button regardless of whether the target letter occurred on the local or the global level. This task leads to a prominent selection negativity for the target letters in the 200–350 ms range over temporoposterior scalp sites in the control subjects. A group of patients with left-hemispheric (LH) lesions (tumours) in the temporoparietal region showed a reduction of the selection negativity to the target letters on the local level, while the right hemisphere (RH) patients displayed a smaller negativity for targets on the global level. This pattern of results corroborates the view of a hemispheric specialization for local (left hemisphere) and global (right hemisphere) information (after data of Heinze *et al.* 1997).

component disappeared. Here, however, the sensory-evoked P1 component was enlarged for global versus local attention. Increased regional cerebral blood flow in the posterior fusiform gyrus was observed bilaterally in PET data during selective attention to either global or local targets, but neither blood flow nor the P1 component showed any tendency toward hemispheric difference for global versus local attention. This indicates that selective filtering at an early perceptual level takes place under selective but not under divided-attention conditions.

Face perception

Evidence for a distinct neural system subserving recognition of faces was first provided by prosopagnosic patients with mostly right-sided lesions in the occipitotemporal region (Milders and Perrett 1993). Some patients were specifically impaired to identify familiar faces; others showed selective deficits for recognition of gaze direction (Campbell *et al.* 1990*b)* or lip-reading (Campbell *et al.* 1996*a,b).* To account for these selective deficits, neuropsychological models have attempted to fractionate face recognition into several subfunctions (see Chapter 1, this volume). For example, in the model of Bruce and Young (1986), facial features are analysed and specified during an initial phase of structural encoding. The products of this stage are then fed into various independent modules that are concerned with analysis of facial expression and speech as well as face recognition. Such models have been supported by findings in neuropsychological patients as well as by primate studies. In humans, functional imaging studies using PET and fMRI revealed bilateral but right predominant activation in the posterior fusiform gyrus for faces as opposed to other objects or textures (Haxby *et al.* 1999; Halgren *et al.* 1999; Kanwisher *et al.* 1998; Clark *et al.* 1998).

Electrophysiological studies in humans add further information on the exact time course of the neural activity reflecting face processing. Using subdural electrodes, a surface negative potential at a latency of 200 ms (N200) was recorded from regions of the left and right fusiform and inferior temporal gyri in response to the presentation of faces but not to any other complex stimuli such as scrambled faces, cars, or butterflies (Allison *et al.* 1994*a,b).* Jeffreys (1993; Jeffreys and Tukmachi 1992; Jeffreys *et al.* 1992) described the so-called vertex positive scalp peak at a latency of 150–200 ms, which preferentially responds to faces. Bentin *et al.* (1996) recorded a negative potential over posterior temporal sites at a latency of 172 ms (N170) that was selectively evoked by faces. In fact, the temporal N170 and the vertex positive peak are probably one and the same component, the different labels merely reflecting the topographical distribution of the dipole. The N170 was reported to be delayed by face inversion and significantly larger to isolated eyes, indicating that N170 might reflect eye-specific instead of whole face-processing. This topic was followed up further in a recent study addressing the effects of gaze direction in images of faces. Human faces and isolated eyes served as stimuli with eyes either directed at the subject or away from the subject (Fig. 3.9). Subjects viewed the stimuli flashed upon a video screen in random order and searched for target elements (dots) present only in a minority of the stimuli, while 148 channels of MEG and 32 channels of EEG were recorded. Both isolated eyes and faces showed a very early effect of gaze direction beginning at around 120 ms. This effect could be localized by minimum norm and dipole localization methods to the inferior posterior surface of the temporal lobe. This result can be taken as evidence that gaze direction is analysed very early and independently of the whole facial gestalt within secondary visual areas.

In another recent study, Münte *et al.* (1998) assessed the electrophysiological differences between matching successively presented pairs of faces (frontal and side-views) for their identity and for their expression (Fig. 3.10). They found that identity matching affected a frontocentral negativity in the 200–400 ms range, whereas the electrophysiological signs of expression matching manifested themselves much later and had a parietal distribution.

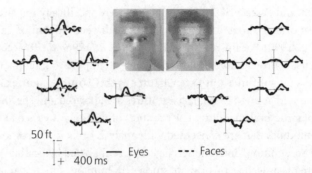

50 ft

400 ms — Eyes --- Faces

Fig. 3.9 Data from an experiment addressing the perception of gaze direction. Stimuli were either faces with only the eye portion visible as shown in the figure, or unmanipulated faces (not shown). The face stimuli either looked directly at the observer or away from her/him. The MEG (148-channel whole-head device) and the ERP (32 channels) responses to the different classes of stimuli were recorded. The figure shows the difference waves obtained by subtracting the waveforms to the faces with straight eyes from the faces with diverted eyes for six MEG sensors over the left and six MEG sensors over the right temporo-occipital scalp. The data show a gaze-direction effect as early as 120 ms that could be localized to the fusiform gyrus by dipole-fitting and minimum norm procedures (unpublished data from Noppeney, Heinze, Scheich, and Münte).

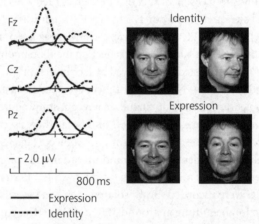

Fz

Cz

Pz

Identity

Expression

— 2.0 μV

800 ms

——— Expression

------- Identity

Fig. 3.10 Data from a study addressing the processing of faces for identity and expression. In the identity-matching conditions, pairs of faces photographed from different angles were shown with a stimulus-onset-asynchrony of 1000 ms. The second face of a pair either matched or did not match the first face in terms of identity of the depicted person. In the expression-matching condition, pairs of faces with either different or the same expression were shown. The ERP data are difference waves obtained by subtracting the matching faces from those to the mismatching faces. There is a clear temporal and topographical distinction of the processing of identity and expression, with the former effect being larger for frontal (Fz) and central (Cz) midline electrodes, whereas the latter displayed a parietal (Pz) maximum (after data from Münte et al. 1998).

Thus, together with functional imaging data, ERPs now provide a quite detailed picture of face-processing in humans. Initial feature analysis and encoding, including the analysis of gaze, seems to take place in secondary visual areas in the fusiform and inferotemporal gyri at latencies between 100 and 200 ms. Later stages of analysis, such as the determination of a person's identity, are carried out by anterior temporal and possibly frontal brain area at latencies beyond 200 ms. Even later, and probably involving multiple brain regions, analysis of emotional expression is carried out. These data in turn can now form the basis for the investigation of prosopagnosic patients of various kinds.

High-frequency induced activity in the visual system

A novel measure derived from electrophysiological data is the so-called induced gamma activity (Tallon-Baudry *et al.* 1997*a*, 1998; Keil *et al.* 1999; Müller *et al.* 1996). This is activity with a frequency of about 40 Hz occurring in a non-time-locked fashion in response to sensory stimulation or cognitive tasks. It has to be distinguished from the evoked 40 Hz activity that can be computed from the EEG by conventional averaging. By contrast, induced gamma activity is not revealed by classical averaging techniques. Rather the time-varying spectra of the EEG tapered by a moving window of a fixed duration have to be computed. Alternatively, the decomposition of the signal can be achieved by wavelet transforms. In general, stimulus-induced gamma activity occurs mainly in the 200–400 ms time window after a stimulus in auditory, somatosensory, and visual tasks. Besides a very general, and therefore more or less meaningless, interpretation of the gamma response as the correlate of *cognitive processing*, a more appealing hypothesis has emerged, mainly from the group of Bertrand and Tallon-Baudry. These authors maintain that the gamma response might constitute the electrophysiological substrate of the binding process. This places the work on induced gamma activity into the context of the hypothesis that coordinated rhythmic discharges in different areas of a neural network serve as one basis of cortical information processing (Singer and Gray 1995).

In one task (see Fig. 3.11) subjects viewed Kanisza-like figures forming either an illusory triangle, no triangle or a real triangle. Only the two triangle conditions (real and illusory) gave rise to a temporary increase of activity in the gamma band around 230 ms. This activity could be mapped to the occipital cortex (Tallon-Baudry *et al.* 1997*b*). It was thus proposed that the increased gamma activity might indicate the perception of a coherent object. In a related study, Rodriguez *et al.* (1999) could show that only patterned stimuli that elicited the perception of a face (Mooney faces) were associated with gamma band activity around 230 ms. Top–down processes guiding perception also differentially elicit induced gamma activity (Tallon-Baudry *et al.* 1998).

Integrating results from temporal and spatial imaging studies

Recent years have seen an explosion of the functional imaging literature on visual processing. Obviously, it is much easier and straightforward to precisely locate activation

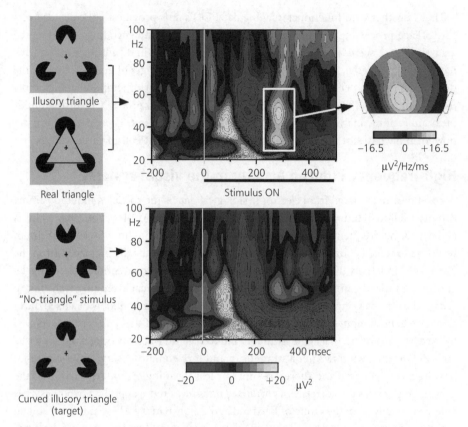

Fig. 3.11 Induced gamma-band responses obtained in an experiment using illusory and real triangles as well as illusory non-triangles. Only the stimuli giving rise to the perception of a triangle were associated with increased gamma-band activity (marked by white box in upper part of the figure) in the 240–300 ms range which was maximal over temporo-occipital scalp regions (after data from Tallon-Baudry *et al.* 1997*b*).

patterns in PET and fMRI than it is to locate ERPs and event-related magnetic fields. On the other hand, the time resolution of imaging methods is much poorer than that of ERPs, even for modern rapid-presentation event-related fMRI. Moreover, the current techniques of functional imaging rely on blood flow and oxygen level measures, which are only an indirect measure of neural activity. The question therefore arises as to how spatial and temporal imaging methods can be combined to yield a more complete view of the human visual system.

In a combined study of visuospatial attention ^{15}O-labelled water PET and ERPs were used in healthy subjects (Heinze *et al.* 1994). This paradigm used a rapid presentation of bilateral stimulus arrays, only one side of which had to be attended. A typical contralateral P1 component represented the earliest electrophysiological sign of spatial attention. This component could be modelled by a dipole located to the posterior part of the fusiform gyrus. The PET data showed an activation at precisely the same location. In addition, other areas, including the cingulate gyrus, were active. Thus, in spite of the very different nature of the signals detected with ERPs and PET, tonic attention-related blood flow changes and transient electrophysiological signals were co-localized. This study has been replicated in several variants including one using fMRI instead of PET (Mangun *et al.* 1998). In this latter study, because of the better signal-to-noise ratio of fMRI, it was possible to investigate the intersubject variability in extrastriate spatial attention effects, and to qualitatively compare this to variations in ERP attention effects. The activations in single subjects replicated the group-averaged PET findings.

As spatial and temporal imaging methods rely on very different signals, it is perhaps not surprising and maybe not even desirable that results do not always converge perfectly in both types of study. Consider, for example, a recent experiment by Martinez *et al.* (1999). Again, as a test of visuospatial attention, subjects were required to discriminate patterned targets within distractor arrays. Such a paradigm is similar to conditions under which Motter (1993) found neural correlates of focal attentive processes in areas V1 and V2 as well as area V4 in behaving macaque monkeys. His monkeys had to perform a stimulus feature analysis and selective spatial processing within a field of competing stimuli. In the Martinez *et al.* (1999) study, fMRI revealed activations in several areas including the striate cortex. The earliest component of the ERP that showed an attentional modulation occurred at 70–75 ms and could be mapped into extrastriate visual areas, while earlier activity (around 50 ms) was unresponsive to spatial attention. The authors therefore hypothesized that the V1-activation seen in the fMRI might reflect the feedback of information from later stages of processing to primary visual cortex.

Even though the experimental and logistical requirements for combined spatial and temporal imaging are immense, the very few studies available so far underscore the utility of such an approach. Moreover, the electrophysiological signals from the visual system often have a circumscribed topographical distribution and therefore lend themselves to localization with dipole models or alternative techniques. This makes the visual system ideal for developing combined spatiotemporal imaging strategies.

Conclusion

Event-related brain potentials, event-related magnetic fields, and induced activity are used to track the fate of a visual stimulus on its way through the cortex. The exquisite temporal resolution of the electrophysiological methods in conjunction with our recent ability to combine temporal and spatial imaging modalities will provide an even more fine-grained picture of visual processing in the future. We will then be able to delineate the neuronal underpinnings of the many peculiar syndromes originating in the visual system, including central achromatopsia, motion blindness, simultanagnosia (Balint's syndrome), prosopagnosia, neglect, and object agnosias.

Acknowledgements

The authors' own research is supported by grants from the DFG.

References

Allison, T., Begleiter, A., McCarthy, G., Roessler, E., Nobre, A.C., and Spencer, D.D. (1993). Electrophysiological studies of color processing in human visual cortex. *Electroencephalogr. Clin. Neurophysiol.* **88** (5), 343–55.

Allison, T., Ginter, H., McCarthy, G., Nobre, A.C., Puce, A., Luby, M., and Spencer, D.D. (1994a). Face recognition in human extrastriate cortex. *J. Neurophysiol.* **71** (2), 821–5.

Allison, T., McCarthy, G., Nobre, A., Puce, A., and Belger, A. (1994b). Human extrastriate visual cortex and the perception of faces, words, numbers, and colors. *Cereb. Cortex* **4** (5), 544–54.

Anderson, S.J., Holliday, I.E., Singh, K.D., and Harding, G.F. (1996). Localization and functional analysis of human cortical area V5 using magneto-encephalography. *Proc. R. Soc. Lond. B, Biol. Sci.* **263** (1369), 423–31.

Anllo-Vento, L. and Hillyard, S.A. (1996). Selective attention to the color and direction of moving stimuli: electrophysiological correlates of hierarchical feature selection. *Percept. Psychophys.* **58** (2), 191–206.

Anllo-Vento, L., Luck, S.J., and Hillyard, S.A. (1998). Spatio-temporal dynamics of attention to color: evidence from human electrophysiology. *Hum. Brain Mapp.* **6** (4), 216–38.

Bentin, S., Allison, T., Puce, A., and Perez, E. (1996). Electrophysiological studies of face perception in humans. *J. Cogn. Neurosci.* **8**, 551–65.

Bodis-Wollner, I. (1992). Sensory evoked potentials: PERG, VEP, and SEP. *Curr. Opin. Neurol. Neurosurg.* **5** (5), 716–26.

Bruce, V. and Young, A. (1986). Understanding face recognition [see comments]. *Br. J. Psychol.* **77** (Pt. 3), 305–27.

Buchner, H., Weyen, U., Frackowiak, R.S., Romaya, J., and Zeki, S. (1994). The timing of visual evoked potential activity in human area V4. *Proc. R. Soc. Lond. B, Biol. Sci.* **257** (1348), 99–104.

Campbell, R., Garwood, J., Franklin, S., Howard, D., Landis, T., and Regard, M. (1990a). Neuropsychological studies of auditory–visual fusion illusions. Four case studies and their implications. *Neuropsychologia* **28** (8), 787–802.

Campbell, R., Heywood, C.A., Cowey, A., Regard, M., and Landis, T. (1990b). Sensitivity to eye gaze in prosopagnosic patients and monkeys with superior temporal sulcus ablation. *Neuropsychologia* **28** (11), 1123–42.

Campbell, R., Brooks, B., De Haan, E., and Roberts, T. (1996a). Dissociating face processing skills: decision about lip-read speech, expression, and identity. *Quart. J. Exp. Psychol. A* **49** (2), 295–314.

Campbell, R., De Gelder, B., and De Haan, E. (1996b). The lateralization of lip-reading: a second look. *Neuropsychologia* **34** (12), 1235–40.

Chelazzi, L. (1995). Neural mechanisms for stimulus selection in cortical areas of the macaque subserving object vision. *Behav. Brain. Res.* **71** (1–2), 125–34.

Clark, V.P., Maisog, J.M., and Haxby, J.V. (1998). fMRI study of face perception and memory using random stimulus sequences. *J. Neurophysiol.* **79** (6), 3257–65.

Downing, C.J. (1988). Expectancy and visual-spatial attention: effects on perceptual quality. *J. Exp. Psychol. Hum. Percept. Perform.* **14**, 188–202.

Driver, J. and Spence, C. (1998a). Cross-modal links in spatial attention. *Phil. Trans. R. Soc. Lond. B, Biol. Sci.* **353** (1373), 1319–31.

Driver, J. and Spence, C. (1998b). Crossmodal attention. *Curr. Opin. Neurobiol.* **8** (2), 245–53.

Duncan, J. (1984). Selective attention and the organization of visual information. *J. Exp. Psychol. Genet.* 113 (4), 501–17.

Eimer, M. (1999). Can attention be directed to opposite locations in different modalities? An ERP study [in process citation]. *Clin. Neurophysiol.* 110 (7), 1252–9.

Eimer, M. and Schröger, E. (1998). ERP effects of intermodal attention and cross-modal links in spatial attention. *Psychophysiology* 35 (3), 313–27.

Eriksen, C.W. and St James, J.D. (1986). Visual attention within and around the field of focal attention: a zoom lens model. *Percept. Psychophys.* 40, 225–40.

Ferrera, V.P. and Lisberger, S.G. (1997). Neuronal responses in visual areas MT and MST during smooth pursuit target selection. *J. Neurophysiol.* 78 (3), 1433–46.

Fink, G.R., Marshall, J.C., Halligan, P.W., and Dolan, R.J. (1999). Hemispheric asymmetries in global/local processing are modulated by perceptual salience. *Neuropsychologia* 37 (1), 31–40.

Gitelman, D.R., Nobre, A.C., Parrish, T.B., LaBar, K.S., Kim, Y.H., Meyer, J.R., and Mesulam, M. (1999). A large-scale distributed network for covert spatial attention: further anatomical delineation based on stringent behavioural and cognitive controls. *Brain* 122 (Pt. 6), 1093–106.

Gomez, G.C., Clark, V.P., Fan, S., Luck, S.J., and Hillyard, S.A. (1994). Sources of attention-sensitive visual event-related potentials. *Brain Topogr.* 7 (1), 41–51.

Halgren, E., Dale, A.M., Sereno, M.I., Tootell, R.B., Marinkovic, K., and Rosen, B.R. (1999). Location of human face-selective cortex with respect to retinotopic areas. *Hum. Brain Mapp.* 7 (1), 29–37.

Harter, M.R. and Aine, C.J. (1986). Discussion of neural-specificity model of selective attention: a response to Hillyard and Mangun and to Naatanen. *Biol. Psychol.* 23 (3), 297–311.

Harter, M.R. and Guido, W. (1980). Attention to pattern orientation: negative cortical potentials, reaction time, and the selection process. *Electroencephalogr. Clin. Neurophysiol.* 49 (5–6), 461–75.

Haxby, J.V., Ungerleider, L.G., Clark, V.P., Schouten, J.L., Hoffman, E.A., and Martin, A. (1999). The effect of face inversion on activity in human neural systems for face and object perception [see comments]. *Neuron* 22 (1), 189–99.

Heinze, H.J. and Münte, T.F. (1993). Electrophysiological correlates of hierarchical stimulus processing: dissociation between onset and later stages of global and local target processing. *Neuropsychologia* 31 (8), 841–52.

Heinze, H.J., Münte, T.F., Gobiet, W., Niemann, H., and Ruff, R.M. (1992). Parallel and serial visual search after closed head injury: electrophysiological evidence for perceptual dysfunctions. *Neuropsychologia* 30 (6), 495–514.

Heinze, H.J., Mangun, G.R., Burchert, W., Hinrichs, H., Scholz, M., Münte, T.F., Gos, A., Scherg, M., Johannes, S., and Hundeshagen, H. (1994). Combined spatial and temporal imaging of brain activity during visual selective attention in humans. *Nature* 372 (6506), 543–6.

Heinze, H.J., Matzke, M., Dorfmueller, G., and Smid, H.G. (1997). Flexibility in the structure of human information processing. *Advan. Neurol.* 73, 359–75.

Heinze, H.J., Hinrichs, H., Scholz, M., Burchert, W., and Mangun, G.R. (1998). Neural mechanisms of global and local processing. A combined PET and ERP study. *J. Cogn. Neurosci.* 10 (4), 485–98.

Hietanen, J.K., Perrett, D.I., Oram, M.W., Benson, P.J., and Dittrich, W.H. (1992). The effects of lighting conditions on responses of cells selective for face views in the macaque temporal cortex. *Exp. Brain Res.* 89 (1), 157–71.

Hillyard, S.A. and Anllo–Vento, L. (1998). Event-related brain potentials in the study of visual selective attention. *Proc. Natl. Acad. Sci. USA.* 95, 781–7.

Hillyard, S.A. and Mangun, G.R. (1986). The neural basis of visual selective attention: a commentary on Harter and Aine. *Biol. Psychol.* 23 (3), 265–79.

Hillyard, S.A. and Münte, T.F. (1984). Selective attention to color and location: an analysis with event-related brain potentials. *Percept. Psychophys.* **36** (2), 185–98.

Hillyard, S.A., Simpson, G.V., Woods, D.L., Van Voorhis, S., and Münte, T.F. (1984). Event-related brain potentials and selective attention to different modalities. In *Cortical integration* (ed. F. Reinoso-Suarez and C. Ajmone-Marsan), pp. 395–413. Raven Press, New York.

Jeffreys, D.A. (1993). The influence of stimulus orientation on the vertex positive scalp potential evoked by faces. *Exp. Brain Res.* **96** (1), 163–72.

Jeffreys, D.A. and Tukmachi, E.S. (1992). The vertex-positive scalp potential evoked by faces and by objects. *Exp. Brain Res.* **91** (2), 340–50.

Jeffreys, D.A., Tukmachi, E.S., and Rockley, G. (1992). Evoked potential evidence for human brain mechanisms that respond to single, fixated faces. *Exp. Brain Res.* **91** (2), 351–62.

Kanwisher, N., Tong, F., and Nakayama, K. (1998). The effect of face inversion on the human fusiform face area. *Cognition* **68** (1), B1–11.

Keil, A., Iler, M.M., Ray, W.J., Gruber, T., and Elbert, T. (1999). Human gamma band activity and perception of a Gestalt. *J. Neurosci.* **19** (16), 7152–61.

Kimchi, R. (1992). Primacy of wholistic processing and global/local paradigm: a critical review. *Psychol. Bull.* **112** (1), 24–38.

Kramer, A.F., Weber, T.A., and Watson, S.E. (1997). Object-based attentional selection—grouped arrays or spatially invariant representations?: comment on Vecera and Farah (1994). *J. Exp. Psychol. Gen.* **126** (1), 3–13.

Lamb, M.R., Robertson, L.C., and Knight, R.T. (1990). Component mechanisms underlying the processing of hierarchically organized patterns: inferences from patients with unilateral cortical lesions. *J. Exp. Psychol. Learn. Mem. Cogn.* **16** (3) 471–83.

Luck, S.J. and Ford, M.A. (1998). On the role of selective attention in visual perception. *Proc. Natl. Acad. Sci., USA* **95** (3), 825–30.

Luck, S.J. and Hillyard, S.A. (1990). Electrophysiological evidence for parallel and serial processing during visual search. *Percept. Psychophys.* **48** (6), 603–17.

Luck, S.J. and Hillyard, S.A. (1994*a*) Electrophysiological correlates of feature analysis during visual search. *Psychophysiology* **31** (3), 291–308.

Luck, S.J. and Hillyard, S.A. (1994*b*) Spatial filtering during visual search: evidence from human electrophysiology. *J. Exp. Psychol. Hum. Percept. Perform.* **20** (5), 1000–14.

Luck, S.J. and Hillyard, S.A. (1995). The role of attention in feature detection and conjunction discrimination: an electrophysiological analysis. *Int. J. Neurosci.* **80** (1–4), 281–297.

Luck, S.J., Hillyard, S.A., Mouloua, M., and Hawkins, H.L. (1996). Mechanisms of visual-spatial attention: resource allocation or uncertainty reduction? *J. Exp. Psychol. Hum. Percept. Perform.* **22** (3), 725–37.

Luck, S.J., Girelli, M., McDermott, M.T., and Ford, M.A. (1997). Bridging the gap between monkey neurophysiology and human perception: an ambiguity resolution theory of visual selective attention. *Cogn. Psychol.* **33** (1), 64–87.

Mangun, G.R. and Hillyard, S.A. (1990). Allocation of visual attention to spatial locations: tradeoff functions for event-related brain potentials and detection performance. *Percept. Psychophys.* **47** (6), 532–50.

Mangun, G.R. and Hillyard, S.A. (1991). Modulations of sensory-evoked brain potentials indicate changes in perceptual processing during visual-spatial priming. *J. Exp. Psychol. Hum. Percept. Perform.* **17** (4), 1057–74.

Mangun, G.R., Buonocore, M.H., Girelli, M., and Jha, A.P. (1998). ERP and fMRI measures of visual spatial selective attention. *Hum. Brain Mapp.* **6** (5–6). 383–9.

Martinez, A., Anllo-Vento, L., Sereno, M.I., Frank, L.R., Buxton, R.B., Dubowitz, D.J., Wong, E.C., Hinrichs, H., Heinze, H.J., and Hillyard, S.A. (1999). Involvement of striate and extrastriate visual cortical areas in spatial attention. *Nat. Neurosci.* 2 (4), 364–9.

Mesulam, M.M. (1990). Large-scale neurocognitive networks and distributed processing for attention, language, and memory. *Ann. Neurol.* 28 (5), 597–613.

Milders, M.V. and Perrett, D.I. (1993). Recent developments in the neuropsychology and physiology of face processing. *Baillières Clin. Neurol.* 2 (2), 361–88.

Morgan, S.T., Hansen, J.C., and Hillyard, S.A. (1996). Selective attention to stimulus location modulates the steady-state visual evoked potential. *Proc. Natl Acad. Sci., USA* 93 (10), 4770–4.

Motter, B.C. (1993). Focal attention produces spatially selective processing in visual cortical areas V1, V2, and V4 in the presence of competing stimuli. *J. Neurophysiol.* 70 (3), 909–19.

Müller, M.M., Bosch, J., Elbert, T., Kreiter, A., Sosa, M.V., Sosa, P.V., and Rockstroh, B. (1996). Visually induced gamma-band responses in human electroencephalographic activity—a link to animal studies. *Exp. Brain Res.* 112 (1), 96–102.

Müller, M.M., Picton, T.W., Valdes-Sosa, P., Riera, J., Teder-Salejarvi, W.A., and Hillyard, S.A. (1998a). Effects of spatial selective attention on the steady-state visual evoked potential in the 20–28 Hz range. *Brain Res. Cogn. Brain Res.* 6 (4), 249–61.

Müller, M.M., Teder-Sälejärvi, W., and Hillyard, S.A. (1998 b). The time course of cortical facilitation during cued shifts of spatial attention [see comments]. *Nat. Neurosci.* 1 (7), 631–4.

Münte, T.F., Ridao-Alonso, M.E., Preinfalk, J., Jung, A., Wieringa, B.M., Matzke, M., Dengler, R., and Johannes, S. (1997). An electrophysiological analysis of altered cognitive functions in Huntington disease. *Arch. Neurol.* 54 (9), 1089–98.

Münte, T.F., Brack, M., Grootheer, O., Wieringa, B.M., Matzke, M., and Johannes, S. (1998). Brain potentials reveal the timing of face identity and expression judgments. *Neurosci. Res.* 30 (1), 25–34.

Münte, T.F., Urbach, T.P., Düzel, E., and Kutas, M. (2000). Event-related brain potentials in the study of human cognition and neuropsychology. In *Handbook of neuropsychology* 2nd edn. Vol. 1. (ed. F. Boller and J. Grafman), pp. 139–236. Elsevier, Amsterdam.

Oram, M.W. and Perrett, D.I. (1992). Time course of neural responses discriminating different views of the face and head. *J. Neurophysiol.* 68 (1), 70–84.

Plendl, H., Paulus, W., Roberts, I.G., Botzel, K., Towell, A., Pitman, J.R., Scherg, M., and Halliday, A.M. (1993). The time course and location of cerebral evoked activity associated with the processing of colour stimuli in man. *Neurosci. Lett.* 150 (1), 9–12.

Posner, M. I. (1980). Orienting of attention. *Q. J. Exp. Psychol.* 32, 3–25.

Robertson, L.C., Lamb, M.R., and Knight, R.T. (1988). Effects of lesions of temporal–parietal junction on perceptual and attentional processing in humans. *J. Neurosci.* 8 (10), 3757–69.

Robertson, L.C., Lamb, M.R., and Knight, R.T. (1991). Normal global–local analysis in patients with dorsolateral frontal lobe lesions. *Neuropsychologia* 29 (10), 959–67.

Rodriguez, E., George, N., Lachaux, J.P., Martinerie, J., Renault, B., and Varela, F.J. (1999). Perception's shadow: long-distance synchronization of human brain activity [see comments]. *Nature* 397 (6718), 430–3.

Singer, W. and Gray, C.M. (1995). Visual feature integration and the temporal correlation hypothesis. *Ann. Rev. Neurosci.* 18, 555–86.

Smid, H.G., Jakob, A., and Heinze, H.J. (1999). An event-related brain potential study of visual selective attention to conjunctions of color and shape. *Psychophysiology* 36 (2), 264–79.

Spence, C. and Driver, J. (1996). Audiovisual links in endogenous covert spatial attention. *J. Exp. Psychol. Hum. Percept. Perform.* 22 (4), 1005–30.

Spence, C. and Driver, J. (1997). Audiovisual links in exogenous covert spatial orienting. *Percept. Psychophys.* 59 (1), 1–22.

Stein, B.E., Meredith, M.A., and Wallace, M.T. (1993). The visually responsive neuron and beyond: multisensory integration in cat and monkey. *Prog. Brain Res.* 95, 79–90.

Tallon-Baudry, C., Bertrand, O., Delpuech, C., and Permier, J. (1997*a*). Oscillatory gamma-band (30–70 Hz) activity induced by a visual search task in humans. *J. Neurosci.* 17 (2), 722–34.

Tallon-Baudry, C., Bertrand, O., Wienbruch, C., Ross, B., and Pantev, C. (1997*b*). Combined EEG and MEG recordings of visual 40 Hz responses to illusory triangles in human. *Neuroreport* 8 (5), 1103–07.

Tallon-Baudry, C., Bertrand, O., Peronnet, F., and Pernier, J. (1998). Induced gamma-band activity during the delay of a visual short-term memory task in humans. *J. Neurosci.* 18 (11), 4244–54.

Teder-Sälejärvi, W.A., Münte, T.F., Sperlich, F.J., and Hillyard, S.A. (1999). Intramodal and crossmodal spatial attention to auditory and visual stimuli. An event-related potential (ERP) study. *Brain Res. Cogn. Brain Res.* 8 (3), 343–7.

Uusitalo, M.A., Virsu, V., Salenius, S., Nasanen, R., and Hari, R. (1997). Activation of human V5 complex and rolandic regions in association with moving visual stimuli. *Neuroimage* 5 (4 Pt. 1), 241–50.

Valdes-Sosa, M., Bobes, M.A., Rodriguez, V., and Pinilla, T. (1998). Switching attention without shifting the spotlight object-based attentional modulation of brain potentials. *J. Cogn. Neurosci.* 10 (1), 137–51.

Van Essen, D.C. (1995). Behind the optic nerve: an inside view of the primate visual system. *Trans. Am. Ophthalmol. Soc.* 93, 123–33.

Van Essen, D.C., Anderson, C.H., and Felleman, D.J. (1992). Information processing in the primate visual system: an integrated systems perspective. *Science* 255 (5043), 419–23.

Vecera, S.P. and Farah, M.J. (1994). Does visual attention select objects or locations? *J. Exp. Psychol. Gen.* 123 (2), 146–60.

Vecera, S.P. and Farah, M.J. (1997). Is visual image segmentation a bottom–up or an interactive process? *Percept. Psychophys.* 59 (8), 1280–96.

Verleger, R., Heide, W., Butt, C., Wascher, E., and Kompf, D. (1996). On-line brain potential correlates of right parietal patients' attentional deficit. *Electroencephalogr. Clin. Neurophysiol.* 99 (5), 444–57.

Watanabe, J. and Iwai, E. (1996). Neuronal activity in monkey visual areas V1, V2, V4 and TEO during fixation task. *Brain Res. Bull.* 40 (2), 143–50.

White, C.T. and White, C.L. (1995). Reflections on visual evoked cortical potentials and selective attention: methodological and historical. *Int. J. Neurosci.* 80 (1–4), 13–30.

Yantis, S. (1992). Multielement visual tracking: attention and perceptual organization. *Cognit. Psychol.* 24, 295–340.

Part 3

Imaging studies: functional magnetic resonance imaging and positron emission tomography

Chapter 4

Functional magnetic resonance imaging and positron emission tomography studies of motion perception, eye movements, and reading

Mark W. Greenlee

Introduction

Functional brain imaging is a rapidly growing area of cognitive neuroscience. fMRI of the visual system is a specialized field, in which methods from neurophysiology, cognitive neuroscience, and psychophysics are combined to study activation of the visual cortex and related cortical areas. This Chapter focuses on recent findings from studies of visual motion processing, eye movements, and reading. As such it serves as a selective introduction to an expanding research area, a survey of which would surpass the aim of this Chapter.

The analysis of retinal image motion is an important feature of all biological visual systems. For example, object motion can be used to segment figure from ground. The relative paths of moving objects with respect to each other and the observer provide important cues for target localization in depth (i.e. motion parallax). Image motion is also evoked by the observer's own eye, head and body movements. Such wide-field motions should be distinguished from local motion related to actual object displacements. Thus, the analysis of object motion involves retinal and extraretinal sources of information. Therefore, it comes as little surprise that biological visual systems have developed elaborated mechanisms for the precise encoding of object motion (Reichardt 1961; van Santen and Sperling 1985) and that a complex hierarchy of cortical areas has evolved to analyse image motion. Damage to the motion-specific cortical areas leads to an impairment in visual motion processing (see Chapter 7, this volume).

Visual motion-processing is believed to be primarily a function of the dorsal visual pathway (Zeki 1974, 1978; Van Essen *et al.* 1981; Albright 1984; Albright *et al.* 1984). Information about image motion passes to cortical regions in the parietal cortex as part of an analysis of spatial relationships between objects in the environment and the viewer (Andersen 1995, 1997; Colby 1998). Signals from the parietal cortex project to the frontal eye fields (FEF) in prefrontal cortex (lateral part of area 6) and are used in the preparation of saccadic and smooth-pursuit eye movements (Schiller *et al.* 1979; Bruce *et al.* 1985; Lynch 1987; Krauzlis and Stone 1999; Tehovnik *et al.* 2000). Thus, an elaborated hierarchy of visual and visuomotor areas underlies the analysis of visual motion. Functional imaging studies in human observers should provide essential information about which areas contribute to our percept of visual motion and to our oculomotor responses to visual motion.

In this chapter we review brain-imaging studies that have investigated cortical responses to visual motion. We also review the evidence for the existence of cortical areas responding during oculomotor tasks, such as those requiring saccades or smooth pursuit. Finally, we review studies that explore the cortical control of reading and evidence for the involvement of cortical areas in reading disabilities. The aim of all of these studies is to determine the extent to which these cortical responses, as indexed by stimulus-evoked changes in blood flow and tissue oxygenation, are specific to the form of visual cognition under investigation. We first review the current findings on functional imaging of human cortical responses to visual motion. We consider the effects related to stimulus properties such as spatiotemporal frequency, contrast, direction, speed, and motion coherence. The results of many groups suggest that several cortical areas respond selectively to visual motion. Different visual areas also respond to complex optic flow fields. Afterwards, we review the literature on task-related changes in the blood oxygen level-dependent (BOLD) response to visual motion. These findings suggest that changes in the subject's attention can modify the BOLD response to visual stimulation. Attention to different aspects of moving stimuli can lead to differences in the response. The role of pursuit eye movements in motion perception and the resultant pattern of BOLD responses are also considered. The task-dependent effects of pro- and anti-saccades, variations in the amplitude and frequency of saccades, and the difference between saccadic eye movements and smooth pursuit are also reviewed. Finally, we discuss results related to reading and disorders of reading. Other reviews on these topics have been recently published (Greenlee 2000; Kanwisher and Wojciulik 2000; Culham *et al.* 2001).

Positron emission tomography studies of motion perception

Several groups have used positron emission tomography (PET) to study changes in regional cerebral blood flow (rCBF) evoked when subjects viewed visual motion. Zeki *et al.* (1991) used PET with the short-life radioactive tracer $H_2^{15}O$ to map cortical responses to random dot motion. The dot stimuli moved with a speed of 6°/second in one of eight directions. They found significant responses to visual motion in the human homologue of area V5/V5a. Watson *et al.* (1993) and Dupont *et al.* (1994) could replicate and expand these findings.

The haemodynamic correlates of the cortical response to optic flow fields were investigated in a study by De Jong *et al.* (1994) with $H_2^{15}O$-PET. In their study, six subjects viewed simulated optic flow fields (consisting of small bright dots on a dark background) under binocular viewing conditions. Comparisons were made between displays with 100% coherent motion (radial expansion from a virtual horizon) and 0% coherent motion (same dots and speed gradients, but random direction). The average speed was 7.6°/s (coherent motion) and 17.8°/s (random condition). The reported Talairach coordinates (based on the stereotactic atlas of Talairach and Tournoux 1988) correspond to the human V5/V5a complex (MT/MST, also referred to as MT+) in the border region between areas 19 and 37, to the inferior cuneus in area 18 (the human homologue of V3), to the insular cortex, and to the lateral extent of the posterior precuneus in occipitoparietal cortex (areas 19/7). In a further PET study, Cheng *et al.* (1995) asked 10 subjects to monocularly view an 80° (virtual) field, while luminous dots moved coherently in one of eight directions. The control conditions consisted either of incoherent motion sequences or mere fixation. The authors used electrooculography (EOG) to control for eye movements during the PET scans. The results indicate that several visual areas respond to visual motion stimuli. Some of the occipitotemporal (V5/V5a, BA 19/37) and occipitoparietal (V3A, BA 7) responses were more pronounced during coherent motion perception, i.e. a condition under which all dots move in one direction. These pioneering PET studies of motion perception suggested at an early phase in this research that several extrastriate and associational visual areas respond selectively to visual motion. The stage is now set for comprehensive functional magnetic resonance imaging (fMRI) studies of human cortical processing of visual motion.

fMRI studies of motion perception

The anatomical location of V5/MT in human cortex

Anatomical MRI with sulci labelling has pointed to the ascending limb of the inferior temporal sulcus as the location of area MT/V5 in humans (Dumoulin *et al.* 2000). Although there is some variation among individual subjects regarding the position and form of this segment of the ITS (Anderson *et al.* 1996), there is considerable agreement across healthy brains.

The BOLD signal

fMRI is a relatively new procedure for assessing changes in brain activation (Roland 1993; Orrison *et al.* 1995; Hennig l998; Logothetis *et al.* 1999, 2001). The first fMRI measures were performed in 1990 in the rat (Ogawa *et al.* 1990). Belliveau *et al.* (1991) conducted the first fMRI measures in humans with the exogenous paramagnetic contrast agent gadolinium, which was given as an intravenous bolus during visual stimulation. Endogenous contrast effects have been found with the circulating blood haemoglobin. Deoxyhaemoglobin is paramagnetic in nature, whereas oxyhaemoglobin is diamagnetic. Perfusion-induced changes in the local amounts of these two forms of haemoglobin yield variations in the T2*-weighted MR-signal. This effect is called BOLD (blood-oxygen-level-dependent) contrast, since deoxyhaemoglobin acts to locally reduce the net transverse magnetization. Changes in T2* contrast following brief visual stimulation have been studied by different groups (Ernst and Hennig 1994; Boynton *et al.* 1996; Janz *et al.* 1997; Logothetis *et al.* 1999). The time course of the T2*-signal can be correlated with the visual stimulus. Voxels containing activated visual cortex can be identified by setting a correlation threshold between the stimulus and response time courses (Friston *et al.* 1995). A three-dimensional voxel cluster can be identified by demanding neighbourhood relationships: only clusters of predefined volume are selected for further study. Figure 4.1 shows an average time course of activated voxels that were located in the brain of a subject who viewed motion. Two things are apparent in this

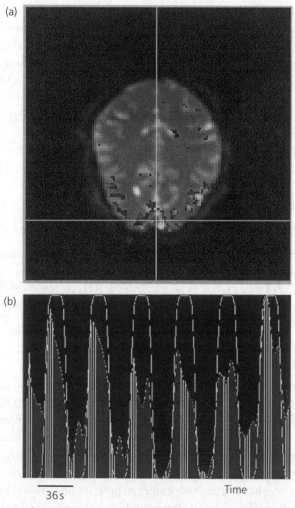

(a)

(b)

36 s

Time

Fig. 4.1 Time course of activation in visual cortex following visual motion stimulation. (a) T2* weighted echo planar image with activated voxels. (b) Time course of T2* signal for six 36 s activation periods followed by 36 s rest periods. For more details see text.

figure: (1) only a small subset of voxels are positively correlated above a predefined correlation threshold with the time course of stimulation, and (2) the time course of the T2*-signal is shifted by approximately 4–6 s. This shift reflects the delays associated with the haemodynamic response function. The time constant of the recovery is 2–3 times longer than the onset delay and, as such, represents a serious limitation in the temporal resolution of the BOLD signal. The exact relationship between the underlying neural activity (in the form of pre-and postsynaptic potentials and action potentials) and the BOLD response is only poorly understood (Logothetis *et al.* 2001; Heeger *et al.* 2000).

Stimulus-specific responses in visual cortex: contrast

In one of the first studies of fMRI in visual cortex, Tootell *et al.* (1995*b*) showed that the human V5 complex showed a selective response to motion, the amplitude of which already saturated at very low values of contrast (around 5%). Tootell *et al.* (1995*b*) mapped BOLD responses in striate and extrastriate visual areas to visual motion stimuli (expanding–contracting radial gratings). They found that the human V5/V5a (also referred to as MT/MST) region and V3a (Tootell *et al.* 1997) respond well to low stimulus contrast levels. Boynton *et al.* (1999) explored the contrast response in visual cortex to stimuli that varied in contrast. They found contrast-dependent BOLD responses that were correlated with the contrast discrimination performance of the subjects. Fahle *et al.* (2001) mapped visual contrast responses on to inflated cortical representations and found monotonic increases in the BOLD response with stimulus contrast that saturated at 10% contrast levels. These studies suggest that the BOLD response can, indeed, index the stimulus-evoked neural response to sensory events.

Direction-specific responses

Motion stimuli can be defined by the spatiotemporal characteristics of the display components. For example, kinetic patterns can be defined by alternate columns of dots, each moving in opposite directions, thereby forming so-called motion borders. Responses to kinetically defined borders were described early on by Reppas *et al.* (1997) and van Oostende *et al.* (1997). Surprisingly, the V5/V5a (MT+) area did not respond selectively to motion-defined contours, although it did respond to the global motion in the stimuli. Van Oostende *et al.* (1997) describe the kinetic occipital (KO) region in the lateral extrastriate cortex, which responded selectively to kinetic contours. This ventral posterior visual area appears to respond to borders defined by the relative directions of moving dots. As such, this area might be involved in the analysis of image motion related to self-motion of the observer (see below).

Several extensive studies have been conducted on the effects of direction and speed of frontoplanar dot motion, using PET and fMRI methods (Dupont *et al.* 1994, 1997; van Oostende *et al.* 1997; Cornette *et al.* 1998; Orban *et al.* 1998). Subjects performed psychophysical tasks of direction and speed discrimination during scanning. Careful documentation of the visual areas responding to various forms of dot motion suggests that, in addition to V5/V5a, several extrastriate areas (e.g. lingual gyrus and cuneus) show selective responses to the direction and speed of visual motion. These responses are enhanced when subjects perform psychophysical tasks in the scanner (see below). As mentioned above, Orban and colleagues identified an area in the ventral portion of extrastriate cortex, which they refer to as the KO cortex (Dupont *et al.* 1994; van Oostende *et al.* 1997). KO responds well to motion-defined borders within complex motion displays.

Visual motion is not only defined by displacement of luminance contours, but can also be defined by the displacement of contrast, texture, or flickering contours (Smith 1994). This latter form of visual motion has been referred to as second-order motion. fMRI has been recently used to explore the cortical regions underlying the processing of second-order motion. Smith *et al.* (1998) compared BOLD responses to motion stimuli yielding first- and second-order motion. Using retinotopic mapping techniques to define area borders, these authors showed that most striate and extrastriate regions responded to both types of motion. Smith *et al.* (1998) found that the lateral posterior region corresponds to the KO region reported by van Oostende *et al.* (1997). Smith *et al.* (1998) refer to this area as V3b, and show that it responds well to second-order motion. Selective activation to second-order motion of plaids has been found in V3 using PET (Wenderoth *et al.* 1999). Significant activations in striate and extrastriate cortex to colour- and motion-defined patterns have also been reported (Skiera *et al.* 2000). The results of these studies suggest that several visual areas are involved in the analysis of visual motion. Structure from motion can be evoked by patterns of motion coherence, and these motion borders elicit activation in some of these areas. A critical feature of a motion detector is its directional selectivity, i.e. the extent to which the activity of the detector is affected by the direction of the stimulus. Since any given voxel will contain neurons coding all possible stimulus directions, fMRI methods will not necessarily be able to reveal the microstructure of motion analysis. However, a given area might show evidence for direction-specific interactions, like motion opponency, which point to the existence of direction-specific coding strategies. Evidence for this phenomenon is outlined next.

Selectivity for stimulus speed/drift frequency and motion opponency

A counterphase flickering sinewave grating can be constructed by superimposing two equal contrast gratings of the same spatial frequency and orientation that drift at the same speed but in opposite directions. By comparing responses to drifting and counterphase flickering stimuli, Heeger *et al.* (1999) showed that the MT+ region exhibited lower responses to flickering than to drifting gratings. The differences in BOLD responses led the authors to suggest the presence of 'motion opponency' in area MT+, which would reflect mutual inhibition of neurons tuned to opposite directions. Further evidence for motion opponency was found in a comparison of single-unit responses in the primate V5 region (Heeger *et al.* 1999). The effects of motion opponency could underlie the higher responses found for coherently moving dot patterns compared to random dot motion. A small, but reliable, effect of motion coherence level was reported by Rees *et al.* (2000) for the V5/MT+ area, the KO area, V3a, and the anterior cingulate gyrus. In a study using retinotopic mapping and grating stimuli, Singh *et al.* (2000) compared BOLD responses in visual areas to drifting and counterphase flickering gratings. By varying the spatial and temporal frequency of the gratings, these authors could determine the modulation-transfer function for these stimuli. Their results are in general agreement with single-unit studies (Foster *et al.* 1985; Levitt *et al.* 1994; Gegenfurtner *et al.* 1997) that show spatial frequency bandpass tuning functions in V1 and lowpass functions in V2, V3, V3A, and V5. The temporal frequency tuning curves of these visual areas show a remarkable similarity, with bandpass functions peaking around 9 Hz. Motion opponency could be examined by calculating the ratio of responses to the drifting and counterphase flickering gratings. This comparison yielded values between 1.0 and 1.5, the largest ratios being in V5. These ratios are lower than those reported by Heeger *et al.* (1999), but do support the idea of motion opponency in some higher visual areas including V5. Speed-dependent BOLD responses in V5 and V3a have been shown for luminance- and colour-contrast dot motion, with maximal responses occurring between 5 and 10°/s depending on the area and stimulus type (Chawla *et al.* 1999*a*; see below).

Motion adaptation, aftereffects

Prolonged stimulation to drifting gratings leads to a decline in the perceived speed and contrast of moving gratings (Thompson 1981; Müller and Greenlee 1994; Mather *et al.* 1998). Prior adaptation to unidirectional motion prolongs the decay of the BOLD response in V5/V5a, and this effect has been related to the perceptual motion aftereffect (Tootell *et al.* 1995*b*). Culham *et al.* 1999 studied the storage of the motion aftereffect with fMRI. They reported storage-related activity in MT/V5, but this activity was less than that evoked by real motion. Following prolonged motion adaptation, a stationary test stimulus evokes pronounced activation in MT/V5, an area that is usually silent to stationary stimuli (Tootell *et al.* 1995*a*). This close correlation between BOLD responses and perceptual phenomena, such as that of the motion aftereffect, suggests that fMRI can, indeed, reflect processes closely coupled to the neural analysis of visual motion. However, Huk *et al.* (2001) have suggested that these earlier studies did not account for the modulatory effects of directed attention (see below). After correcting for the effects of attention, the authors showed that a direction-selective component of the fMRI response following motion adaptation was still evident. In a recent fMRI study in anaesthetized monkeys, Tolias *et al.* (2001) showed that all early visual areas exhibit adaptation effects that are directionally selective, suggesting that motion adaptation effects are not restricted to V5/MT.

Biological motion

Biological motion refers to motion sequences arising from complex three-dimensional displacements of body parts including motions of limbs, eyes, and mouths. Brain-imaging studies have been conducted to explore the cortical basis of biological motion processing. In a PET study with light-point figures (Johansson 1975), Bonda *et al.* (1996) explored responses to coherent versus random motion sequences. Compared to random motion, body movements evoked greater activity in the STS region and the amygdala. Subjects had to perform a postscan memory test, which might explain the involvement of the amygdala and entorhinal cortex. Responses to the movements of the eyes and mouth were compared to that evoked by a radial grating (Puce *et al.* 1998). The number of significantly activated voxels was compared for the different stimuli in selected regions of interest. They found that radial gratings evoked a large activation in V5 but little or no activation in the superior temporal sulcus (STS) region. In contrast, mouth and eye motion evoked activation in the STS but less activation in V5/MT+. Responses in the STS to optic flow stimuli have also been reported (see below). Taken together, these studies suggest the existence of a cortical area that preferentially responds to biological motion. It remains open whether these responses are related to the analysis of visual motion as such or to the preparation for possible imitation (such as the activity described in 'mirror neurons'; see Iacoboni *et al.* 2001).

Task-related activation in motion-sensitive areas

Effects of attention

The effects of selective and divided attention have been studied using both PET and fMRI methods. In an early PET study, Corbetta *et al.* (1991) had subjects attend either to the speed, colour, or shape of sparse, randomly moving blocks. Two conditions were compared. In the *selective attention condition*, subjects were instructed to attend to one of the three stimulus dimensions and the stimuli differed only along that dimension. In the *divided attention condition*, the stimuli could differ along any one of the three dimensions and the subjects had to detect whether or not a change occurred. In the selective attention condition, the authors found a shift in activation depending on the stimulus dimension to which the subject attended. When subjects attended to the speed of the moving stimuli the activation occurred in lateral occipitotemporal cortex (probably in the V5/V5a region, but also in more anterior regions in Brodmann areas (BA) 21 and BA22).

The subject's attention level has been shown to affect the BOLD response in fMRI experiments. In an fMRI study on the effects of selective attention on the response to visual motion, subjects viewed complex motion displays, in which random dot motion was sequentially interleaved with motion containing a circular annulus of coherently moving dots (Beauchamp *et al.* 1997). The subjects were instructed either to attend to the central fixation point, to both the location and speed of the dots within the annulus, or only to the colour of the dots within the annulus. The BOLD signal in the human homologue of V5/V5a was highest for the condition with attention to both speed and location, and the response decreased to 60 and 45% of this value when attention was shifted to the dot colour or to the fixation point, respectively.

Independent evidence for the claim that shifts of attention can modulate the response to visual motion was presented by O'Craven *et al.* (1997). They instructed subjects to attend either to moving or static random dots (black dots moving among static white dots). This dynamic stimulus remained constant during the entire MR-image acquisition period. Following instructions, subjects attended either to the static or the dynamic dots. The authors found a modulation in the BOLD signal depending on which instruction set the subjects followed. Attention to the dynamic components of the displays led to larger responses in the V5/V5a region. Alternating attention to left or right grating targets led to modulations in the BOLD response (Gandhi *et al.* 1999). The effect was about 25% of the stimulus-evoked response (driven by left–right physical alternation of the grating stimulus). Similar effects have been reported for spatial attention to flickering bar stimuli presented in one of the four visual quadrants (Tootell *et al.* 1998).

Using fMRI, Shulman *et al.* (1999) studied the effects of direction-cueing on cortical activation in a coherent motion paradigm. Comparing block and event-related designs, these authors could isolate response components related to the processing of the cue information (neutral, one of four directions), to the preparation of a motor response (button press when coherent motion was present, no response when absent), and to the processing/detection of noise and noise plus coherent motion. Since subjects responded only on trials where they thought they saw coherent motion, the design could not disentangle the BOLD signals related to the motor aspects of the response from the visual processing of the coherent motion. V5/MT+ and area V3B/KO showed little effect of motion coherence (Fig. 6 in Shulman *et al.* 1999). Interestingly, V5/MT+ responded during the cue period, although only stationary dots and a static cue were present. This anticipatory response suggests that expectation can lead to significant haemodynamic responses despite the absence of adequate stimuli (cf. Kastner *et al.* 1999), and as such points to substantial 'top–down' modulation in early visual areas. Cued trials also led to larger responses during the noise + motion periods (Fig. 7 in Shulman *et al.* 1999). The use of spatial cues (left, right) in association with the parametric effect of motion coherence level was employed by Rees *et al.* (2000). Overall, these authors report a linear increase in BOLD signal with increasing motion coherence.

In summary, the effects of attention tend to enhance the BOLD signal in association with the visual stimulus. The effects reported so far vary between 25 and 50% of the stimulus-evoked response. Similar effects have been reported for static patterns (Kastner *et al.* 1998). Based on the results of the studies reviewed above, attention appears to modulate a stimulus-evoked response, but it has not been shown to evoke responses in otherwise silent areas. Evidence reported by Smith *et al.* (2000) suggests that attention might act to reduce spontaneous activity in non-attended regions of the visual field, thereby increasing the signal-to-noise ratio within the attended region.

Caveat: Can attention modulate activation in primary visual cortex (area VI)?

Although there is considerable controversy concerning the role of attention in the response in primary visual cortex to visual stimuli, recent work by Martinez *et al.* (1999, 2001) suggests that attention can indeed modulate V1 activity. These authors compared responses to eccentrically presented, complex stimuli (plaid background with nine superimposed white crosses), when the subjects were instructed to attend to the left or right visual hemifield. The subject's task was to detect the presence of a 'T' among the crosses. The fMRI responses increased over retinotopically defined visual cortex when subjects shifted attention to that location and this increase was also evident in the late components of event-related potentials (ERPs) measured in separate sessions in the same subjects. This late modulation of the visually evoked response suggests that spatially directed attention has a top–down influence over processing in primary visual cortex. Further evidence for the role of attention in modulating responses in visual cortex is reviewed in Chapter 3, this volume.

Discrimination of direction, speed, and colour of moving stimuli

Several research groups have investigated the effects of task performance on cortical activation with the PET camera or MR-scanner. Such approaches require the subjects to make psychophysical judgements and button-press responses while they view visual motion sequences. In a PET study, Orban *et al.* (1998) studied changes in rCBF while subjects performed speed discrimination tasks. They reported no increment in response in the motion-sensitive V5/MT+ region while subjects performed speed discrimination. In contrast, areas 19 and 20 showed significant response enhancements during speed discrimination compared to simple motion detection trials.

As mentioned above, Chawla *et al.* (1999*a*) reported the results of three subjects who viewed stimuli defined by colour or luminance contrast. They found speed-dependent responses in V3a and V5 (see also Singh *et al.* 2000). In a further study, Chawla *et al.* (1999*b*) cued subjects to attend to the speed or colour of moving dot stimuli in an event-related design. Their results indicate that cued attentional shifts to the speed of the stimuli enhanced responses in V5/MT+ and attentional shifts to the colour of the dots enhanced the response in V4. Although these effects are small, they suggest a top–down influence of baseline activation in neural circuits in extrastriate visual areas (compare above).

In a similar fashion, Huk and Heeger (2000) reported that area V5 responded more while subjects performed speed discrimination compared to when they performed either direction or contrast discriminations. The stimulus speeds varied around 8°/s for the speed discrimination and 0°/s for the direction discrimination (lower threshold for motion). They found higher responses in MT when the subjects were discriminating the speed of the stimuli. The interpretation of the results is not straightforward, since different speed ranges were used for the different tasks. The lack of enhanced MT activation in the Orban *et al.* (1998) study compared to the presence of an effect in the Huk and Heeger (2000) study could be related to differences in the methods used to assess brain activity (PET versus fMRI).

Optic flow stimuli

Wide-field motion evoked by eye, head, or body movements has been referred to as optic flow (Koenderink 1986). BOLD responses to optic flow stimuli have been studied by Rutschmann *et al.* (2000). Their subjects viewed dynamic, random-dot kinematograms (RDK) dichoptically. Different speeds ranging from 4 to 13°/sec were used to simulate random, expansion–contraction and rotational motion fields. They also varied the binocular disparity of the flow fields. In two conditions, dichoptic flow fields with and without disparity were presented. Little response selectivity was found in the striate and immediate extrastriate regions. Areas in the cuneus, putatively corresponding to the dorsal parts of V3 and V3a, responded somewhat better to the random walk stimuli than to the other three conditions. The V5/V5a complex showed little sensitivity to the flow patterns of the motion stimulation. In contrast, area KO in the ventral region of V3 appeared to show the greatest selectivity to optic flow. This area also exhibited slightly larger responses to the condition with disparity gradients in the optic flow fields. The results indicate that striate (V1) and extrastriate areas (V2, V3/V3a) respond robustly to optic flow. However, with the exception of a more pronounced response in V3/V3a to random walk, Rutschmann *et al.* found little evidence for response selectivity with respect to flow type and disparity in these early visual areas. In a large PET study, Beer *et al.* (2002) reported a similar selectivity to optic flow stimuli in area KO/V3b.

fMRI responses to random-dot motion sequences, in which noise fields were compared to rotation, expansion, and simulated three-dimensional motion, have been reported (Paradis *et al.* 2000). V5/MT+ responded well in the random noise–static comparison, but little additional activation was found when the random noise was compared to the coherent motion conditions. Selective enhancement of the V5/MT+ area during coherent rotational or expansion/contraction motion sequences has been demonstrated by Morrone *et al.* (2000). However, these enhanced responses could only be obtained when the stimuli rapidly alternated between one of two directions, suggesting that these responses might be more related to the processing of sudden direction changes and not to optic flow as such.

Effects of eye movements on visual-motion responses

An obvious source of experimental error in imaging studies of visual processing is the extent to which the subjects move their eyes during the scanning period. Although movements of the head are restrained by various methods and the effects of head motion can be partially eliminated by postacquisition motion correction (Cox 1996; Woods *et al.* 1998*a,b*), the effects of eye movements have been largely ignored in the past. Some form of prescan training has been employed in the hope that the subjects conform to the instructions during the entire scan period. Our experience suggests that this is often not the case especially for long scan periods. The effects of pursuit during motion perception (Barton *et al.* 1996) and a comparison between saccades and pursuit (Petit *et al.* 1997) without eye position monitoring have been published. In the next section we outline studies that have attempted to quantify the effect of eye movements on resultant BOLD responses. Some of these investigations proceed to describe cortical areas underlying the control of saccadic and pursuit eye movements.

Disturbances in eye movement control and double vision are among the most common symptoms following head injury.

fMRI studies of eye movements

Several groups have analysed the cortical responses evoked during saccadic eye movements. To a lesser extent, a few studies have examined the responses evoked during smooth-pursuit eye movements. Below, we review these findings and point out the methodical shortcomings of several studies, which are related to the restraints imposed by the magnetic field in the MR-scanner.

Saccadic eye movements

Saccadic eye movements serve to bring a visual object of interest to the foveal region of the eye. Saccades are fast eye movements, which are both voluntary and ballistic in nature. The brain programmes the saccadic metrics (direction, amplitude) before the neural command signals are sent to the oculomotor nuclei in the brainstem for saccade execution. Before a saccade occurs, attention must be disengaged from a previously attended target, the saccade target must be selected, and the spatial location of this target must be estimated. Several cortical and subcortical regions are involved in the generation of saccades. Among these regions are the frontal eye fields (FEF; Bruce and Goldberg 1985), the dorsolateral prefrontal cortex (Funahashi *et al.* 1991; Pierrot-Deseilligny *et al.* 1991), the supplementary eye fields (Schlag and Schlag-Rey 1987), the posterior parietal cortex (Gnadt and Andersen 1988; Barash *et al.* 1991*a,b*; Pierrot-Deseilligny *et al.* 1991), the primary visual cortex, the basal ganglia (Hikosaka and Wurtz 1985*a,b*), and the superior colliculus (Schiller *et al.* 1979).

Recent functional imaging studies have explored the cortical areas underlying the control of saccadic eye movements in humans (Petit *et al.* 1993; Paus *et al.* 1995; Luna *et al.* 1998; Darby *et al.* 1996; Bodis-Wollner *et al.* 1997; Sweeney *et al.* 1996; Perry and Zeki 2000). In most of these studies, eye movements could not be adequately measured during the scanning sessions. Attempts to use electrooculography have not been very successful, due to the currents induced into the recording equipment during gradient switching (see Felblinger *et al.* 1996). The exact pattern of eye movements contributing to the cortical activity during imaging thus remained undetermined in these studies.

Changes in the BOLD response related to the task performed could reflect saccade preparation. A favourite paradigm used to compare task effects is the pro- versus anti-saccade tasks. A visual target appearing to the left, say, will evoke a short latency pro-saccade. This saccade can, however, be suppressed and the subject can be instructed to look in the opposite direction, thus performing an anti-saccade (Everling and Fischer 1998). The imaging literature is controversial with respect to differences in responses evoked by pro- and anti-saccades. In a PET study by Paus *et al.* (1993) and a more recent fMRI study by Muri *et al.* (1998), no significant differences in FEF activity between these two tasks could be found. In a recent study, Kimmig *et al.* (2001) compared responses in

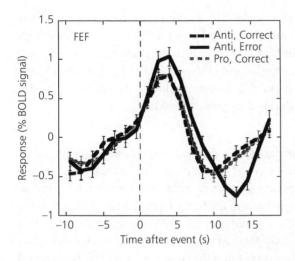

Fig. 4.2 Average time course of the BOLD response in the frontal eye fields (FEF) in three subjects who performed a pro- or anti-saccade task (from Cornelissen *et al.* 2002). Correct and incorrect trials are denoted by the different symbols.

pro- and anti-saccade tasks and report significant differences in the FEF in premotor cortex, as well as differences in the dorsal cuneus and parietal cortex, for these two types of task. These same authors developed a fibre-optic limbus tracking system that is compatible with the magnetic resonance scanning environment. Using this system, Kimmig *et al.* (1999) reported differences in the pattern of BOLD responses evoked by saccades versus pursuit.

Event-related fMRI of saccadic eye movements

Most of the studies reported in the last section used the so-called 'block-design' to study responses related to saccadic eye movements. Usually, these paradigms require the subjects to hold fixation for a prolonged period, say, 30 seconds, and then start performing saccadic eye movements over a 30 second period. This on–off design has the obvious limitation that responses related to the preparation and execution of saccades cannot be disentangled. The event-related design (Buckner *et al.* 1996) has been introduced to overcome these limitations. Here single-trial events are separated in time and each target onset is triggered by the gradient system of the scanner. The subject performs a single saccade, holds fixation at the peripheral location for, say, 3 seconds, then returns to the centre after the target disappears and the central fixation spot reappears. By repeating this procedure 10 to 20 times for each condition, the responses in saccade-related areas can be examined. In the study of Cornelissen *et al.* (2002), the subjects were cued to perform pro- or anti-saccades depending on a colour change of the central fixation spot just prior to fixation offset and target onset. A change from blue to green signalled a pro-saccade, whereas a change from blue to red indicated that the subject should perform an anti-saccade. The responses to these two conditions are shown in Fig. 4.2 and indicate that pro- and anti-saccades evoked similar activity in the FEF region in prefrontal cortex. Further evaluation of correctly performed and erroneous pro- and anti-saccades indicated some differences related to task performance (Cornelissen *et al.* 2002). Connolly *et al.* (2000) compared activation in prefrontal and parietal areas during pro- and anti-saccades. These activations were compared to those arising during pro- and anti-pointing to a visual target with gaze remaining straight ahead. The authors report a substantial overlap between areas responding in both tasks, with additional voxels activated during the pointing and anti-tasks. The FEF appears to respond not only during saccade execution, but also during the suppression of saccadic behaviour (required during their pointing task).

Summary

Block-design and event-related methods have also been used to study the effect of task components related to the relative on- and offsets of the fixation and target stimuli. Performance in the so-called 'gap' paradigm has recently been compared to that found for the 'step' paradigm. In the gap paradigm the fixation point is extinguished 200 ms prior to target onset. This stimulus onset asynchrony (SOA) allows the fixation system to 'unfixate' and begin preparation for the next saccade. In the step condition, the fixation stimulus remains on for a short period after the target stimulus has been presented. These different conditions led to different distributions of saccadic reaction times, where more 'express saccades' occur in the gap but not in the overlap conditions. An ongoing set of experiments in our laboratory (Özyurt *et al.* 2001) explores possible differences in the BOLD response patterns to these two types of oculomotor tasks. The initial results suggest that there exist differences in the pattern of BOLD activation for these slightly different saccade tasks. Memory-guided saccades are voluntary eye movements to the remembered locations of previously presented visual targets. The FEF appear to be more active during memory-guided compared to visually guided tasks (Greenlee *et al.* 2001). In a variant of the memory-guided saccade task, Sereno *et al.* (2001) had subjects perform centrifugal saccades to remembered locations along a virtual circle in clockwise and counterclockwise directions. The repetitive nature of this task allowed the authors to apply Fourier methods to extract the phase and amplitude of the cyclic BOLD response. The phase of this response provided evidence for a retinotopic organization in an area in the intraparietal sulcus, which they refer to as the putative lateral intraparietal (LIP) area.

Pursuit eye movements

Recent electrophysiological and neuroanatomical studies in monkeys suggest that there is a large overlap in the neural control of (small) saccades, fixation, and pursuit (see Krauzlis and Stone 1999). Smooth pursuit allows us to maintain our gaze on a target, despite the fact that the target is in motion. The mechanisms underlying the perception of visual motion and those controlling resultant pursuit appear to be closely related, at least during the initial stages of pursuit programming (Lisberger and Movshon 1999). Few studies have looked at the effects of pursuit eye movements on the responses in visual and oculomotor areas. Kimmig *et al.* (1999) showed that the activity in the FEF was greater during saccades than during pursuit, whereas MT+ (V5/V5a) responded better during pursuit than during saccades. Petit *et al.* (1997)

found differences in the location of activation in the FEF related to the type of eye movement performed. Pursuit was associated with activation in the lateral and saccades with activation in the more medial parts of the FEF. Further support for a subdivision of labour in the FEF for saccades and pursuit has been reported by Rosano *et al.* (2002). Freitag *et al.* (1998) found that the response in V5/V5a to moving dot stimuli increased during pursuit compared to fixation. Dukelow *et al.* (2001) first isolated area MST by identifying ipsilateral responses to eccentric motion displays and then characterized this area's response to visual or self-guided pursuit. The subjects had to pursue either a moving target or an image of their own finger, which they waved in front of their face in the dark. Eye movements were not measured in the scanner, so the intrusion of saccades cannot be ruled out. Nevertheless, the subjects showed selective responses during pursuit and these responses were most pronounced in an area anterior, but adjacent, to MT/V5. These studies point to an extraretinal input into the V5/V5a region, suggesting that this area might be involved in the analysis of object and self-motion (Greenlee 2000). The results of these oculomotor studies indicate that several cortical regions are involved in the programming and execution of saccadic and pursuit eye movements. There is mounting evidence that these different types of eye movements have separate, but also partially overlapping, representations in neocortex. We next outline studies that have explored cortical responses measured during the complex visuooculomotor behaviour required for reading.

fMRI studies of reading

Reading is an important social skill, which, unlike spoken language, has to be acquired in a controlled learning setting over a prolonged period of time during the first years of schooling. Indeed, civilized societies devote considerable resources to ensure that their children learn to read and write with an acceptable level of competence. Which areas of the human brain underlie the ability to read and which of these areas are involved in learning how to read? What goes wrong in the brain functioning of children who, despite normal or above normal intelligence, cannot read at a level appropriate for their age cohort? Which brain functions are impaired in patients with acquired dyslexia following cortical stroke (see Chapter 7, this volume)? Clearly, there are no simple answers to these questions, since the skill of reading is itself a multimodal activity involving the coordination and interaction between visual, auditory, oculomotor, and language areas in the brain. Several brain-imaging studies have looked at reading and disorders of reading (dyslexia) in otherwise healthy subjects. Below we give a brief (and selective) overview of recent studies that have explored the brain associated with reading, with learning how to read, and with reading disabilities. For recent reviews see Shaywitz *et al.* (1998), Pugh *et al.* (2000), and Habib (2000).

Normal reading

Reading is a complex oculomotor task, in which the reader shifts his or her gaze sequentially along stationary text. Psychophysical analysis of the visual components of reading has been conducted in a series of papers by Legge and co-workers (e.g. Legge *et al.* 2001). It is usually assumed that orthographic analysis of the individual letters that make up the words is performed by early visual detectors that respond to orientation, spatial frequency, and contrast of the letter elements. Lexical access is a cognitive process, whereby the reader extracts individual words from the letter strings and compares these strings to long-term memory representations of words (i.e. mental lexical) in the respective language. Phonological analysis and access can be compared by having subjects read lists containing proper words (with low and high occurrence frequencies), pseudohomophones (compound words with meaning), and pseudowords (pronounceable non-words; cf. Simos *et al.* 2002). Language-specific responses are evoked by reading of meaningful words and these activations are primarily located in the posterior part of the left temporal gyrus. Reading pseudowords led to less activation in this area. Reading of both types of words led to additional activation in the superior temporal gyrus, suggesting a phonological analysis in this cortical region (Pugh *et al.* 1996). The oculomotor component of reading will lead to additional activations in parietal and prefrontal regions (see above). Keller *et al.* (2001) explored fMRI responses to reading sentences of high and low syntactic complexity where these sentences contained words with either high or low lexical frequency. The authors found the largest responses for sentences containing low-frequency words with high syntactic complexity. Significant frontal lobe responses were also evident in the left hemisphere.

Mirror-script reading and procedural learning

To ensure his privacy and ward off plagiarism, Leonardo Da Vinci wrote his notes in mirror script with his left hand (Richter 1975). Left-handed writers apparently perform mirror writing with greater ease (Tucha *et al.* 2000). The ability to read mirror script can be learned and, given a sufficient amount of training, mirror script can be read without difficulty. Learning how to read mirror script is a prototypical procedural learning task. The performance of untrained subjects on this task is correlated with measures of visuospatial ability (Schmidtke *et al.* l996). Several neuropsychological studies have employed this paradigm to study procedural learning in patients. Normal learning was found in 20 patients with prefrontal lesions (Schmidtke *et al.* 1998). These results suggest that areas beyond those in the frontal-striatal loops are involved in learning how to read mirror script. Other factors involve visual priming of otherwise unfamiliar visual patterns, an increase in the capacity to perform the required mental rotation or inversion, an improvement of working memory capacity required to maintain, combine, and verify decoded letters, and direct recognition of mirror-reversed letters or letter groups.

Three recent fMRI studies examined the patterns of cortical activation in reading spatially transformed versus plain text. Goebel *et al.* (1998) reported significant increases of BOLD signal along the intraparietal sulcus bilaterally, in the left superior parietal lobule (SPL), the left occipitotemporal cortex, and at the posterior bank of the left precentral sulcus. In a study of Poldrack *et al.* (1998), similar, bilateral activation was found in the posterior SPL, the occipital cortex, parts of the inferior temporal cortex, along the intraparietal sulcus, and also in the cerebellum and pulvinar. The authors suggest that reading of transformed script involves a parietal 'visuospatial transformation' area and an occipitotemporal 'object recognition' area.

Kassubek *et al.* (2001) studied 10 healthy subjects while they read visually presented single plain-script and mirror-script words. fMRI responses in naive subjects on day 1 were compared to those acquired on day 2 after an intensive training period of mirror-script reading. Their results indicate that striate and extrastriate visual areas, associative parietal cortex (BA7 and BA40, superior and inferior parietal lobulus), and the prefrontal cortex (BA6) were bilaterally active during plain- and mirror-script reading. Activation in the primary visual cortex (BA17) was stronger during plain script reading compared to mirror-script reading (which is related to a word-length effect—longer words were used in the plain script task). The reverse pattern, i.e. significantly stronger activation during mirror-reading, was seen in BA7 and BA40 (parietal associative cortex) and in BA6 (FEF). After training, FEF and parietal area BA7 bilaterally and right BA40 exhibited a decrease of activation during mirror reading, suggesting their involvement in learning. The training-dependent deactivation of areas that were relatively more active during initial performance indicates that procedural learning of the mirror-reading task is accompanied by a decrease in the demand on the attentional system, on the control of eye movements, and on visuospatial transformation processes. In a follow-up study, Poldrack and Gabrieli (2001) discriminated between skill learning and priming effects arising during multiple training sessions of mirror-script reading. They found decreased activity in several areas related to repetition priming, as well as increases and decreases in activation related to learning. Their findings suggest that procedural learning involves a widespread neural activation of several memory systems.

These studies are provocative, since they suggest that a widely distributed network of visual and oculomotor/motor areas is involved in reading and the ability to learn to read new types of script (such as mirror-script). As such, they suggest that disturbances in reading performance might involve a complex interaction between visual, oculomotor, grapheme–phoneme conversion, language, and learning-related areas in the human brain. The next section outlines selected studies related to problems of reading.

fMRI responses in dyslexia

The phenomenon of dyslexia is characterized by an inability to read at a reasonable level in otherwise normally intelligent and educated persons. Habib (2000) focuses on the problem of grapheme–phoneme transformation in his summary statement: 'Neuropsychological studies have provided considerable evidence that the main mechanism leading to these children's learning difficulties is phonological in nature, namely, a basic defect in segmenting and manipulating the phoneme constituents of speech.' This so-called 'temporal processing impairment' theory of dyslexia has received considerable attention in the dyslexia literature (Pugh *et al.* 2000; Habib 2000).

Brain-imaging approaches to dyslexia have concentrated mostly on BOLD responses, but some recent work also suggests microanatomical differences in persons with reading impairments. Diffusion-tensor imaging suggests differences in the microstructure of white matter in the left temporoparietal region in dyslexics (Klingberg *et al.* 2000). The correlation between reading ability and the anisotropy value within the area of interest suggests that dyslexia is associated with a disturbance in the left-hemispheric anterior–posterior connectivity.

In a recent fMRI study, Temple *et al.* (2000) explored BOLD responses in eight adults with dyslexia and compared their results to those of 10 age-matched controls on rapid versus slow auditory pitch discrimination. Significant activation in the left prefrontal cortex (BA46/9) was evident in the rapid/slow presentation contrasts in the normal readers. This activation was absent in the dyslexics. The results point to a malfunction of the left temporal–prefrontal cortical loop in sound discrimination in adult dyslexics. Training of rapid sound sequences led to a left prefrontal response in two of three dyslexics.

Shaywitz *et al.* (1998) compared BOLD responses in occipitotemporal and prefrontal areas (Broca's area) during tasks involving the simple discrimination of letter-case strings (bbBb, bBbb) and non-word rhymes. They compared the responses of normal readers with those of subjects with impaired reading abilities. These authors found an overactivation in Broca's area and underactivation in the angular gyrus during non-word rhyming. The authors interpret their findings as evidence for a malfunction between orthographic and phonological processes.

Several groups have explored possible visual-related bases for dyslexia using psychophysical and fMRI techniques. Evidence for and against the so-called 'magnocellular deficit' in dyslexia can be found in the literature. Eden *et al.* (1996) reported significantly lower BOLD responses in MT/V5 in dyslexics (compared to controls) during motion perception. Demb *et al.* (1998*a*) reported elevated psychophysically determined speed discrimination thresholds in dyslexics and suggest that this joint impairment (i.e. deficit in speed discrimination and reading impairment) might be related to disturbances in the magnocellular input to the visual cortex. In support of this view, Demb *et al.* (1998*b*) found fMRI response differences for magnocellular-type stimuli in the MT+ area. Their results suggest that persons with a reading impairment showed lower BOLD responses overall and a less steep slope in the estimated contrast response functions (BOLD response versus stimulus contrast). They further report a correlation between BOLD response in area V5/MT and reading rate (with a sample size of 5 dyslexics and 5 controls). These findings need to be confirmed with larger sample sizes, but they do suggest that there could be a visual component in dyslexia related to a disturbance of the magnocellular projection from LGN to primary visual cortex (see review by Eden and Zeffiro 1998). Such a disturbance could lead to subnormal activation of motion-selective regions in extrastriate visual cortex. The results reviewed here suggest that fMRI can be used to analyse the cortical responses evoked during reading. As reading demands the coordinated effort of a widespread multimodal representation of form and content, the brain responses will necessarily be widespread and complex in nature. By decomposing these tasks into subcomponents, research in this area might be able to dissociate the neural mechanisms underlying each aspect of reading. Such newly gained knowledge might help provide a better understanding of the pathology underlying reading disorders.

Summary

In summary, we have reviewed brain imaging studies of visual motion processing, of oculomotor control, and of reading. The brain-imaging studies all point to V5/MT as an area in the occipitotemporal junction that is involved in several aspects of visual motion encoding. Earlier visual areas, such as V3a and the kinetic occipital area (KO), also exhibit motion-selective responses. These areas appear to contribute to the analysis of motion-defined boundaries required to segment complex visual scenes into figure and ground. Once this segmentation has taken place, visual attention can focus processing capacity to a selected visual target. Focal attention modulates the amplitude of the BOLD signal evoked by these selected stimuli. Attention not only enhances responses to selected targets, but can also enhance responses to selected dimensions of a single target, such as its colour or motion characteristics.

Once a moving target has been segmented from a background and selected as a target for attention, it can be pursued by the observer. Smooth pursuit is associated with activation in motion-selective visual areas, but also in areas in premotor cortex related to the control of eye movements. Task difficulty is a critical variable in oculomotor paradigms. The eye fields in prefrontal cortex can be activated during simple pro- and anti-saccade tasks, and the magnitude of this activity appears to be, at least to some extent, dependent on the task the subject is performing.

Reading is a complex task that requires visual, oculomotor, and language processing. Brain imaging has been employed to study these areas and to explore differences related to reading ability. Dyslexia is a disturbance of reading ability in otherwise healthy and intelligent individuals. It is our hope that, with the help of fMRI, cognitive neuroscience will be able to provide new insights into the multiple processes underlying visual cognition and disorders of visual cognition.

Acknowledgements

The author thanks the Deutsche Forschungsgemeinschaft (grants: SFB 517, C9, European Graduate School for Neurosensory Systems) for their support and Jale Özyurt and Roland M. Rutschmann for valuable comments on this manuscript.

References

Albright, T.D. (1984). Direction and orientation selectivity of neurons in visual area MT of the macaque. *J. Neurophysiol.* **52**, 1106–130.

Albright, T.D., Desimone, R., and Gross, C.G. (1984). Columnar organization of directionally selective cells in visual area MT of the macaque. *J. Neurophysiol.* **51**, 16–31.

Andersen, R.A. (1995). Encoding of intention and spatial location in the posterior parietal cortex. *Cereb. Cortex* 5, 457–69.

Andersen, R.A. (1997). Neural mechanisms of motion perception in primates. *Neuron* 18, 865–72.

Anderson, S.J., Holliday, I.E., Singh, K.D., and Harding, G.F.A. (1996). Localization and functional analysis of human cortical area V5 using magnetoencephalography. *Proc. R. Soc. Lond.* 263, 423–31.

Barash, S., Bracewell, R.M., Fogassi, L., Gnadt, J.W., and Andersen, R.A. (1991*a*). Saccade-related activity in the lateral intraparietal area. II. Spatial properties. *J. Neurophysiol.* 66, 1109–24.

Barash, S., Bracewell, R.M., Fogassi, L., Gnadt, J.W., and Andersen, R.A. (1991*b*). Saccade-related activity in the lateral intraparietal area. I. Temporal properties; comparison with area 7a. *J. Neurophysiol.* 66, 1095–108.

Barton, J.J.S., Simpson, T., Kiriakopoulos, E., Stewart, C., Crawley, A., Guthrie, B., Woods, M., and Mikulis, D. (1996). Functional MRI of lateral occipitotemporal cortex during pursuit and motion perception. *Ann. Neurol.* 40, 387–98.

Beauchamp, M.S., Cox, R.W., and DeYoe, E.A. (1997). Graded effects of spatial and featural attention on human area MT and associated motion processing areas. *J. Neurophysiol.* 78, 516–20.

Beer, J., Blakemore, C., Previc, F.H., and Liotti, M. (2002). Areas of the human brain activated by ambient visual motion, indicating three kinds of self-movement. *Exp. Brain Res.* 143 (1), 51–6.

Belliveau, J.W., Kennedy, D.N. Jr, McKinstry, R.C., Buchbinder, B.R., Weisskoff, R.M., Cohen, M.S., Vevea, J.M., Brady, T.J., and Rosen, B.R. (1991). Functional mapping of the human visual cortex by magnetic resonance imaging. *Science* 254 (5032), 716–19.

Bodis-Wollner, I., Bucher, S.F., Seelos, K.C., Paulus, W., Reiser, M., and Oertel, W.H. (1997). Functional MRI mapping of occipital and frontal cortical activity during voluntary and imagined saccades. *Neurology* 49, 416–20.

Bonda, E., Petrides, M., Ostry, D., and Evans, A. (1996). Specific involvement of human parietal systems and the amygdala in the perception of biological motion. *J. Neurosci.* 16 (11), 3737–44.

Boynton, G.M., Engel, S.A., Glover, G.H., and Heeger, D.J. (1996). Linear systems analysis of functional magnetic resonance imaging in human V1. *J. Neurosci.* 16, 4207–21.

Boynton, G.M., Demb, J.B., Glover, G.H., and Heeger, D.J. (1999). Neuronal basis of contrast discrimination. *Vision Res.* 39, 257–69.

Bruce, C.J. and Goldberg, M.E. (1985). Primate frontal eye fields. I. Single neurons discharging before saccades. *J. Neurophysiol.* 53, 603–35.

Bruce, C.J., Goldberg, M.E., Stanton, G.B., and Bushnell, M.C. (1985). Primate frontal eye fields: 2. Physiological and anatomical correlates of electrically evoked eye movements. *J. Neurophysiol.* 54, 714–34.

Buckner, R.L., Bandettini, P.A., O'Craven, K.M., Savoy, R.L., Petersen, S.E., Raichle, M.E., and Rosen, B.R. (1996). Detection of cortical activation during averaged single trials of a cognitive task using functional magnetic resonance imaging. *Proc. Natl Acad. Sci., USA* 93, 14878–83.

Chawla, D., Buechel, C., Edwards, R., Howseman, A., Josephs, O., Ashburner, J., and Friston, K.J. (1999*a*). Speed-dependent responses in V5: a replication study. *Neuroimage* 9, 508–15.

Chawla, D., Rees, G., and Friston, K.J. (1999*b*). The physiological basis of attentional modulation in extrastriate visual areas. *Nat. Neurosci.* 2, 671–6.

Cheng, K., Fujita, H., Kanno, I., Miura, S., and Tanaka, K. (1995). Human cortical regions activated by wide-field visual motion: an $H_2^{15}O$ PET study. *J. Neurophysiol.* 74, 413–27.

Colby, C.L. (1998). Action-oriented spatial reference frames in cortex. *Neuron* 20, 15–24.

Connolly, J.D., Goodale, M.A., Desouza, J.F., Menon, R.S., and Vilis, T. (2000). A comparison of frontoparietal fMRI activation during anti-saccades and anti-pointing. *J. Neurophysiol.* 84, 1645–55.

Corbetta, M., Miezin, F.M., Dobmeyer, S., Shulman, G.L., and Petersen, S.E. (1991). Selective and divided attention during visual discriminations of shape, color and speed: functional anatomy by positron emission tomography. *J. Neurosci.* 11, 2383–402.

Cornelissen, F.W., Kimmig, H., Schira, M., Broerse, A., Rutschmann, R.M., Maguire, R.P., Den Boer, J.A., and Greenlee, M.W. (2002). Event-related fMRI responses in the human frontal eye fields in a mixed pro- and antisaccade task. *Exp. Brain Res.* 145, 270–4.

Cornette, L., Dupont, P., Rosier, A., Sunaert, S., Van Hecke, P., Michiels, J., Mortelsmans, L., and Orban, G.A. (1998). Human brain regions involved in direction discrimination. *J. Neurophysiol.* 79, 2749–65.

Cox, R.W. (1996). AFNI: software for analysis and visualization of functional magnetic neuroimages. *Comput. Biomed. Res.* 29, 162–73.

Culham, J.C., Sheng, H., Dukelow, S. and Verstraten, F.A.J. (2001). Visual motion and the human brain: what has neuroimaging told us? *Acta Psychologia* 107, 69–94.

Culham, J.C., Dukelow, S.P., Vilis, T., Hassard, F.A., Gati, J.S., Menon, R.S., and Goodale, M.A. (1999). Recovery of fMRI activation in motion area MT following storage of the motion aftereffect. *J. Neurophysiol.* 81 (1), 388–93.

Darby, D.G., Nobre, A.C., Thangaraj, V., Edelman, R., Mesulam, M.M., and Warach, S. (1996). Cortical activation in the human brain during lateral saccades using EPISTAR functional magnetic resonance imaging. *Neuroimage* 3, 53–62.

de Jong, B.M., Shipp, S., Skidmore, B., Frackowiak, R.S.J., and Zeki, S. (1994). The cerebral activity related to the visual perception of forward motion in depth. *Brain* 117, 1039–54.

Demb, J.B., Boynton, G.M., Best, M., and Heeger, D.J. (1998*a*). Psychophysical evidence for a magnocellular pathway deficit in dyslexia. *Vision Res.* 38, 1555–9.

Demb, J.B., Boynton, G.M., and Heeger, D.J. (1998*b*). Functional magnetic resonance imaging of early visual pathways in dyslexia. *J. Neurosci.* 18, 6939–51.

Dukelow, S.P., DeSouza, J.F., Culham, J.C., van den Berg, A.V., Menon, R.S., and Vilis, T. (2001). Distinguishing subregions of the human MT+ complex using visual fields and pursuit eye movements. *J. Neurophysiol.* 86, 1991–2000.

Dumoulin, S.O., Bittar, R.G., Baker, C.L. Jr, Le Goualher, G., Pike, B., and Evans, A.C. (2000). A new anatomical lankmark for reliable indentification of the Human area V5/MT: a quantitative analysis fo sulcal patterning. *Cereb. Cortex* 10, 454–563.

Dupont, P., Orban, G.A., De Bruyn, B., Verbruggen, A., and Mortelsmans, L. (1994). Many areas in the human brain respond to visual motion. *J. Neurophysiol.* 72, 1420–4.

Dupont, P., De Bruyn, B., Vandenberghe, R., Rosier, A.M., Michiels, J., Marchal, G., Mortelsmans, L., and Orban, G. (1997). The kinetic occipital region in human visual cortex. *Cereb. Cortex* 7, 283–92.

Eden, G.F. and Zeffiro, T.A. (1998). Neural systems affected in developmental dyslexia revealed by functional neuroimaging. *Neuron* 21 (2), 279–82.

Eden, G.F., VanMeter, J.W., Rumsey, J.M., Maisog, J.M., Woods, R.P., and Zeffiro, T.A. (1996). Abnormal processing of visual motion in dyslexia revealed by functional brain imaging. *Nature* 382, 66–9.

Ernst, T. and Hennig, J. (1994). Observation of a fast response in functional MR. *Mag. Reson. Med.* 32, 146–9.

Everling, S. and Fischer, B. (1998). The antisaccade: a review of basic research and clinical studies. *Neuropsychologia* 36, 885–99.

Fahle, M., Rosik, L., Repnow, M., and Terwey, B. (2001). Contrast independence of fMRI signals induced by luminance-defined figure-ground segregation. *Perception* 30 (suppl.), 10.

Felblinger, J., Müri, R.M., Ozdoba, C., Schroth, G., Hess, C.W., and Boesch, C. (1996). Recordings of eye movements for stimulus control during fMRI by means of electro-oculographic methods. *Mag. Reson. Med.* 36, 410–14.

Foster, K.H., Gaska, J.P., Nagler, M., and Pollen, D.A. (1985). Spatial and temporal frequency selectivity of neurones in visual cortical areas V1 and V2 of the macaque monkey. *J. Physiol.* 365, 331–63.

Freitag, P., Greenlee, M.W., Lacina, T., Scheffler, K., and Radü, E.W. (1998). Effect of eye movements on the magnitude of fMRI responses in extrastriate cortex during visual motion perception. *Exp. Brain Res.* 119, 409–14.

Friston, K.J., Holmes, A.P., Grasby, P.J., Williams, S.C.R., and Frackowiak, R.S.J. (1995). Analysis of fMRI time-series revisited. *Neuroimage* 2, 45–53.

Funahashi, S., Bruce, C.J., and Goldman-Rakic, P.S. (1991). Neuronal activity related to saccadic eye movements in the monkey's dorsolateral prefrontal cortex. *J. Neurophysiol.* 65, 1464–83.

Gandhi, S.P., Heeger, D.J., and Boynton, G.M. (1999). Spatial attention affects brain activity in human primary visual cortex. *Proc. Natl Acad. Sci., USA* 96, 3314–19.

Gegenfurtner, K.R., Kiper, D.C., and Levitt, J.B. (1997). Functional properties of neurons in macaque area V3. *J. Neurophysiol.* 77, 1906–23.

Gnadt, J.W. and Andersen, R.A. (1988). Memory related motor planning activity in posterior parietal cortex of macaque. *Exp. Brain Res.* 70, 216–20.

Goebel, R., Khorram-Sefat, D., Muckli, L., Hacker, H., and Singer, W. (1998). The constructive nature of vision: direct evidence from functional magnetic resonance imaging studies of apparent motion and motion imagery. *Eur. J. Neurosci.* 10, 1563–73.

Greenlee, M.W. (2000). Human cortical areas underlying the perception of optic flow: brain imaging studies. *Int. Rev. Neurobiol.* 44, 269–92.

Greenlee, M.W., *et al.* (2001). Event-related fMRI of the saccadic system. *Perception* 30 (suppl.), 11.

Habib, M. (2000). The neurological basis of developmental dyslexia: an overview and working hypothesis. *Brain* 123, 2373–99.

Heeger, D.J., Boynton, G.M., Demb, J.B., Seidemann, E., and Newsome, W.T. (1999). Motion opponency in visual cortex. *J. Neurosci.* 19 (16), 7162–74.

Heeger, D.J., Huk, A.C., Geisler, W.S., and Albrecht, D.G. (2000). Spikes versus BOLD: what does neuroimaging tell us about neuronal activity? *Nat. Neurosci.* 3, 631–3.

Hennig, J. (1998). Radio waves. In *Functional imaging. Principles and methodology* (ed. G.K. von Schulthess and J. Hennig), pp. 267–390. Lippincott–Raven, Philadelphia.

Hikosaka, O. and Wurtz, R.H. (1985a). Modification of saccadic eye movements by GABA-related substances. II. Effects of muscimol in monkey substantia nigra pars reticulata. *J. Neurophysiol.* 53, 292–308.

Hikosaka, O. and Wurtz, R.H. (1985b). Modification of saccadic eye movements by GABA-related substances. I. Effect of muscimol and bicuculline in monkey superior colliculus. *J. Neurophysiol.* 53, 266–91.

Huk, A.C. and Heeger, D.J. (2000). Task-related modulation of visual cortex. *J. Neurophysiol.* 83, 3525–36.

Huk, A.C., Ress, D., and Heeger, D.J. (2001). Neuronal basis of the motion aftereffect reconsidered. *Neuron* 32, 6–8.

Iacoboni, M., Koski, L.M., Brass, M., Bekkering, H., Woods, R.P., Dubeau, M.C., Mazziotta, J.C., and Rizzolatti, G. (2001). Reafferent copies of imitated actions in the right superior temporal cortex. *Proc. Natl Acad. Sci., USA* 98, 13995–9.

Janz, C., Speck, O., and Hennig, J. (1997). Time-resolved measurements of brain activation after a short visual stimulus: new results on the physiological mechanisms of the cortical response. *NMR Biomed.* 10, 222–9.

Johansson, G. (1975). Visual motion perception. *Sci. Am.* 232, 76–88.

Kanwisher, N. and Wojciulik, E. (2000). Visual attention: insights from brain imaging. *Nat. Rev. Neurosci.* 1, 91–100.

Kassubek, J., Schmidtke, K., Kimmig, H., Lucking, C.H., and Greenlee, M.W. (2001). Changes in cortical activation during mirror reading before and after training: an fMRI study of procedural learning. *Brain Res. Cogn. Brain Res.* 10, 207–17.

Kastner, S., De Weerd, P., Desimone, R., and Ungerleider, L.G. (1998). Mechanisms of directed attention in the human extrastriate cortex as revealed by functional MRI. *Science* 282, 108–11.

Kastner, S., De Weerd, P., and Ungerleider, L.G. (1999). Increased activity in human visual cortex during directed attention. I The absence of visual stimulation. *Neuron* 22, 751–61.

Keller, T.A., Carpenter, P.A., and Just, M.A. (2001). The neural bases of sentence comprehension: a fMRI examination of syntactic and lexical processing. *Cereb. Cortex* 11, 223–37.

Kimmig, H., Greenlee, M.W., Huethe, F., and Mergner, T. (1999). MR-Eyetracker: a new method for eye movement recording in functional magnetic resonance imaging (fMRI). *Exp. Brain Res.* 126, 443–9.

Kimmig, H., Greenlee, M.W., Gondan, M., Schira, M., and Mergner, T. (2001). Relationship between saccadic eye movements and cortical activity as measured by fMRI: quantitative and qualitative aspects. *Exp. Brain Res.* 141, 184–94.

Klingberg, T., Hedehus, M., Temple, E., Salz, T., Gabrieli, J.D., Moseley, M.E., and Poldrack, R.A. (2000). Microstructure of temporo-parietal white matter as a basis for reading ability: evidence from diffusion tensor magnetic resonance imaging. *Neuron* 25, 493–500.

Koenderink, J.J. (1986). Optic flow. *Vision Res.* 26, 161–79.

Krauzlis, R.J. and Stone, L.S. (1999) Tracking with the mind's eye. *Trends Neurosci.* 22 (12), 544–50.

Legge, G.E., Mansfield, J.S., and Chung, S.T. (2001). Psychophysics of reading. XX. Linking letter recognition to reading speed in central and peripheral vision. *Vision Res.* 41, 725–43.

Levitt, J.B., Kiper, D.C., and Movshon, J.A. (1994). Receptive fields and functional architecture of macaque V2. *J. Neurophysiol.* 71, 2517–42.

Lisberger, S.G. and Movshon, J.A. (1999). Visual motion analysis for pursuit eye movements in area MT of macaque monkeys. *J. Neurosci.* 19, 2224–46.

Logothetis, N., Guggenberger, H., Peled, S., and Pauls, J. (1999). Functional magnetic resonance imaging of the monkey brain. *Nat. Neurosci.* 2, 555–62.

Logothetis, N.K., Pauls, J., Augath, M., Trinath, T., and Oeltermann, A. (2001). Neurophysiological investigation of the basis of the fMRI signal. *Nature* 412, 150–7.

Luna, B., Thulborn, K.R., Strojwas, M.H., McCurtain, B.J., Berman, R.A., Genovese, C.R., and Sweeney, J.A. (1998). Dorsal cortical regions subserving visually guided saccades in humans: an fMRI study. *Cereb. Cortex* 8, 40–7.

Lynch, J.C. (1987). Frontal eye field lesions disrupt visual pursuit. *Exp. Brain Res.* 68, 437–41.

Martinez, A. Anllo-Vento, L., Sereno, M.I., Frank, L.R., Buxton, R.B., Dubowitz, D.J., Wong, E.C., Hinrichs, H., Heinze, H.J., and Hillyard, S.A. (1999). Involvement of striate and extrastriate visual cortical areas in spatial attention. *Nat. Neurosci.* 2, 364–9.

Martinez, A. DiRusso, F., Anllo-Vento, L., Sereno, M.I., Buxton, R.B., and Hillyard, S.A. (2001). Putting spatial attention on the map: timing and localization of stimulus selection processes in striate and extrastriate visual areas. *Vision Res.* 41, 1437–57.

Mather, G., Verstraten, F., and Anstis, S. (1998). *The motion aftereffect: a modern perspective.* MIT Press, Boston, Massachusetts.

Morrone, M.C., Tosetti, M., Montanaro, D., Fiorentini, A., Cioni, G., and Burr DC. (2000). A cortical area that responds specifically to optic flow, revealed by fMRI. *Nat. Neurosci.* 3, 1322–8.

Müller, R. and Greenlee, M.W. (1994). Effect of contrast and adaptation on the perception of the direction and speed of drifting gratings. *Vision Res.* **34**, 2071–92.

Muri, R.M., Heid, O., Nirkko, A.C., Ozdoba, C., Felblinger, J., Schroth, G., and Hess, C.W. (1998). Functional organisation of saccades and antisaccades in the frontal lobe in humans: a study with echo planar functional magnetic resonance imaging. *J. Neurol., Neurosurg., Psychiatry* **65**, 374–7.

O'Craven, K.M., Rosen, B.R., Kwong, K.K., Triesman, A., and Savoy, R.L. (1997). Voluntary attention modulates fMRI activity in human MT-MST. *Neuron* **18**, 591–8.

Ogawa, S., Lee, T.M., Kay, A.R., and Tank, D.W. (1990). Brain magnetic resonance imaging with contrast dependent on blood oxygenation. *Proc. Natl Acad. Sci., USA* **87**, 9868–72.

Orban, G.A., Dupont, P., De Bruyn, B., Vandenberghe, R., Rosier, A., and Mortelsmans, L. (1998). Human brain activity related to speed discrimination tasks. *Exp. Brain Res.* **122**, 9–22.

Orrison, W.W. Jr, Levine, J.D., Sanders, J.A., and Hartshorne, M.F. (1995) *Functional brain imaging.* Mosby, St. Louis.

Özyurt, J., DeSouza, P., West, P., Rutschmann, R.M., Greenlee, M.W. (2001). Comparison of cortical activity and oculomotor performance in the gap and step paradigms. *Perception* **30**, (Suppl.), 101–2.

Paradis, A.L., Cornilleau-Peres, V., Droulez, J., Van De Moortele, P.F., Lobel, E., Berthoz, A., Le Bihan, D., and Poline, J.B. (2000). Visual perception of motion and 3-D structure from motion: an fMRI study. *Cereb. Cortex* **10**, 772–83.

Paus, T., Petrides, M., Evans, A.C., and Meyer E. (1993). Role of the human anterior cingulate cortex in the control of oculomotor, manual, and speech responses: a positron emission tomography study. *J. Neurophysiol.* **70**, 453–69.

Paus, T., Marrett, S., Worsley, K.J., and Evans, A.C. (1995). Extraretinal modulation of cerebral blood flow in the human visual cortex: implications for saccadic suppression. *J. Neurophysiol.* **74**, 2179–83.

Perry, R.J. and Zeki, S. (2000). The neurology of saccades and covert shifts in spatial attention: an event-related fMRI study. *Brain* **123**, 2273–88.

Petit, L., Orssaud, C., Tzourio, N., Salamon, G., Mazoyer, B., and Berthoz A. (1993). PET study of voluntary saccadic eye movements in humans: basal ganglia–thalamocortical system and cingulate cortex involvement. *J. Neurophysiol.* **69**, 1009–17.

Petit, L., Clark, V.P., Ingeholm, J., and Haxby, J.V. (1997). Dissociation of saccade-related and pursuit-related activation in human frontal eye fields as revealed by fMRI. *J. Neurophysiol.* **77**, 3386–90.

Pierrot-Deseilligny, C., Rivaud, S., Gaymard, B., and Agid, Y. (1991). Cortical control of reflexive visually-guided saccades. *Brain* **114**, 1473–85.

Poldrack, R.A. and Gabrieli, J.D. (2001). Characterizing the neural mechanisms of skill learning and repetition priming: evidence from mirror reading. *Brain* **124**, 67–82.

Poldrack, R.A., Desmond, J.E., Glover, G.H., and Gabrieli, J.D. (1998). The neural basis of visual skill learning: an fMRI study of mirror reading. *Cereb. Cortex* **8**, 1–10.

Puce, A., Allison, T., Bentin, S., Gore, J., and McCarthy, G. (1998). Temporal cortex activation in humans viewing eye and mouth movements. *J. Neurosci.* **18**, 2188–99.

Pugh, K.R. , *et al.* (1996). Cerebral organization of component processes in reading. *Brain* **119**, 1221–38.

Pugh, K.R., Mencl, W.E., Jenner, A.R., Katz, L., Frost, S.J., Lee, J.R., Shaywitz, S.E., and Shaywitz, B.A. (2000). Functional neuroimaging studies of reading and reading disability (developmental dyslexia). *Ment. Retard. Dev. Disbil. Res. Rev.* **6**, 198–206.

Rees, G., Friston, K., and Koch, C. (2000). A direct quantitative relationship between the functional properties of human and macaque V5. *Nat. Neurosci.* **3**, 716–23.

Reichardt, W. (1961). Autocorrelation: a principle for the evaluation of sensory information by the central nervous system. In *Sensory communication* (ed. W.A. Rosenblith), MIT Press, pp. 303–17. Cambridge, Massachusetts.

Reppas, J.B., Niyogi, S., Dale, A.M., Sereno, M.I., and Tootell, R.B.H. (1997). Representation of motion boundaries in retinotopic human visual cortical areas. *Nature* **388**, 175–9.

Richter, J.P. (1975). *The notebooks of Leonardo Da Vinci*. Dover Books, London.

Roland, P. (1993). *Brain activation*. Wiley, New York.

Rosano, C., Krisky, C.M., Welling, J.S., Eddy, W.F., Luna, B., Thulborn, K.R., and Sweeney, J.A. (2002). Pursuit and saccadic eye movement subregions in human frontal eye field: a high-resolution fMRI investigation. *Cereb. Cortex* **12**, 107–15.

Rutschmann, R.M., Schrauf, M., and Greenlee, M.W. (2000). Brain activation during dichoptic presentation of optic flow stimuli. *Exp. Brain Res.* **134**, 533–7.

Schiller, P.H., True, S.D., and Conway, J.L. (1979). Effects of frontal eye field and superior colliculus ablations on eye movements. *Science* **206**, 590–2.

Schlag, J. and Schlag-Rey, M. (1987). Evidence for a supplementary eye field. *J. Neurophysiol.* **57**, 179–200.

Schmidtke, K., Handschu, R., and Vollmer, H. (1996). Cognitive procedural learning in amnesia. *Brain Cogn.* **32** (3), 441–67.

Schmidtke, K., Manner, H., and Vollmer, H. (1998). Deficits of procedural learning in focal prefronto-striatal lesions and Huntington's disease. *Neurol.* **245**, 354.

Sereno, M.I., Pitzalis, S., and Martinez, A. (2001). Mapping of contralateral space in retinotopic coordinates by a parietal cortical area in humans. *Science* **294**, 1350–4.

Shaywitz, S.E., Pugh, K.R., Fulbright, R.K., *et al.* (1998). Functional disruption in the organization of the brain for reading in dyslexia. *Proc. Natl Acad. Sci., USA* **95**, 2636–41.

Shulman, G.L., Ollinger, J.M., Akbudak, E., Conturo, T.E., Snyder, A.Z., Petersen, S.E., and Corbetta, M. (1999). Areas involved in encoding and applying directional expectations to moving objects. *J. Neurosci.* **19** (21) 9480–96.

Simos, P.G., Breier, J.I., Fletcher, J.M., Foorman, B.R., Castillo, E.M., and Papanicolaou, A.C. (2002). Brain mechanisms for reading words and pseudowords: an integrated approach. *Cereb. Cortex* **12**, 297–305.

Singh, K.D., Smith A.T., and Greenlee, M.W. (2000). Spatiotemporal frequency and direction sensitivities of human visual areas measured using fMRI. *Neuroimage* **12**, 550–64.

Skiera, G., Petersen, D., Skalej, M., and Fahle, M. (2000). Correlates of figure–ground segregation in fMRI. *Vision Res.* **40**, 2047–56.

Smith, A.T. (1994). The detection of second-order motion. In *Visual detection of motion* (ed. A.T. Smith and R. Snowden), Chapter 6. Academic Press, New York.

Smith, A.T., Greenlee, M.W., Singh, K.D., Kraemer, F.M., and Hennig, J. (1998). The processing of first- and second-order motion in human visual cortex assessed by functional magnetic resonance imaging (fMRI). *J. Neurosci.* **18**, 3816–30.

Smith, A.T., Singh, K.D., and Greenlee, M.W. (2000). Attentional suppression of activity in the human visual cortex. *Neuroreport* **11** (2), 271–7.

Sweeney, J.A., Mintun, M.A., Kwee, S., Wiseman, M.B., Brown, D.L., Rosenberg, D.R., and Carl, J.R. (1996). Positron emission tomography study of voluntary saccadic eye movements and spatial working memory. *J. Neurophysiol.* **75**, 454–68.

Talairach, J. and Tournoux, P. (1988). *Co-planar stereotaxic atlas of the human brain*. Thieme Verlag, Stuttgart.

Tehovnik, E.J., Sommer, M.A., Chou, I.H., Slocum, W.M., and Schiller, P.H. (2000). Eye fields in the frontal lobes of primates. *Brain Res. Brain Res. Rev.* **32** (2–3), 413–48.

Temple, E., Poldrack, R.A., Protopapas, A., Nagarajan, S., Salz, T., Tallal, P., Merzenich, M.M., and Gabrieli, J.D. (2000). Disruption of the neural response to rapid acoustic stimuli in dyslexia: evidence from functional MRI. *Proc. Natl Acad. Sci., USA* **97**, 13907–12.

Thompson, P. (1981). Velocity after-effects: the effects of adaptation to moving stimuli on the perception of subsequently seen moving stimuli. *Vision Res.* 21, 337–45.

Tolias, A.S., Smirnakis, S.M., Augath, M.A., Trinath, T. and Logothetis, N.K. (2001). Motion processing in the macaque: revisited with functional magnetic resonance imaiging. *J. Neurosci.* 21, 8594–601.

Tootell, R.B., Reppas, J.B., Dale, A.M., Look, R.B., Sereno, M.I., Malach, R., Brady, T.J., and Rosen, B.R. (1995a). Visual motion aftereffect in human cortical area MT revealed by functional magnetic resonance imaging. *Nature* 375, 139–41.

Tootell, R.B., Reppas, J.B., Kwong, K.K., Malach, R., Born, R.T., Brady, T.J., Rosen, B.R., and Belliveau, J.W. (1995b). Functional analysis of human MT and related visual cortical areas using magnetic resonance imaging. *J. Neurosci.* 15, 3215–30.

Tootell, R.B.H., Mendola, J.D., Hadjikhani, N.K., Ledden, P.J., Liu, A.K., Reppas, J.B., Sereno, M.I., and Dale, A.M. (1997). Functional analysis of V3A and related areas in human visual cortex. *J. Neurosci.* 17, 7060–78.

Tootell, R.B., Hadjikhani, N., Hall, E.K., Marrett, S., Vanduffel, W., Vaughan, J.T., and Dale, A.M. (1998). The retinotopy of visual spatial attention. *Neuron*, 21, 1409–22.

Tucha, O. Aschenbrenner, S., and Lange, K.W. (2000). Mirror writing and handedness. *Brain Lang.* 73, 432–41.

Van Essen, D.C., Maunsell, J.H.R., and Bixby, J.L. (1981). The middle temporal visual area in the macaque: myeloarchitecture, connections, functional properties and topographic organization. *J. Comp. Neurol.* 199, 293–326.

van Oostende, S., Sunaert, S., Van Hecke, P., Marchal, G., and Orban, G.A. (1997). The kinetic occipital (KO) region in man: an fMRI study. *Cereb. Cortex* 7, 690–701.

van Santen, J.P. and Sperling, G. (1985). Elaborated Reichardt detectors. *J. Opt. Soc. Am. A* 2, 300–21.

Watson, J.D.G., Myers, R., Frackowiak, R.S.J., Hajnal, J.V., Woods, R.P., Mazziotta, J.C., Shipp, S., and Zeki, S. (1993). Area V5 of the human brain: evidence from a combined study using positron emission tomography and magnetic resonance imaging. *Cereb. Cortex* 3, 79–84.

Wenderoth, P., Watson, J.D., Egan, G.F., Tochon-Danguy, H.J., and O'Keefe, G.J. (1999). Second order components of moving plaids activate, extrastriate cortex: a positron emission tomography study. *NeuroImage* 9, 227–34.

Woods, R.P., Grafton, S.T., Holmes, C.J., Cherry, S.R., and Mazziotta, J.C. (1998a). Automated image registration: I. General methods and intrasubject, intramodality validation. *J. Comput. Assist. Tomogr.* 22, 139–52.

Woods, R.P., Grafton, S.T., Watson, J.D., Sicotte, N.L., and Mazziotta, J.C. (1998b). Automated image registration: II. Intersubject validation of linear and nonlinear models. *J. Comput. Assist. Tomogr.* 22, 153–65.

Zeki, S.M. (1974). Functional organization of a visual area in the posterior bank of the superior temporal sulcus of the rhesus monkey. *J. Physiol.* (Lond.) 236, 549–73.

Zeki, S. (1978). Uniformity and diversity of structure and function in rhesus monkey prestriate visual cortex. *J. Physiol.* 277, 273–90.

Zeki, S., Watson, J.D.G., Lueck, C.J., Friston, K.J., Kennard, C., and Frackowiak, R.S.J. (1991). A direct demonstration of functional specialization in human visual cortex. *J. Neurosci.* 11, 641–9.

Part 4

Lesion studies in trained monkeys and humans (transcranial magnetic stimulation)

Chapter 5

Lesions in primate visual cortex leading to deficits of visual perception

William H. Merigan and Tatiana Pasternak

Introduction

The primate cortical visual pathways offer an attractive animal model for relating the function of individual nerve cells to the behaviour of the organism. The anatomical structures and connections of this pathway have been explored in detail with both anatomical and physiological methods (Hubel and Wiesel 1968), and clear linkages have been shown between the physiological response of individual cells in this system and the behaviour of the entire animal (Britten *et al.* 1996). Other features that make this an attractive model are the retinotopic organization of many of the cortical areas (Felleman and Van Essen 1991), the possibility of dividing visual cortex into functionally different 'dorsal and ventral' or 'colour/form and motion' parallel pathways (Ungerleider and Mishkin 1982), and the growing evidence, largely from functional magnetic resonance imaging (fMRI), that the visual cortices of humans and non-human primates are remarkably similar (Sereno *et al.* 1995; Logothetis *et al.* 1999).

Figure 5.1 shows a diagram of selected anatomical areas and connections in the macaque cortical visual pathway (adapted from Croner and Albright 1999). This representation emphasizes two prominent features of the cortical visual pathways that are not evident in traditional diagrams (e.g. Merigan and Maunsell 1993): (1) the general progression from larger to smaller cortical areas, and (2) the relatively small size of the dorsal stream at the level of area MT, relative to the ventral stream at the level of area V4 (Lennie 1998). The diagram has been arranged to emphasize the separation of the cortical pathway beyond area V2 into a dorsal and ventral stream of processing (Ungerleider and Mishkin 1982; see also Deyoe *et al.* 1994). Various authors have called these streams the 'motion' and 'colour and form' (Maunsell and Newsome 1987) or 'how' and 'what' (Goodale and Milner 1992) pathways in order to reflect the different visual functions they may be involved in. Receptive field (RF) size increases, and retinotopy decreases, in each successive cortical area of both the dorsal and ventral streams.

Despite the modularity of cortical areas, there is great complexity in the interconnections at the level of individual neurons. The dense network of feedforward, feedback,

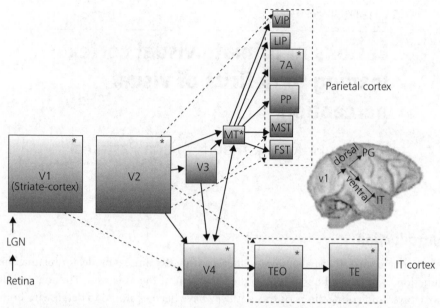

Fig. 5.1 Diagram of major macaque cortical visual areas. Individual cortical areas are shown as blocks, roughly proportional in size to the extent of the visual area (Felleman and Van Essen 1991). The grey arrows show some of the more prominent ascending (these pathways are also reciprocal) projections from the retina to the highest level areas of the dorsal and ventral pathways. Asterisks indicate cortical areas that have been lesioned in some of the studies examined in this review. The dotted and dashed arrows show some of the minor 'bypassing' pathways (Felleman and Van Essen 1991; Nakamura *et al.* 1993*b*) that could be responsible for some sparing of vision after V2 and V4 (dotted arrows) or MT (dashed arrows) lesions (Nakamura *et al.* 1993*b*). LGN, lateral geniculate nucleus; V1, visual area 1; V2, visual area 2; V3, visual area 3; V4, visual area 4; MT, middle temporal area; TEO, TEO area of inferotemporal cortex; TE, TE area of inferotemporal cortex; FST, fundus of the superior temporal sulcus; MST, medial superior temporal area; PP, posterior parietal area; 7A, visual area 7A; LIP, lateral intraparietal area; VIP, ventral intraparietal area. (Adapted from Croner and Albright (1999).)

and lateral connections (Boussaoud *et al.* 1990; Tanaka *et al.* 1990; Felleman and Van Essen 1991; Rockland and Van Hoesen 1994; Gilbert *et al.* 1996) makes it difficult to determine how the function of individual neurons contributes to the overall capabilities of the system. Fortunately, a wide and growing array of methodologies, including recordings from single cells in animals performing behavioural tasks (e.g. Britten *et al.* 1992*b*; Rainer and Miller 2000), fMRI (e.g. Logothetis *et al.* 1999), selective reversible and permanent inactivation (e.g. Yamasaki and Wurtz 1991; Li *et al.* 1999; Rudolph and Pasternak 1999), and computational studies (e.g. Dan *et al.* 1996; Shadlen *et al.* 1996; Rolls *et al.* 1997), is being brought to bear upon this question, and this use of converging approaches is illuminating visual neural function in a way that no subset of methodologies could. The present chapter represents a selective, critical analysis of the contribution of one of these methodologies, lesions of visual neurons, to our understanding of the function of the visual pathways. The literature on such inactivation is extensive, and earlier work has already been reviewed (Gross 1973; Dean 1982). Our analysis will emphasize more recent studies that have examined the effects of striate and extrastriate lesions in the primate.

Methods of inactivation

There are many techniques for inactivating neural tissue, some permanent and some transitory, and each has its own advantages and disadvantages. Permanent lesions are made by aspiration, thermocoagulation, or injections of neurotoxic agents. Of these methods, the use of neurotoxic agents, such as ibotenic acid, is by far the most preferred, since it permits the creation of cell-body-specific lesions that spare fibres of passage (Schwarcz *et al.* 1979). This approach has proven important in regions of the nervous system where damaging fibres of passage may contribute to the observed deficit (Meunier *et al.* 1999). An important advantage of permanent inactivation is that the lesion is morphologically stable over a long period of time. This makes it possible to determine the precise extent and severity of the lesion after completion of the experiment by histological mapping (e.g. Yamasaki and Wurtz 1991) or by MRI (Pasternak and Merigan 1994; Merigan 2000). This stability also avoids the complex time course that can occur with pharmacological inactivations as cortex returns to normal after an injection, or if repeated injections produce diminishing inactivation. On the other hand, a potential disadvantage of permanent lesions is that the nervous system could reorganize in response to the lesion, resulting in a change in the magnitude or the nature of the induced deficit (e.g. Newsome and Paré 1988; Yamasaki and Wurtz 1991; Rudolph and Pasternak 1999). Another limitation of neurotoxic lesions is that to inactivate very large areas of the brain (e.g. inferotemporal cortex) would require an impractically large number of injections. For such inactivations, aspiration (e.g. Huxlin *et al.* 2000*b*) or cooling (see below) is more common. The majority of studies of the perceptual effects of neural inactivation in the macaque have used permanent lesions.

Transitory inactivation of nervous tissue is typically achieved by the local injection of pharmacological blocking agents that affect only cell bodies, such as muscimol (Dias and Segraves 1999; Li *et al.* 1999; Martin and Ghez 1999) or γ-aminobutyric acid (GABA; Malpeli 1999). Other commonly used reversible methods of inactivation, such as injections of lidocaine (Malpeli 1999) and the application of cold to the cortical surface (e.g. Fuster *et al.* 1981; Horel *et al.* 1984; Quintana *et al.* 1989), are less selective, since they inactivate both cell bodies and fibres. These methods offer rapid and reversible inactivation of neural tissue, with recovery within minutes after GABA and lidocaine injections, and after hours with muscimol injection, and a time course controlled by the investigator in the application of cold. Such transitory inactivation is used to minimize the problem of reorganization in the nervous system, because the time of inactivation can be quite brief. This method is also advantageous because control observations can be taken just before, and in some cases again just after, the inactivation. Such controls are important in examining perceptual effects, because visual performance is often practice-dependent and, when control observations are taken before the lesion is made, the postlesion observations often involve a more experienced, or in some cases, a more discouraged, subject. One limitation of the use of pharmacological methods is that the area inactivated by a single injection is relatively small (Hupé *et al.* 1999; Malpeli 1999) and extending this region requires multiple injections at different locations. Another limitation is the relatively short duration of the effect, which limits the length of the testing sessions and extent of psychophysical measures. A methodological concern with cooling studies is that a gradient of partial cooling extends from the site of targeted cooling, and it is important to determine if this gradient, which sometimes reaches cells that were meant to be spared from inactivation, contributes to the neural deficit. Although temporary inactivation has been extensively used to study the visual system (e.g. Malpeli *et al.* 1981; Girard *et al.* 1991; Ferrera *et al.* 1994*a*), there are few instances in which it has been used to study perceptual effects in macaques.

Methodological concerns in lesion studies

The use of lesions to study brain organization has a long and productive history, with many of the first insights into the function of different brain regions resulting from lesion studies (e.g. Cowey and Gross 1970; Passingham 1972; Kluver and Bucy 1997). However, lesions remain a controversial approach to understanding neural function (Gregory 1961; Dean 1982), perhaps because it appears counterintuitive to explore the function of a complex system by damaging it (think of studying the function of an audio-amplifier by removing resistors). Fortunately, careful design of the lesion study, and sensitivity to potential errors in interpretation can help in making lesion studies informative. On the other hand, because of the complexity of experimental protocols used to study lesion effects, it is easy to mistakenly either overestimate or underestimate the perceptual role of the missing neurons.

Underestimation of the effects of a lesion

Underestimation of the effects of a neural lesion can result from only partial damage to a cortical area or recovery from a lesion due to reorganization of the brain. Incomplete lesions will produce minimal lesion effects if the spared neurons can mediate the tested abilities. This can be particularly critical when lesions are made in retinotopic areas, since survival of a small region could give quite normal function in some parts of the visual field. A good solution to this problem is to make lesions over only a portion of the visual field, and then confine stimulus presentation to the affected region, by using controlled fixation. The visual field extent of the lesion can be verified by physiological recording (Merigan *et al.* 1991) or by behavioural mapping (Merigan and Pham 1998).

Substantial, and in some cases complete, recovery of function has been reported after brain lesions at a variety of locations including the oculomotor system (Schiller *et al.*

1980), the somatosensory system (Merzenich *et al.* 1983), and the extrastriate cortical visual system (Newsome and Paré 1988; Rudolph and Pasternak 1999). This recovery may include several factors that evolve over time. First, there is often a recovery of local neural processing that immediately follows the lesion, suggesting an unmasking of pre-existing functional connections (Das and Gilbert 1995). Following this, there can be an improvement over the first few days after the lesion that may be due to resolution of the oedema, gliosis, and acute nerve injury that follow a lesion (Horgan and Finn 1997). Finally, there is often a long-term (sometimes practice-dependent) reorganization of the nervous system that can substitute for the function of the lesioned area (Florence and Kaas 1995; Eysel and Schweigart 1999).

Overestimation of the effects of a lesion

Overestimation of the effects of a cortical lesion could be due to unintended damage to neurons beyond those targeted, or to a profound, but non-specific, change in some more general aspect of neural function. There can be unintended damage to neigh-bouring cortical areas, if the lesion extends beyond the planned size. It is also possible to inadvertently lesion fibres passing through or near a lesioned area. A particularly important example of this is unintended damage to optic radiation fibres caused by experimental lesions of parietal or temporal cortex in macaques, or by stroke or neuro-surgery in human patients. The extent of optic radiation damage can be assessed by examining degeneration in the lateral geniculate nucleus (LGN; Ungerleider and Brody 1977; Huxlin *et al.* 2000*b*), and such degeneration is often substantial. If degeneration in the LGN is present, it could cause scattered dense scotomata across the visual field, making interpretation of parietal or temporal lobe lesions difficult.

A second way in which lesions can cause an overestimate of the role of a cortical region in a given perceptual function is by causing a generalized and non-specific change in the behaviour used to evaluate neural function. Such unwanted effects as loss of motivation, impaired motor function, or attentional deficits must be ruled out before other interpretations of neural lesions can be made. This can best be done by using a range of perceptual tasks and stimuli—some likely to be affected by the lesion and some likely to be spared.

Early visual cortex

Area V1

Primary visual cortex (also known as striate cortex or V1), is the first cortical stage of the primate visual pathways, and the recipient of the great majority of fibres from the retino-geniculate pathway. This is a very large cortical area with precise retinotopy, and has the smallest RFs of any visual cortical area (Hubel and Wiesel 1968). V1 neurons show several emergent selectivities (properties not seen at earlier stages of the visual system) such as orientation, direction, and disparity tuning. In addition, orientation- and colour-tuned cells are grouped within V1 in orientation columns and blobs, respectively (Hubel *et al.* 1976). A small number of fibres from the retinogeniculate pathway bypass V1 and terminate directly in V2 (Bullier and Kennedy 1983; also see Chapter 3, this volume and Fig. 5.1). There are also minor projections from subcortical structures, such as the pulvinar, that bypass V1 and project directly to extrastriate cortical areas (Levitt *et al.* 1995), and such fibres may help mediate residual function after lesions of area V1.

Although the anatomical segregation of neural classes that becomes the ventral and dorsal streams (see Fig. 5.1) begins in area V1, these pathways are closely intertwined within V1 (Lund 1988; Casagrande 1994), and lesion studies have not had the precision to tease apart their functional contribution. Thus, V1 lesions affect both pathways producing a profound effect on visual performance, leading to regions of the visual field that have such dense loss of vision that they are termed scotomata. Most of the studies described in this section of the review have tried to determine the characteristics of any slight residual vision within these scotomata.

That V1 lesions cause severe visual loss was first discovered in human subjects, in whom head injuries suffered in the Russo–Japanese war of 1905 or the First World War of 1917 caused visual field defects (e.g. Glickstein 1988; Grusser and Landis 1991; Glickstein and Fahle 2000). Such defects rarely show substantial change in extent or density over the succeeding years. Monkey studies also show severe visual loss after V1 lesions (Weiskrantz and Cowey 1967; Miller *et al.* 1980; Merigan *et al.* 1993), although the completeness of this loss was questioned after some monkeys with V1 lesions appeared to orient toward visual stimuli (e.g. Humphrey and Weiskrantz 1967; see Chapter 9, this volume). Recent interest in the effects of V1 lesions has been generated largely by two developments—the growing recognition that humans may show some residual vision (termed 'blindsight') after V1 lesions (Weiskrantz 1986) and the observation of activity in extrastriate cortical areas after lesions of striate cortex in monkeys and humans (Rodman *et al.* 1989; Ffytche *et al.* 1996).

The interpretation of many macaque studies of the effects of V1 lesions is aided by histological verification that V1 was completely destroyed (e.g. Miller *et al.* 1980), and that the LGN showed no evidence of spared sectors (some remaining cells in the LGN are to be expected, given that neurons in this nucleus project to other targets besides striate cortex). Such evidence is not available for humans with 'blindsight', making interpretation of their residual vision more uncertain. In macaque studies, following complete (i.e. histologically verified) removal of the striate cortex, the profound visual loss is accompanied by survival of some rudimentary vision. Destriated monkeys can detect rapid flicker (Humphrey and Weiskrantz 1967; Chapter 9, this volume), discriminate blue from yellow and red from green (Schilder *et al.* 1972; Keating 1979), track moving lights (Humphrey and Weiskrantz 1967), discriminate simple forms (Keating and Horel 1976; Dineen and Keating 1981), and even successfully grasp two objects placed side by side (Humphrey and Weiskrantz 1967; see Chapter 9, this volume). However interesting these residual abilities are, of course, they represent minor sparing in a virtually complete loss of vision.

Studies of residual vision in humans after striate cortex lesions (Grusser and Landis 1991) show many of the same surviving visual abilities as shown in the above studies in monkeys. For example, subjects can make eye movements (Poppel 1973) or reach (Weiskrantz 1986) towards punctate targets, they show some preservation of motion thresholds, especially in peripheral vision, they can discriminate large changes in stimulus orientation (Weiskrantz 1986), and they can detect stimuli on the basis of chromatic change (Stoerig and Cowey 1992).

It is likely that different visual pathways are responsible for different aspects of the minimal vision that survives V1 lesions. For example, the minimal colour vision that survives V1 lesions may depend on colour-opponent neurons, making it likely that this ability reflects the function of primate beta ganglion cells projecting through the pulvinar (Cowey et al. 1994). On the other hand, coarse localization after V1 lesions may be maintained by non-colour-opponent cortical projections from the superior colliculus (Walker et al. 1995). There is also evidence that in monkeys with V1 lesions, light–dark discrimination, one of the simplest possible visual tasks, can be maintained even by a very minimal visual pathway, the accessory optic tract (Pasik and Pasik 1973).

Area V2

Area V2 is a large cortical area that receives most of its ascending input from area V1, and sends substantial projections to areas V3, middle temporal (MT), and V4. This area consists of a series of elongated regions that can be labelled by cytochrome oxidase (Olavarria and Van Essen 1997) or the antibody Cat 301 (Deyoe et al. 1990) and that are termed thick, thin, and interstripes. The thick stripes appear to be an early component of the dorsal pathway, and they contain cells projecting to area MT that are selective for direction of motion and disparity (Shipp and Zeki 1985; Roe and Tso 1997; see Chapter 3, this volume). The thin stripes and interstripes are seen as an early component of the ventral stream, show selectivity for colour and orientation, and project to area V4 (Felleman et al. 1997), but some fibres project directly to TEO bypassing V4 (Nakamura et al. 1993a). Physiological RFs in V2 are larger than in V1, and some response properties are more complex than those of V1. For example, V2 cells respond well to illusory contour stimuli (von der Heydt and Peterhans 1989) and to stimuli of moderately complex form (Kobatake and Tanaka 1994).

Numerous earlier studies have described lesions made in prestriate cortex, of which V2 is a component (i.e. anterior to area V1). However, this is a difficult region to study with lesions, because it consists of several highly retinotopic areas (V2, V3, V3a, and V4), and the extent of damage to each of these areas, as well as possible sparing of some portion of the visual field of each area, cannot be determined without physiological mapping. A second problem is that, in the macaque, area V2 is closely apposed to area V1, representing the same portion of the visual field, making it almost impossible to lesion area V2 without partially lesioning area V1. The best solution to this problem is to physiologically map the damage to V1 and V2, and place test stimuli in a part of the visual field that corresponds to complete V2 damage, with no V1 damage (Merigan et al. 1993).

One study that was able to verify that visual testing was done only within the affected part of the visual field in V2 (Merigan et al. 1993), found results consistent with the physiology of V2 neurons. While contrast sensitivity for orientation discrimination (measured with gratings defined by luminance or colour) was depressed by V2 lesions, contrast sensitivity for discriminating the direction of motion, tested with rapidly moving stimuli, was unaffected (Fig. 5.2).

The selectivity of this effect is surprising since the lesions were large relative to the size of cytochrome oxidase compartments, thus involving both thick, thin and interstripes,

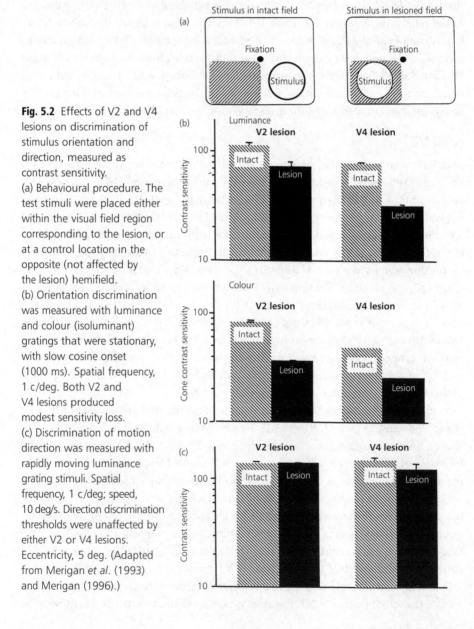

Fig. 5.2 Effects of V2 and V4 lesions on discrimination of stimulus orientation and direction, measured as contrast sensitivity.
(a) Behavioural procedure. The test stimuli were placed either within the visual field region corresponding to the lesion, or at a control location in the opposite (not affected by the lesion) hemifield.
(b) Orientation discrimination was measured with luminance and colour (isoluminant) gratings that were stationary, with slow cosine onset (1000 ms). Spatial frequency, 1 c/deg. Both V2 and V4 lesions produced modest sensitivity loss.
(c) Discrimination of motion direction was measured with rapidly moving luminance grating stimuli. Spatial frequency, 1 c/deg; speed, 10 deg/s. Direction discrimination thresholds were unaffected by either V2 or V4 lesions. Eccentricity, 5 deg. (Adapted from Merigan *et al.* (1993) and Merigan (1996).)

and most likely disrupting both ventral and dorsal pathways. However, as can be seen in Fig. 5.1, there is a large projection from V1 directly to MT that might be partly responsible for the spared sensitivity for the direction of grating motion after V2 lesions. V2 lesions also profoundly disrupted two complex form discriminations—one discrimination that involved the collinearity of dots and another that required perceptual grouping of line segments (Fig. 5.3(a), (b)). These disruptions of moderately complex spatial perception were retinotopically matched to the location and extent of the lesion, appeared permanent, and could not be accounted for by the small reduction in visual sensitivity. This profile of visual loss, combined with the selective disruption of visual sensitivity, suggests comparison to the ventral pathway lesions described below.

Ventral pathway

The ventral pathway has been termed the 'colour and form' pathway (Maunsell and Newsome 1987) because both colour and shape selectivity are prominent in the physiological responses of V4 (Zeki 1983b; Desimone et al. 1985; Kobatake and Tanaka 1994) and inferotemporal (IT) cortex neurons (Gross et al. 1969; Tanaka 1992), the two major components of the ventral pathway. This section will provide an overview of the perceptual effects of lesions in these two areas.

Like areas V1 and V2, area V4 is a highly retinotopic cortical area, although the receptive fields of its neurons are larger and slightly more irregular than those of areas V1 and V2 (Lennie 1998). As mentioned above, the thin- and interstripes of V2 project to V4, and there is some evidence of a modular organization within V4 that reflects these inputs (Xiao et al. 1999). However, to date, no lesion studies have had the precision to separately study these modules.

Perception of simple forms: stimulus orientation

This section summarizes the growing evidence that V4 and IT lesions can elevate thresholds for some simple form discriminations. This evidence may appear at odds with earlier conclusions that mid- and high-level ventral pathway lesions produce minimal, if any, effects on many basic visual thresholds, as well as on physiologically measured evoked responses in areas V1 and V2 (Dean 1975; Kulikowski et al. 1994; Cowey et al. 1998).

Merigan (1996) examined the effects of V4 lesions on contrast thresholds for detection and discrimination of the orientation and direction of motion of simple sinusoidal gratings (see Fig. 5.2). While orientation discrimination thresholds were elevated, direction discrimination thresholds were not affected. The stimuli used in this study to test orientation thresholds were stationary with a slow onset, whereas those used to test direction thresholds drifted at 10°/s. Subsequently, detection thresholds were also measured for the low and high temporal frequency stimuli, and V4 lesions affected only the low temporal frequency thresholds. This selective deficit for thresholds measured with low temporal frequency gratings may be a reflection of damage to projections from parvocellular neurons, which are highly responsive to low temporal frequencies (Merigan and Maunsell 1993) and which are normally present in area V4 (Ferrera et al. 1994b).

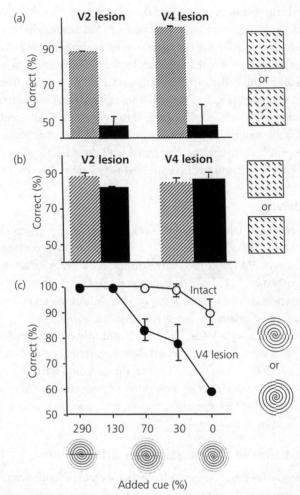

Fig. 5.3 Effects of V2 and V4 lesions on the discrimination of complex texture and illusory contours. Performance in the lesioned portion of the visual field was compared to that in the intact field (see Fig. 5.2(a)). (a) Grouping. The monkeys discriminated the orientation of pop-outs composed of three misoriented line segments within the two textures. This discrimination required grouping of the three line segments to form a vertical or horizontal pop-out. Performance was at chance level in the visual field locus that corresponded to the lesion. (b) Detection. Detection control for the discrimination illustrated in (a). The monkey reported the presence or absence of a single misoriented line segment. Little postlesion deficit was found in this detection task. (c) Illusory contours. The monkeys discriminated between the orientations of the two illusory contours. The discrimination illustrated to the right was measured with varying amounts of added cue (illustrated below abscissa), which at the maximum (290%), turned the task into an orientation discrimination for a 'real' contour. The cued discrimination was not affected by the V4 lesion. However, when the contour was illusory (0% cue), monkeys could not perform the discrimination above chance level at the lesion location. Eccentricity, 5 deg. (Adapted from Merigan (2000).)

Later, Rudolph and Pasternak (1999) explicitly studied the selectivity of V4 and MT lesions for orientation versus direction discriminations measured with both higher and lower spatial and temporal frequencies. They found that V4 lesions resulted in deficits in contrast thresholds for discriminating orientation (Fig. 5.4), while those for discriminating the direction of motion of gratings of the same spatial and temporal frequencies were unaffected (Fig. 5.5). The elevation of thresholds for orientation discrimination was most pronounced at higher spatial and lower temporal frequencies. Thus, V4 lesion effects were limited to orientation discrimination measured with lower temporal and higher spatial frequency gratings. These authors also found elevated signal/noise ratios for orientation, but not direction, discrimination when the gratings were masked by spatial noise (Fig. 5.5). Schiller and Lee (1994) also measured the effects of V4 lesions on contrast thresholds with luminance and chromatic checkerboards (draughtboards), rather than with gratings, and found a sensitivity deficit.

A similar selectivity for contrast sensitivity measured with orientation thresholds versus direction thresholds was seen by Merigan after bilateral IT lesions (Fig. 5.6). Again, contrast thresholds for orientation discrimination were markedly affected by the lesion, while those measured with direction discrimination were intact. This result suggests that, like V4 lesions, area IT lesions may also selectively disrupt orientation discriminations. It is noteworthy that, in an earlier study, IT lesions did not appear to affect contrast thresholds when the monkeys were required only to detect the presence of the grating, rather than to identify its orientation (Cowey *et al.* 1998).

The effects of lesions of the ventral pathway on the precision of orientation discrimination have been studied by several groups. DeWeerd *et al.* (1996) examined orientation difference thresholds in monkeys with longstanding V4 lesions, and found elevations of thresholds for gratings defined by texture and by illusory contours. Deficits for luminance-defined gratings were either absent or very small. A similar observation that orientation difference thresholds for luminance gratings are spared by V4 lesions was made by Rudolph and Pasternak (1999).

Relatively modest deficits in the accuracy of orientation discrimination have also been observed following lesions of IT cortex. Dean (1978) used luminance-defined gratings to examine orientation difference thresholds in monkeys with IT lesions and found consistent threshold elevations. In a more recent study, Vogels *et al.* (1997) tested orientation discrimination in monkeys with unilateral IT lesions involving areas TE and TEO, combined with transection of callosal connections. Orientation discrimination was measured with two tasks—one involving the comparison of simultaneously presented orientations and the other the comparison of successively presented oriented stimuli. The accuracy of orientation discrimination measured in a simultaneous discrimination paradigm was largely unaffected. However, when orientation discrimination was measured with the task that required the monkeys to remember the orientation of a previously presented stimulus, area IT lesions caused a great disruption.

(a) Behavioural procedure: same/different orientations

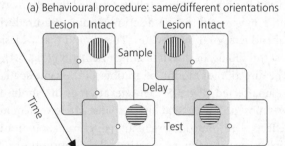

(b) Orientation: contrast sensitivity

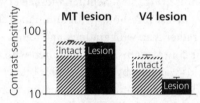

(c) Orientation: noise masking

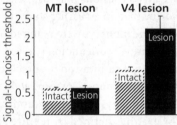

Fig. 5.4 Effects of V4 and MT lesions on orientation discrimination. (a) Psychophysical testing procedure. Monkeys fixated a small spot for 1 s to initiate the trial. The orientation of the sample was chosen at random from a set of six orientations and the orientation of the test was the same as, or orthogonal to, that of the sample. (b) Contrast sensitivity. Only the contrast of the sample was varied; the test was set to 51% contrast. Spatial frequency, 1 c/deg; temporal frequency (counterphase flicker), 5 Hz. (c) Signal-to-noise thresholds. The grating was masked by adding 3 × 3 pixel two-dimensional noise. The noise levels masking the sample were varied. The test grating contained no noise and was set to 51% contrast, and the task was identical to that shown in (b). The area V4 lesion reduced contrast sensitivity and elevated signal/noise thresholds, while MT/MST lesions had no significant effect on orientation discrimination. Lesions of areas V4 and MT/MST were unilateral and were made by multiple injections of ibotenic acid. Representative data are shown for a single monkey with a V4 lesion and from another with an MT/MST lesion. The MT/MST lesion data were adapted from Rudolph and Pasternak (1999). The V4 lesion data were adapted from Rudolph (1997, University of Rochester, doctoral dissertation).

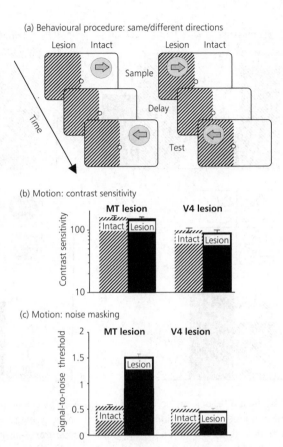

Fig. 5.5 Effects of MT and V4 lesions on direction discrimination. (a) Psychophysical testing procedure. Monkeys fixated a small spot for 1 s to initiate the trial. Sample and test stimuli (arrows indicate drifting gratings) appeared successively in the same location. The offset of sample and the onset of test were separated by a 200 ms delay. Fixation was maintained until the test stimulus disappeared. The monkey indicated whether the test was either same as, or different from, the sample by pressing the right or left button, respectively. One of eight possible directions of motion was selected at random as a sample stimulus and the test stimulus moved either in the same or the opposite direction. Thresholds were measured by varying the visibility of the motion. (b) Contrast sensitivity (1/contrast thresholds × 100). Contrast thresholds were measured in the intact and the lesioned portions of the visual field. Spatial frequency, 1 c/deg; speed, 5 deg/s (temporal frequency, 5 Hz). The contrast or signal-to-noise of the sample was varied. The test remained at 51% contrast with no masking noise. Neither V4 nor MT lesions permanently altered contrast sensitivity. (c) Signal-to-noise thresholds measured by varying the proportion of pixels in the grating that assumed random intensities. The noise level of the sample stimulus was varied. The test grating contained no noise and was set to 51% contrast. Spatial and temporal (speed) frequency, target size, and position are the same as in (b). The MT/MST lesion elevated signal-to-noise thresholds for discriminating differences in direction. The V4 lesion had no measurable effect on direction discrimination thresholds. The MT/MST lesion data were adapted from Rudolph and Pasternak (1999). The V4 lesion data were adapted from Rudolph (1997, University of Rochester, doctoral dissertation).

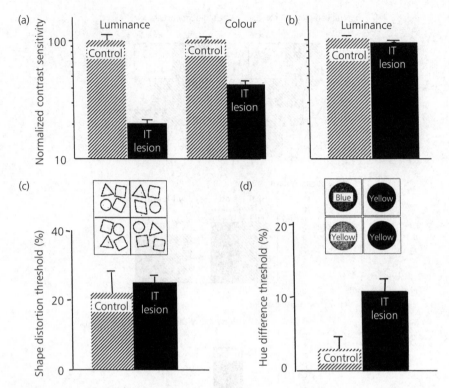

Fig. 5.6 Effects of bilateral IT lesions. (a) Normalized contrast sensitivity (control set to 100) for orientation discrimination measured with luminance and chromatic gratings. Both measures showed at least a twofold threshold elevation. (b) Normalized contrast sensitivity measured with direction discrimination. Sensitivity was not significantly reduced by the lesion.
(c) Shape distortion thresholds, tested by having the monkey choose which of the four stimulus panels contained a distorted shape. In the stimulus shown, the upper right panel contains a 40% distorted square. Distortion thresholds were not significantly elevated by the IT lesion.
(d) Hue discrimination in which the monkey chose the odd colour. Three of the stimuli were of the same colour, but were of random brightness to remove apparent brightness as a cue to the colour discrimination. Hue thresholds were substantially elevated by the IT lesions. For all panels, hatched bars represent stable thresholds before the lesion, and filled bars stable thresholds after the lesion. ((a), (b) Unpublished. (c), (d) Adapted from Huxlin *et al.* (2000*b*).)

These results indicate that lesions of the components of the ventral pathway can selectively elevate contrast or noise-masked thresholds for discriminating the orientation of simple gratings, as well as disrupt orientation discrimination measured with more complex stimuli. There is some evidence that these effects are more pronounced for stimuli of higher spatial and lower temporal frequencies. Furthermore, loss under the same conditions of testing was not seen after lesions of the main component of the dorsal pathway, area MT (see below; also Fig. 5.4).

Perception of complex form

Involvement of the ventral pathway in the perception of complex forms was initially suggested by physiological findings of shape selectivity in IT cortex (Gross *et al.* 1979). These results led to an extensive series of studies of the effects of IT lesions on form and other discriminations (e.g. Cowey and Gross 1970), which generally supported the idea that IT lesions affected shape discriminations. Subsequent physiological studies confirmed the extraordinary shape selectivity of IT neurons for such features as faces and hands (Desimone *et al.* 1984) as well as moderate shape tuning in V4 neurons (Kobatake and Tanaka 1994; Gallant *et al.* 1996; Pasupathy and Connor 1999).

Lesions of area V4

Many studies have shown that V4 lesions cause transitory disruption of moderately difficult shape discriminations. Walsh and his colleagues (1992*a*) found little effect of V4 lesions on a square–triangle discrimination, but did find an increase in the number of trials needed to relearn more complex form discriminations, including rotated letters and numbers. Heywood and Cowey (1987) reported that monkeys with V4 lesions required an increased number of trials to reach criterion (90% correct) on shape and face discriminations that had been trained before the lesions were made.

Other studies have found strong evidence for permanent shape discrimination deficits after V4 lesions. DeWeerd *et al.* (1996) reported consistent and pronounced deficits in orientation difference thresholds, using contours created by illusory contours, or texture differences. On the other hand, orientation thresholds for luminance, colour, or motion shear contours showed much less effect.

Heywood *et al.* (1992) examined visual search for the odd stimulus among nine stimuli presented on each trial. Monkeys with V4 lesions could perform the task when the odd stimulus differed in colour from the distractors, but when form discrimination was tested with alphanumeric characters, the discrimination ability was severely impaired.

Subsequently, Merigan (2000) used the approach of extended testing, one discrimination at a time, to try to uncover stimuli that could not be discriminated after V4 lesions. A wide range of line–element segmentation and grouping tasks, three-dimensional object discriminations (see Figs 5.3(a),(b) and 5.7), and discriminations involving illusory contours (see Fig. 5.3(c)), were tested under conditions designed to identify any residual discrimination ability that survived the lesion. Those discriminations that could not be easily performed at the visual field locus of the lesion were subsequently presented with added visual cues that were intensified or eliminated, under a staircase procedure, to aid discrimination. Also, these discriminations were initially presented at the edge of the affected portion of the visual field, and gradually moved toward the lesioned location dependent on the performance of the monkey. Despite these efforts, the monkeys were never able to relearn the grouping, illusory contour, and three-dimensional form discriminations. Those discriminations, unlike many

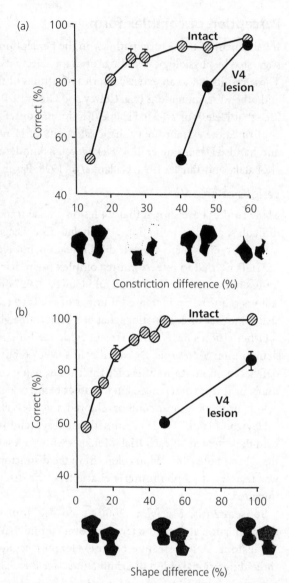

Fig. 5.7 Effect of V4 lesion on the discrimination of three-dimensional shapes. Pairs of three-dimensional shapes were presented side by side at a location corresponding to a V4 lesion (filled symbols) or at a control location (open symbols). The monkey reported whether the two shapes were the same or different. (a) The shapes differed in the amount of constriction of their midsection (waist). Pairs of stimuli below the abscissa illustrate the range tested from slight to large constriction differences. The V4 lesion greatly elevated the three-dimensional shape threshold. (b) The shapes differed in the shape of their cross-section from circular to pentagonal. Pairs of stimuli below the abscissa show the range tested from small to large shape differences. The V4 lesion markedly elevated the three-dimensional shape threshold. Eccentricity, 4 deg. (Adapted from Merigan and Pham (1998).)

similar texture discriminations, appeared to depend on the visual processing provided by V4, and could not be performed, even after extensive training, in its absence.

Schiller (1995) also found permanent form discrimination deficits, with an approach that combined several concurrent discriminations of relatively simple shapes. Following a V4 lesion, shape-matching was severely disrupted at the lesion location, and required extensive training to partially recover. Adding a new object profoundly affected matching performance for several days. Finally, the matching procedure was made less predictable by varying either the size of the sample stimulus or by transforming the match stimuli and, under these conditions, matching dropped to near chance levels.

These results demonstrate an enduring deficit in shape discrimination or shape-matching after V4 lesions that, in the studies that used controlled fixation testing, was confined to the region of the visual field corresponding to the lesion.

Lesions of IT cortex

Numerous studies have compared the effects of IT cortex and prestriate (largely V4) lesions on form discriminations (Gross 1973), and they have found a disruption of both initial learning and relearning of discriminations. For example, Cowey and Gross (1970) studied the effects of IT and prestriate lesions, and found deficits in both the initial learning and the retention of form discriminations after both IT and V4 lesions with both single and concurrently presented sets of visual stimuli.

Weiskrantz and Saunders (1984) used an unusual intervention to make object discriminations difficult. They trained monkeys to choose one of the two objects in nine pairs of objects, and then altered the appearance of the positive objects by 'transforming' their size, three-dimensional orientation, or the direction of lighting of an intense spotlight. They found that prestriate (largely V4) and IT lesions resulted in similarly large deficits in discriminating both the untransformed and transformed objects. In all cases, however, the monkeys could discriminate the transformed objects given sufficient practice.

The effects of IT lesions on shape perception have also been also examined by measuring thresholds, rather than trials to criterion. Blake *et al.* (1977) measured thresholds for discriminating right angles (90°) from smaller, acute angles after IT lesions. They found that, although monkeys with IT lesions learned the discrimination more slowly, their final thresholds were not elevated. In a recent study, Huxlin *et al.* (2000*b*) tested shape distortion thresholds for simple geometric shapes (see Fig. 5.6(c)) before and after IT lesions. They found a relatively transient disruption in shape distortion thresholds. These results show that, when shape discrimination is assessed by measuring thresholds using procedures that usually involve extensive testing, it does not appear to be permanently disrupted by ventral pathway lesions.

Interpretation of these findings as a selective effect of ventral pathway lesions on the discrimination of complex form requires clear evidence that form discriminations are disrupted, while other discriminations are unaffected. Several of the studies described above have shown such a dissociation. For example, DeWeerd *et al.* (1996) found marked threshold elevations only for those contours that required complex form-processing. Luminance and colour contours, as well as those created by motion shear, were much less affected. Merigan (2000) reported that only a few form discriminations were severely affected by V4 lesions. Others, including the one illustrated in Fig. 5.3(b), were unaffected.

Thus, both V4 and IT lesions can cause an increase in the number of errors committed while learning or relearning complex form discriminations. Permanent disruption of complex form discriminations or elevation of thresholds measured with them, has been more pronounced after V4 than after IT lesions. These results confirm an important role for V4 neurons in complex form discriminations. The failure to find equally severe effects of IT lesions could be due to postlesion reorganization.

The studies described above can be divided into two groups. The first group assessed the effects of lesions by measuring either speed of learning of new discriminations or the postlesion retention of previously learned discriminations that were relatively easy. These studies have commonly reported a disruption in the performance of previously learned discriminations, or slowed learning of new discriminations, followed by subsequent recovery. The second group used more difficult discriminations and in some cases measured visual thresholds. When such studies have involved IT lesions, they have often reported no permanent performance or threshold deficits, while those involving V4 lesions have consistently reported a permanent, but variable, decrease in performance.

Colour vision

It has long been accepted that the ventral cortical pathway in primates is central to colour-processing. This view initially emerged from the findings of Zeki (1983*a,b*) that chromatic selectivity was particularly prominent in area V4 neurons. It was augmented by the later findings of strong colour components in the responses of both V4 (Schein and Desimone 1990) and IT neurons (Komatsu *et al.* 1992; Kobatake and Tanaka 1994). It has also been shown that the input to the colour-responsive regions within V4 comes from colour-tuned regions within V2 (thin stripes), which in turn receive input from the colour-responsive blobs of area V1 (Xiao *et al.* 1999). Based on the physiological evidence of colour selectivity, many studies have looked at the effect of V4 and IT lesions on basic colour discriminations (often hue difference thresholds or visual detection based on colour). A few studies have also examined the effect of V4 lesions on more complex colour discriminations.

Lesions of area V4

V4 lesions frequently cause a transitory disruption of colour vision, as indicated by an increase in the number of errors made while learning or relearning colour discrimination. Walsh and colleagues (1992*b*, 1993) trained monkeys after bilateral V4 lesions to make pairwise discriminations of colours (Munsell patches) and found slower learning of colour discriminations in those monkeys with V4 lesions. In the first experiment of a subsequent study, the same group (Walsh *et al.* 1993) found that monkeys with V4 lesions also showed an increase in the number of trials required to relearn a previously mastered pairwise colour discrimination.

Another way of assessing loss in colour vision involves the use of thresholds as a measure of performance, and numerous studies have examined thresholds for hue and chromatic contrast sensitivity after V4 lesions. No disruption of hue thresholds by bilateral V4 lesions was reported in several studies (Dean 1979; Wild *et al.* 1985; Heywood *et al.* 1988, 1992; Walsh *et al.* 1993; see also Chapter 6, this volume) or later in a study that used controlled fixation testing in monkeys with quadrant V4 lesions (Merigan 1996). An experiment that had earlier found small, but consistent, elevations of hue thresholds after V4 lesions (Heywood and Cowey 1987) was repeated by the same laboratory with somewhat different parameters (Heywood *et al.* 1988, 1992), and found no hue threshold elevations. On the other hand, chromatic contrast sensitivity was tested along red–green and blue–yellow colour axes in four monkeys with unilateral V4 lesions (Merigan 1996), and found to be decreased by about a factor of two. Schiller (1993) also reported a series of threshold measures of colour sensitivity, hue difference, colour saturation, and colour contrast after V4 lesions. Although substantial effects were observed in all of these thresholds, the results are difficult to directly compare with the above studies, because they represent comparisons of stimulus appearance at lesioned and unlesioned visual field locations (see above).

Lesions of IT cortex

The effects of IT lesions on colour-related discriminations can be much more dramatic than those of V4 lesions, but they range in severity, in different studies, from virtually no effect to profound disruption of colour vision. Minimal effects of IT lesions include the slight increase in errors to criterion found in two studies (Heywood *et al.* 1988; Aggleton and Mishkin 1990) for performance of colour discriminations, and the recovery to normal hue difference thresholds after IT lesions in a third study (Dean 1979). The first report of a severe loss of colour vision was that of Heywood and colleagues (1995). This study included three groups of monkeys with different sizes and locations of IT lesions, and the magnitude of colour loss was closely related to the lesion extent. All the monkeys in the group with the largest lesions lost the ability to perform hue discriminations, while colour discrimination loss was found in only two of four in the group with intermediate lesions, and in none of the monkeys in the group with the smallest lesions. This effect was specific to colour, since the same monkeys had no difficulties performing achromatic (grey) discrimination.

From the above results, it appeared that the major factor governing the magnitude of colour vision loss might be the size of the IT lesion. However, a subsequent study (Buckley *et al.* 1997) demonstrated that marked colour effects could be produced even by lesions smaller than those that caused almost no colour loss in the Heywood study. The lesions in the Buckley study included only a portion of IT, but the colour task was more difficult, and the monkeys were profoundly impaired on the colour discrimination.

Recently, Huxlin *et al.* (2000*b*) tested the effects on hue discrimination of bilateral IT lesions similar to the large lesions of the Heywood study. They, too, found a complete loss of the ability to discriminate large hue differences that had been easily learned before the lesions. By adding large luminance cues to the hue discrimination, it was possible to laboriously re-train the lesioned monkeys to make colour discriminations. However, even after extensive training, during which luminance cues were made irrelevant, these monkeys still showed moderate elevations of hue difference thresholds (see Fig. 5.6(d)).

These studies show that colour vision can be profoundly disrupted by IT lesions, provided that the damage is extensive or that relatively difficult discriminations are used to assess the effect. It is not clear why IT lesions can cause such disproportionately greater colour loss than that caused by V4 lesions. It is noteworthy that large IT lesions, of the type that cause the most marked colour vision change, also produce more generalized behavioural effects, such as the 'Kluver–Bucy' syndrome of emotional alterations, as well as some colour preferences that show up as stimulus bias during discrimination testing (Merigan, unpublished). Evidence that IT lesions interact with stimulus biases is described in the next section. Further studies are needed to determine if these are the basis of the greater colour vision alterations after IT lesions.

Finally, one study demonstrated that, even when colour discriminations are not disrupted by V4 or IT lesions, some features of performance may be substantially changed. Walsh and colleagues (2000) found that monkeys with V4 or TEO lesions could perform a colour pop-out discrimination with no apparent deficit. However, these monkeys did not show the normal priming, i.e. a latency advantage when the correct stimulus occurs on consecutive trials. This loss of priming probably reflects a memory deficit, a type of loss that has been little studied after V4 lesions.

In summary, V4 lesions appear to transiently disrupt colour discrimination learning and to slightly elevate chromatic contrast thresholds, but not to permanently disrupt discrimination of hue differences. This result would be surprising if the alternative cortical stream, the dorsal pathway, were completely devoid of colour responsivity. However, recent evidence suggests a more balanced view of the two pathways with respect to colour processing, with the growing awareness of substantial chromatic sensitivity in the dorsal pathway (Dobkins and Albright 1994; Gegenfurtner et al. 1994; Seidemann et al. 1999; Wandell et al. 1999) of both macaque and human. There is evidence that the function of colour-processing in the dorsal pathway may be primarily to subserve the perception of motion meditated by moving colour patterns (Wandell et al. 1999), whereas that in the ventral pathway may be more related to object recognition and segmentation by colour. Thus, differences in the sensitivity of dorsal and ventral pathway chromatic vision (Gegenfurtner et al. 1994) might simply reflect the stimulus conditions (e.g. spatiotemporal profile) most appropriate to the different uses of the colour information (Wandell et al. 1999). In any case, the substantial colour sensitivity found in the dorsal pathway may help account for the failure to find large, permanent colour vision loss after V4 lesions.

Lesions of IT can cause permanent and/or profound losses of colour vision. Such effects typically result from more extensive damage but, for some especially complex colour discriminations, smaller IT lesions can also cause permanent colour loss.

Learning

In recent years, the idea that cortical neurons may be involved in visual learning (e.g. Crist et al. 1997) has become widely accepted. The basis of this view is the consistent finding that perceptual learning has features that could only come from cortical neurons, such as orientation specificity and interocular transfer (Fiorentini and Berardi 1980; Schoups et al. 1995; Ahissar and Hochstein 1996). The fact that such abilities as orientation discrimination and face recognition show perceptual learning (Schoups et al. 1995; Gold et al. 1999) suggests an involvement of the ventral pathway.

Area V4 lesions

The most commonly described learning deficits after V4 lesions, some of which were described above in the sections on colour and form discriminations, are the increased errors that monkeys make while learning colour and form discriminations (Heywood and Cowey 1987; Walsh *et al.* 1993). This increase in errors typically marks slowed learning, with the monkeys eventually reaching criterion performance for the discriminations.

Another deficit in learning after a V4 lesion was reported by Merigan (1996) who found that a monkey could not learn to perform a match-to-sample task in the V4-lesioned quadrant. This learning problem made it impossible to test hue matching at this location. However, an additional monkey was subsequently trained to perform the match-to-sample task with controlled fixation, before the V4 lesion was made, and this monkey had no difficulty with matching to sample or hue discriminations at the lesioned location.

A final example of a visual learning deficit after V4 lesions was reported by Schiller (1995). He found that monkeys with V4 lesions showed devastated performance on a shape-matching task when new stimuli were introduced at the lesion location, followed by very slow learning as they became accustomed to the new stimulus. This effect may involve both learning ability and disruptions of shape discrimination.

IT cortex lesions

As described above, many IT lesion studies reviewed by Gross (1973) showed disruptions in recalling previously learned discriminations and in learning new ones. The deficit in learning new discriminations is well illustrated by a study of pattern learning reported by Gaffan *et al.* (1986) (Fig. 5.8). In this study, monkeys were initially trained to choose one of a pair of stimuli presented on a touch screen, with right–left position randomized on each trial. Each stimulus consisted of a small alphanumeric character superimposed on a larger alphanumeric character, with the colour of the two characters chosen randomly. After bilateral IT lesions were made, new pairs of stimuli were presented, one in each

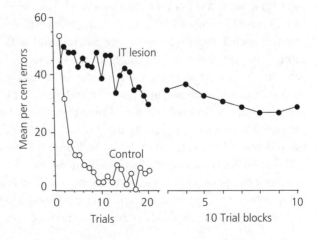

Fig. 5.8 Average percentage errors per trial made by monkeys learning pairwise shape discriminations, either before (open symbols) or after (closed symbols) an IT lesion. Before the lesion, the average errors per trial had decreased to 18% by the third trial, whereas after the IT lesion it remained above 30% until the twentieth trial. (Adapted from Gaffan *et al.* (1986).)

session of 100 trials. Control monkeys learned the discriminations quickly, rapidly reaching approximately 90% correct, whereas monkeys with IT lesions took much longer to reach an equivalent level of performance. Although the magnitude of the deficit was gradually reduced by training within each individual learning set, the deficit was persistent across problems, lasting for the full 60 sets of postoperative learning.

Fortunately, the characteristics of the IT lesion learning deficit have been examined in many studies, so there is now a good understanding of the conditions under which it is found. First, it is apparently confined to visual discriminations, since IT lesions cause no disruption in the learning of discriminations involving audition, touch, or olfaction (Dean 1975). Curiously, however, the disruption of visual learning by IT lesions is related, not to the type of visual stimuli being discriminated, but rather to the difficulty of the discrimination (Gross 1973). Thus, the learning of colour discriminations (Heywood *et al.* 1988) can be as severely impaired as the learning of complex object discriminations (Butler 1969) if the former discrimination is as 'difficult' as the latter (i.e. the number of trials needed to learn the discrimination is as high in normal monkeys).

This observation raises some concerns about the basis of this effect, since we might expect difficulties in discrimination learning to be specific to the complex discriminative features evident in the response of IT neurons. Clearly, it is important to determine whether the visual learning deficit is general to all learning situations. One feature of learning studies is that the monkey is usually required to reverse pre-existing stimulus biases, and it is possible that IT lesions may interfere with this reversal. In the Gaffan *et al.* (1986) study described above, it was noted that the monkeys often strongly preferred one of the pair of stimuli during the first few presentations of a pair. In subsequent testing, the strength of this preference was a good predictor of the number of errors made by the monkey during the remainder of the test session. Thus, it appears that IT lesions reduce the monkey's ability to reverse stimulus preferences, and that this may be a major component of the disruption of learning by such lesions.

The importance of stimulus preferences in IT lesion effects was reflected in an earlier study (Holmes and Gross 1984) that examined the postoperative learning of monkeys with IT lesions using two types of stimulus pairs. The first type were standard form stimuli, in which the two patterns were different and, with these stimuli, the monkeys showed the typical deficit in learning. In the second type of discrimination, the two patterns were identical, but one was rotated by at least 60° from the other. With the latter stimuli, the authors found no learning deficit after IT lesions. This is one of the few instances in which IT-lesioned monkeys showed no visual learning deficit compared to controls, suggesting that the lack of strong stimulus preference when using identical, but rotated, stimuli may have been the reason.

These results suggest that an altered ability to reverse stimulus preferences could be an important component of IT lesion effects. Such an effect could be considered cognitive, but may have an important perceptual component, since one study found that the impaired learning was confined to one part of the visual field. Butler (1969) demonstrated that monkeys with a unilateral lesion of IT showed the visual learning deficit only in the visual field contralateral to the IT lesion. This unusual deficit was revealed by combining a unilateral IT lesion with a split optic chiasm and forebrain commissure so that monocular vision covered only one hemifield. When testing object learning, the designation of correct or incorrect object was made after the animal's first choice, with the object not chosen designated correct for the rest of testing. This required that the monkey reverse any stimulus preference it showed on the first trial and, when the monkeys used the lesioned hemisphere, they required roughly three times as many trials to learn (i.e. reverse their stimulus preference) as when they were using their non-lesioned hemisphere. Since the impaired learning was confined to half of the visual field, it could not be due to a non-visual behavioural change, such as decreased motivation, perseveration, or a general cognitive decline. This conclusion also pertains to the two studies of V4 lesions described above (Schiller 1995; Merigan 1996) that found retinotopic alterations in learning.

Another study that used unusual stimuli also found an atypical effect of IT lesions on the learning and retention of form discriminations (Britten *et al.* 1992*a*). In this study, monkeys were required to learn or retain form discriminations, in which the form was conveyed in one set of stimuli by the usual luminance variation, but in a second set of stimuli by relative motion. With both types of discriminations, the monkeys showed the typical deficit in retention of discrimination performance after IT lesions. IT lesions also caused impaired acquisition of new form discriminations when form was conveyed by luminance variation. However, when form information was conveyed by relative motion, the IT-lesioned monkeys showed no impairment in learning new form discriminations. This study supports the rather general finding that ventral pathway lesions typically spare motion discriminations. However, it also suggests that even form discriminations may be partially spared from the effects of ventral pathway lesions when the form is conveyed by motion.

Finally, we should mention a study that may have important implications for the nature of ventral pathway lesion effects on learning. Manning (1971) found that monkeys with IT lesions learned pattern discriminations as quickly as control monkeys if they received a shock when they made errors in addition to being rewarded with food for correct responses. On the other hand, the same monkeys showed the typical impaired visual pattern learning when they were only rewarded with food for correct responses. It is unlikely that the learning impairment found when no shock was delivered could be attributed entirely to a motivational decrease caused by IT lesions, given that the effect of an IT lesion on learning in the Butler study described above (Butter and Hirtzel 1970) was confined to one part of the visual field. Clearly, more research is needed to examine the implications of this result for both IT lesions and perceptual learning.

In summary, ventral pathway lesions impair visual learning in ways that imply a major perceptual alteration. Stimulus–response learning is especially degraded, although other forms of learning are also affected (Merigan 1996), suggesting that the ventral pathway is central to many forms of visual learning.

Attention

It is well established that visual attention plays an important role in the response of macaque V4 and IT neurons (Maunsell *et al.* 1992; Motter 1993; Connor *et al.* 1997; Chelazzi *et al.* 1998; Reynolds *et al.* 2000). These physiological studies have shown that the response of V4 and IT neurons depends strongly on the visual field location or stimulus type the monkey is attending to. These observations raise the possibility that V4 or IT lesions could alter visual performance by changing the allocation of visual attention to different locations of the visual field or different stimulus types.

One of the first reported attentional effects of ventral pathway lesions was an alteration of search performance in monkeys at the visual field location that corresponded to a V4 lesion (Schiller and Lee 1991). The monkeys viewed 4 to 64 stimuli presented symmetrically around fixation and then made an eye movement to the single odd stimulus. V4 lesions severely disrupted the ability to detect a less salient (smaller, less coarse, etc.) odd stimulus, but had less effect on the ability to detect a more salient (larger, coarser) odd stimulus. This result is consistent with current views that V4 may be part of the circuitry involved in the control of attention.

In a recent paper, DeWeerd and colleagues (1999) described a very different effect of V4 and TEO lesions in macaques that also suggested mediation by altered attention. Monkeys performed an orientation discrimination for a single circular patch of grating, presented a few degrees from a fixation stimulus. Curiously, when three irrelevant circular distractors were placed around the grating patch, orientation thresholds were elevated more at the site of the V4 and TEO lesion than at the control visual field location. Furthermore, as predicted by a model of the role of attention in ventral pathway neural responses (Desimone and Duncan 1995), the degree of threshold elevation was proportional to the contrast of the distractors. This result supports the possibility that V4 lesions can alter perception by disrupting the role of attention in separating visual targets from distractors (Braun 1994).

These findings suggest that attention, an important determinant of visual function that is inherently an element of top–down neural control, may be involved in some aspects of ventral pathway lesion effects. Clearly, further study is needed to determine the role of attention, both in the normal function of visual cortex and following cortical lesions.

Dorsal pathway

The dorsal pathway has been called the 'motion' pathway because of the selectivity of its neurons for the direction of stimulus motion. This property, while present in only limited numbers of neurons in area V1 (Hawken *et al.* 1988), becomes more prominent in area V3 (Felleman and Van Essen 1987; Gegenfurtner *et al.* 1997) and is present in a majority of neurons in area MT (Maunsell and Van Essen 1983; Albright 1984). At subsequent stages of processing in the dorsal pathway, neuronal tuning becomes more complex. Neurons in the middle superior temporal (MST) area show selectivities to expanding versus contracting motion, and clockwise versus counterclockwise rotation (Duffy and

Wurtz 1991; Graziano *et al.* 1994). Neurons in parietal cortex, such as those in areas 7a and lateral inter parietal (LIP), integrate information from several sensory modalities with motor output, as well as constructing an extrapersonal representation of space (Andersen 1997; Read and Siegel 1997; Siegel and Read 1997). This specialization for the processing of motion suggests that lesions early in the dorsal pathway are likely to result in deficits in the ability to perform various types of motion discriminations. The spatial orientation and sensorimotor integration responses of neurons within parietal cortex suggest that damage to this region will cause deficits in behaviours that utilize these properties. Indeed, the data reviewed below support the notion of specialization of the dorsal pathway for processing of image motion. They also suggest that the dorsal pathway is important for the integration of motion information to construct a representation of space that can be used in navigation and other motor behaviours.

Area MT lesions

Area MT has become the area of choice for examining the effects of lesions within the dorsal pathway, primarily because of its high incidence of directionally selective neurons, its clearly defined borders within the superior temporal sulcus (STS) and its precise retinotopy. The first studies involving lesions of areas MT and MST used ibotenic acid, and examined the effects of MT and MST lesions on eye movement responses. Wurtz and his colleagues reported that MT and MST lesions resulted in retinotopically specific deficits in smooth-pursuit eye movements (Newsome *et al.* 1985; Durnsteler *et al.* 1987; Dursteller and Wurtz 1988). The monkeys had been trained to pursue moving targets but, after MT lesions, were unable to match the speed of their smooth-pursuit eye movements to the speed of the target. The animals also had problems adjusting the amplitude of their saccadic eye movements to compensate for target motion, but had no problems making saccades to stationary targets. Since these effects reflected difficulties in matching the velocity of visual targets, without evidence of motor abnormalities, they were interpreted as impaired perception of stimulus velocity. A similar deficit in smooth-pursuit eye movements was later reported (Schiller and Lee 1994). Subsequently, the studies described below examined the effects of damage to area MT on motion perception more directly. In most of these experiments, the monkeys judged differences in the direction or speed of stimulus motion.

Discrimination of stimulus direction

In the first study in this series, Newsome and Paré (1988) examined the perception of image motion with displays in which the proportion of coherently and randomly moving dots was adjusted to measure threshold. The monkeys reported whether the stimulus moved up or down by making a saccade to one of two small targets on the screen. The lesion was made by injecting ibotenic acid into sites in MT that were physiologically identified while the monkey was performing the discrimination task. Severe deficits in motion coherence thresholds were observed when stimuli were placed in the portion of the visual field affected by the lesion. A similar inability to extract coherent motion in the presence of noise was subsequently reported after MT/MST lesions by Pasternak and Merigan (1994), who tested monkeys with bilateral damage to MT/MST produced by multiple injections of ibotenic acid.

More recently, Rudolph and Pasternak (1999) used a match-to-sample task to examine in greater detail the MT lesion-induced inability to extract motion from directional noise. They compared the effects of unilateral MT/MST lesions on the ability of monkeys to discriminate the direction of motion of random-dots or of drifting gratings masked by noise (Figs 5.5(c) and 5.9(a)). On each trial, the monkeys indicated whether the two sequentially presented stimuli, sample and test, moved in the same or in different directions (Fig. 5.5(a)). The delay separating the two comparison stimuli was very brief (200 ms). Thus, the task imposed only minimal requirements on the ability to remember the preceding stimulus. Deficits in direction discrimination were found with both types of stimuli (Fig. 5.5(c), left). On the other hand, no permanent deficits were found in contrast thresholds for discriminating the direction of drifting gratings measured in an identical task (Fig. 5.5(b) left). This selectively increased susceptibility to noise was specific to the domain of motion perception, since the same monkeys showed no deficit in discriminating the orientation of gratings masked by two-dimensional noise (Fig. 5.4). Moreover, visual deficits after V4 lesions, measured with the same tasks, were limited to discriminations of stimulus orientation, and were not found when the monkeys were required to discriminate stimulus direction, even when the motion stimulus was masked by noise (Rudolph 1999; Rudolph and Pasternak 1999; Figs 5.4 and 5.5). These selective results demonstrated the importance of MT/MST neurons for the ability to discriminate motion direction in the presence of noise.

Direction integration

In addition to an increased susceptibility to noise, MT/MST lesions result in deficits in the integration of local motion vectors (Pasternak and Merigan 1994; Rudolph and Pasternak 1996; Bisley and Pasternak 2000). To measure motion integration, individual, randomly positioned dots were displaced in a range of directions, and the speed of stimulus motion, which depended on the size of the displacement, remained constant throughout each session (Fig. 5.9(b)). The maximal range of directions in the random-dot stimulus at which the monkeys could reliably judge the overall direction of motion was taken as a measure of the integration of local directional signals (Williams and Sekuler 1984; Watamaniuk et al. 1989). Unilateral MT/MST lesions resulted in a deficit in motion integration thresholds (see Figs 5.9(b) and 5.10(b)). Although this deficit was most pronounced early in postlesion testing and decreased with continued training, some loss persisted throughout the several years of postlesion testing.

Remembering stimulus direction

The task used by Bisley and Pasternak (2000) required that the monkeys not only process information about stimulus direction, but also remember that direction for a brief period of time. They used the same task that Rudolph and Pasternak (1999; see

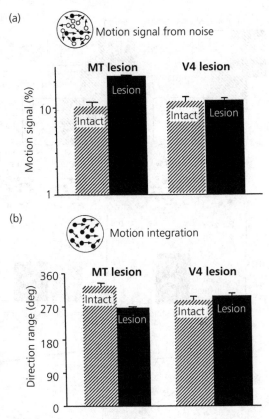

Fig. 5.9 Effect of an MT/MST lesion on discrimination of direction, measured with random-dot stimuli. The behavioural procedure was identical to that shown in Fig. 5.5(a). (a) Motion signal thresholds (motion coherence in the presence of noise). Random-dot stimuli consisted of a fraction of dots moving coherently in a single direction of motion (% motion signal), and the remainder moving in random directions. The MT/MST lesion caused a permanent increase in the percentage of coherently moving dots needed for direction discrimination, while the V4 lesion had no effect. (b) Motion integration (direction range thresholds). Random-dot stimuli consisted of dots displaced in directions chosen from a rectangular distribution. The width of this distribution determined the range of directions within which individual dots moved, and was varied between 0 deg (all dots moving in the same direction) and 360 deg (dots moving in all directions). MT/MST lesions produced permanent, but relatively subtle, deficits in integration thresholds. The V4 lesion had no measurable effect on performance (Adapted from Rudolph and Pasternak (1999) and from Rudolph (1997, University of Rochester, doctoral dissertation).)

above) had used, but extended the delay between the sample and test stimuli (Figs 5.5(a) and 5.10(a)). In addition, they introduced a spatial separation between the two stimuli, placing them in corresponding locations of the intact and the lesioned hemifields. This spatial separation allowed them to measure the contribution of MT/MST to the performance of individual components of the memory task: the encoding of visual motion (sample); its retention (delay); and its retrieval/comparison (test). They found

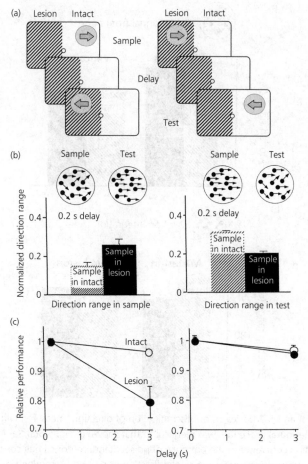

Fig. 5.10 Effect of MT/MST lesions on discrimination and retention of the direction of complex motion. (a) The behavioural procedure was identical to that shown in Fig. 5.5(a), except that the sample and test stimuli were spatially separated, so that one was placed in the lesioned hemifield, and the other in the corresponding location in the intact hemifield. (b) Normalized direction range thresholds ((360-range threshold)/360). The sample stimulus or the test stimulus was composed of dots moving in a range of directions, while the other stimulus contained only coherently moving dots. Thresholds were measured with the sample and test placed on either side of the vertical meridian. 'Sample in intact' indicates that the sample was presented in the intact visual field and the test in the lesioned hemifield. 'Sample in lesion' indicates that the sample was presented in the lesioned, and the test in the intact, hemifield. Delay, 0.2 s. Thresholds were elevated whenever the stimulus containing non-coherent motion was placed in the lesioned field. (c) Effect of delay on performance for two direction range tasks. Thresholds were measured with both stimuli placed in the intact (open symbols) or in the lesioned hemifields (solid circles) (see Fig. 5.5(a)). Range thresholds were measured either by varying the range of directions in the sample, while the test moved coherently, (left plot) or by varying the range of directions in the test, while the sample moved coherently (right plot). Thresholds were normalized to the data measured at 0.2 s delay. Error bars are SEM. A delay-specific deficit was present only when the remembered stimulus (sample) contained a broad range of directions and required integration. (Adapted from Bisley and Pasternak (2000).)

that, when the stimuli consisted of random dots moving in a broad range of directions, MT/MST lesions disrupted the retention of these stimuli, just as they had disrupted their encoding (see Fig. 5.10(c)). However, when the stimulus was coherent, there was no additional deficit due to a longer delay (see Fig. 5.10(c), right plot). On the other hand, the pattern of results was different when they measured direction difference thresholds for coherently moving dots. In this case, lesions of MT/MST only disrupted the retrieval/comparison component of the task, and not the encoding or storage, since a deficit was detectable only when the test, and not the sample stimulus, was placed in the lesion (Fig. 5.11). Also, no additional deficit was found at longer delays. Thus, the

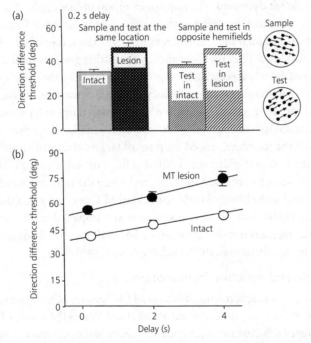

Fig. 5.11 Effects of MT/MST lesions on direction difference thresholds measured with coherently moving random dots. The behavioural procedures were identical to those shown in Figs 5.5(a) and 5.10(a). (a) Thresholds shown on the left were measured with both stimuli, sample, and test, placed either in the intact (light column) or in the lesioned (black column) hemifield (see Fig. 5.5(a)). Thresholds shown on the right were measured with sample and test stimuli spatially separated and placed on either side of the vertical meridian (see Fig. 5.10(a)). 'Test in intact' indicates that the test was presented in the intact field and the sample in the lesion, while 'test in lesion' indicates that the sample was presented in the intact hemifield field and the test stimulus in the lesion. The MT/MST lesion significantly elevated direction threshold only when the test stimulus was placed in the lesioned field. (b) Effect of delay on direction difference thresholds, measured with both sample and test stimuli placed either in the intact (open symbols) or in the lesioned (filled symbols) hemifields (see Fig. 5.1(a)). A threshold elevation was found for stimuli placed within the lesioned location at the 0.2 s delay, and this elevation did not increase significantly at longer delays. (Adapted from Bisley and Pasternak (2000).)

effects of MT/MST lesions depended upon both the demands of the task and the nature of the visual motion stimuli. These results suggest that MT/MST contributes to the retention of visual motion information only if it is involved in its encoding.

Discrimination of stimulus speed

Three studies have examined the discrimination of stimulus speed after MT lesions. Pasternak and Merigan (1994) made bilateral ibotenic acid lesions involving areas MT and MST, and measured the accuracy of speed discrimination using gratings moving at a speed of 2°/s over a range of contrasts. They found a 2–3-fold elevation of speed difference thresholds over a broad range of stimulus contrasts. With additional training (see below), this deficit decreased. The improvement was unlikely to be due to the monkeys relying on cues other than speed, such as differences in temporal frequencies, since the accuracy of discrimination of differences in flicker rates, measured with counterphase gratings, was lower than that measured with drifting gratings (also see Pasternak 1987). Orban *et al.* (1995) used bilateral aspiration to measure the effects of lesions of areas MT and MST in monkeys trained to discriminate differences in speed. They found a loss in the accuracy of speed discrimination over a broad range of base speeds. Schiller and Lee (1994) examined the effect of MT lesions on speed discrimination with an oddity task, in which the monkeys viewed eight small targets arranged around a fixation target, one of which moved with a speed different from the other stimuli. The monkeys were required to saccade to the odd stimulus, and made the most errors when the odd stimulus was placed in the hemifield affected by the MT lesion and when the differences in speed were relatively small. These monkeys were also impaired in discriminating differences in flicker rate, a result that confirms earlier findings after damage to the visual motion system in cats (Pasternak 1987; Pasternak *et al.* 1989).

Relative motion and structure-from-motion

Only a few studies have explored the effects of MT lesions on other aspects of the processing of complex motion. Andersen and Siegel (1989) tested the effects of MT lesions on the perception of relative motion, and found deficits in the detection of motion shear. This deficit was transitory, and they found nearly complete recovery within a few days of continued training. This study also measured the effects of MT lesions on the detection of structure-from-motion in a single monkey, and reported severe deficits that lasted longer, and were more pronounced, than the deficit in perceiving relative motion.

Recovery of function after MT lesions

The data cited above demonstrate that lesions of areas MT/MST lead to selective deficits on a variety of motion discrimination tasks, as well as tests of smooth pursuit eye movements. However, equally striking in the above studies, is the extent to which many lesion-disrupted visual functions recover. The early studies by Wurtz and his colleagues reported essentially complete recovery in smooth pursuit after small MT or MST lesions (Newsome *et al.* 1985; Dursteler *et al.* 1987; Dursteler and Wurtz 1988;

Yamasaki and Wurtz 1991). Subsequently, Yamasaki and Wurtz (1991) examined this recovery in greater detail, and found residual deficits only when the lesion was larger and included both MT and MST. Newsome and Paré (1988) also reported rapid and nearly complete recovery of motion coherence thresholds for discriminating opposite directions of motion.

On the other hand, Pasternak and her colleagues (Rudolph and Pasternak 1999; Bisley and Pasternak 2000), despite finding substantial postlesion improvements on several motion discriminations, generally found permanent, albeit subtle, residual deficits on most studied tasks. Residual vision motion deficits following MT lesions have also been reported by other laboratories (see above), only some of which addressed the question of functional recovery directly (e.g. Andersen 1989). The relatively rapid and complete recovery observed by Wurtz and his colleagues is in stark contrast to the observations of residual deficits detectable years after the lesion. The most likely explanation for this apparent discrepancy is the time at which threshold measurements began in the lesioned portion of the visual field. In studies where recovery was observed within days after the lesion (Dursteler *et al.* 1987; Dursteler and Wurtz 1988; Newsome and Paré 1988; Yamasaki and Wurtz 1991), the damage to a retinotopically localized portion of MT was produced while the monkey was performing a behavioural task in the corresponding portion of the visual field. Thus, immediately after the lesion and in the days that followed, the animal received extensive behavioural training in the damaged visual field. On the other hand, in the experiments by Pasternak and her colleagues (Pasternak and Merigan 1994; Rudolph and Pasternak 1999; Bisley and Pasternak 2000) this type of training occurred many days or even months after the lesion, and improvements in performance became apparent only after the initiation of training on a given task in the affected portion of the visual field (Rudolph and Pasternak 1999). This suggests that a necessary condition for partial or complete recovery after lesions is behavioural training within the lesioned portion of the visual field.

It is generally thought that the partial or complete recovery of a visual function following localized cortical damage reflects the assumption of processing by other cortical areas (e.g. Newsome and Paré 1988; Pasternak and Merigan 1994). It is also possible that motion processing normally involves a wide network of many cortical areas, and that recovery represents an adaptation of those not damaged. However, little is known about the mechanisms underlying recovery of function after extrastriate cortical lesions, although efforts are currently underway in elucidate its histochemical and anatomical basis (e.g. Eysel and Schweigart 1999; Huxlin and Pasternak 1999, 2001; Huxlin *et al.* 2000a).

Lesions of parietal cortex

Within parietal cortex, the neuronal properties of areas LIP and 7a have been studied most extensively. Such studies indicate that neurons in these areas integrate visual, somatosensory, auditory, and vestibular signals that reflect the observer's location (Andersen 1997). They are also active before and during saccadic eye movements (Andersen *et al.* 1990) and hand-reaching movements, and during memory tasks requiring withholding a movement (Snyder *et al.* 1997, 1998). Moreover, the representation of space generated in parietal neurons is continuously updated in conjunction with the impending motor action, and these dynamic transformations are modulated by attention (Colby and Goldberg 1999). In addition, many parietal neurons respond to various types of optic flow motion (Read and Siegel 1997; Siegel and Read 1997; Phinney and Siegel 2000) as well as three-dimensional features of objects (Sakata *et al.* 1994; Taira *et al.* 2000). These properties point to a role for parietal neurons in the integration of sensory signals, and in constructing a representation of extrapersonal space in preparation for motor action.

A relatively small number of lesion studies have been performed in non-human primates to examine the functional contribution of these areas to behaviour. An important role of posterior parietal cortex in spatial aspects of task performance was first shown by Ridley and Ettlinger (1975) and Ratcliff *et al.* (1977). Subsequently, Latto (1986), tested monkeys after bilateral lesions of area 7a and found deficits in the performance of a spatial landmark test. Further evidence for a role of parietal cortex in space coding was reported by Quintana and Fuster (1993), who applied cooling to areas 5 and 7 of the parietal cortex. They found that the monkeys showed decreased speed and accuracy in both reaching and eye movements during the performance of tasks that required the processing and retention of spatial information. More recently, Li *et al.* (1999) reported deficits in memory-guided saccadic eye movements after reversible inactivation of LIP, produced by injections of muscimol. They concluded that LIP neurons play a direct role in processing incoming sensory information to programme saccadic eye movements. Inaccuracy in reaching towards visual targets after lesions of areas 7a, 7b, and LIP was observed by Rushworth *et al.* (1997).

Thus, lesions of parietal cortex appear to disrupt the ability of a subject to coordinate movements relative to him/herself or to other locations in extrapersonal space.

General summary and conclusions

Lesions of cortical visual areas in the macaque have proved to be a powerful and informative method for elucidating the functional specializations of visual cortical areas. Lesions of primary visual cortex cause profound visual loss, whereas lesions higher in the visual pathways cause less dramatic, but selective visual loss. Within the ventral pathway, lesions cause selective loss of orientation-based discriminations, especially those involving borders defined by texture or illusory contour, as well as impaired colour vision and discrimination of complex forms. Lesions of the dorsal pathway disrupt direction and speed discriminations, and there is now evidence that some components of this pathway play a role not only in processing this information, but also in retaining it in memory. Dorsal pathway lesions have also disrupted speed and accuracy in reaching and making eye movements, orienting in space, and discriminations involving motion shear and structure from motion. A number of lesion studies have also produced disruptions of more complex behaviours such as reaching, eye movements, and learning and attention.

Many studies have demonstrated a remarkable degree of recovery after lesions in both the ventral and the dorsal pathways, although the recovery appears to be much more pronounced in the dorsal than in the ventral pathway. This difference may not be as large as it currently seems, because the studies of dorsal pathway lesions that have shown postlesion improvements were better designed to reveal such recovery and to study their time course. However, both the transitory and permanent behavioural effects of lesions are consistent with the description of primate visual cortex as two relatively parallel streams of processing. Ventral pathway lesions disrupt primarily the perception of form and colour, while dorsal pathway lesions affect largely the perception of motion and space.

References

Aggleton, J.P. and Mishkin, M. (1990). Visual impairments in macaques following inferior temporal lesions are exacerbated selectively by additional damage to superior temporal sulcus. *Behav. Brain Res.* **39**, 262–74.

Ahissar, M. and Hochstein, S. (1996). Learning pop-out detection: specificities to stimulus characteristics. *Vision Res.* **36**, 3487–500.

Albright, T.D. (1984). Direction and orientation selectivity of neurons in visual area MT of the macaque. *J. Neurosci.* **4**, 1106–30.

Andersen, R.A. (1989). Visual and eye movement functions of the posterior parietal cortex. *Ann. Rev. Neurosci.* **12**, 377–403.

Andersen, R.A. (1997). Multimodal integration for the representation of space in the posterior parietal cortex. *Phil. Trans. R. Soc. Lond. B, Biol. Sci.* **352**, 1421–8.

Andersen, R.A. and Siegel, R.M. (1989). Motion processing in primate cortex. In *Signal and sense: local and global order in perceptual maps* (ed. G.M. Edelman, W.E. Gall, and W.M. Cowan), pp. 163–84. Wiley, New York.

Andersen, R.A., Bracewell, R.M., Barash, S., Gnadt, J.W., and Fogassi, L. (1990). Eye position effects on visual, memory, and saccade related activity in areas LIP and 7a of macaque. *J. Neurosci.* **10**, 1176–96.

Bisley, J.W. and Pasternak, T. (2000). The multiple roles of visual cortical areas MT/MST in remembering the direction of visual motion. *Cereb. Cortex* **10**, 1053–65.

Blake, L., Jarvis, C.D., and Mishkin, M. (1977). Pattern discrimination thresholds after partial inferior temporal or lateral striate lesions in monkeys. *Brain Res.* **120**, 209–20.

Boussaoud, D., Ungerleider, L.G., and Desimone, R. (1990). Pathways for motion analysis: cortical connections of the medial superior temporal and fundus of the superior temporal visual areas in the macaque. *J. Comp. Neurol.* **296**, 462–95.

Braun, J. (1994). Visual search among items of different salience—removal of visual attention mimics a lesion in extrastriate area V4. *J. Neurosci.* **14**, 554–67.

Britten, K.H., Newsome, W.T., and Saunders, R.C. (1992a). Effects of inferotemporal cortex lesions on form-from-motion discrimination in monkeys. *Exp. Brain Res.* **88**, 292–302.

Britten, K.H., Shadlen, M.N., Newsome, W.T., and Movshon, J.A. (1992b). The analysis of visual motion: a comparison of neuronal and psychophysical performance. *J. Neurosci.* **12**, 4745–65.

Britten. K.H., Newsome, W.T., Shadlen, M.N., Celebrini, S., and Movshon, J.A. (1996). A relationship between behavioral choice and the visual responses of neurons in macaque MT. *Vis. Neurosci.* **13**, 87–100.

Buckley, M.J., Gaffan, D., and Murray, E.A. (1997). Functional double dissociation between two inferior temporal cortical areas: perirhinal cortex versus middle temporal gyrus. *J. Neurophysiol.* **77**, 587–98.

Bullier, J. and Kennedy, H. (1983). Projection of the lateral geniculate nucleus onto cortical area V2 in the macaque monkey. *Exp. Brain Res.* **53**, 168–72.

Butler, C.R. (1969). Is there a memory impairment in monkeys after inferior temporal lesions? *Brain Res.* **13**, 383–93.

Butter, C.M. and Hirtzel, M. (1970). Impairment in sampling visual stimuli in monkeys with inferotemporal lesions. *Physiol. Behav.* **5**, 369–70.

Casagrande, V.A. (1994). A third parallel visual pathway to primate area V1. *Trends Neurosci.* **17**, 305–10.

Chelazzi, L., Duncan, J., Miller, E.K., and Desimone, R. (1998). Responses of neurons in inferior temporal cortex during memory-guided visual search. *J. Neurophysiol.* **80**, 2918–40.

Colby, C.L. and Goldberg, M.E. (1999). Space and attention in parietal cortex. *Ann. Rev. Neurosci.* **22**, 319–49.

Connor, C.E., Preddie, D.C., Gallant, J.L., and Van Essen, D.C. (1997). Spatial attention effects in macaque area V4. *J. Neurosci.* **17**, 3201–14.

Cowey, A. and Gross, C.G. (1970). Effects of foveal prestriate and inferotemporal lesions on visual discrimination by rhesus monkeys. *Exp. Brain Res.* **11**, 128–44.

Cowey, A., Stoerig, P., and Bannister, M. (1994). Retinal ganglion cells labelled from the pulvinar nucleus in macaque monkeys. *Neuroscience* **61**, 691–705.

Cowey, A., Dean, P., and Weiskrantz, L. (1998). Ettlinger at bay: can visual agnosia be explained by low-level visual impairments? In *Comparative neuropsychology* (ed. A.D. Milner) pp. 30–50. Oxford University Press, Oxford.

Crist, R.E., Kapadia, M.K., Westheimer, G., and Gilbert, C.D. (1997). Perceptual learning of spatial localization: specificity for orientation, position, and context. *J. Neurophysiol.* **78**, 2889–94.

Croner, L.J. and Albright, T.D. (1999). Seeing the big picture: integration of image cues in the primate visual system [review]. *Neuron* **24**, 777–89.

Dan, Y., Atick, J.J., and Reid, R.C. (1996). Efficient coding of natural scenes in the lateral geniculate nucleus: experimental test of a computational theory. *J. Neurosci.* **16**, 3351–62.

Das, A. and Gilbert, C.D. (1995). Long-range horizontal connections and their role in cortical reorganization revealed by optical recording of cat primary visual cortex [see comments]. *Nature* **375**, 780–4.

Dean, P. (1975). Effects of inferotemporal lesions on the behavior of monkeys. *Psychol. Bull.* **83**, 41–71.

Dean, R. (1978). Visual cortex ablation and thresholds for successively presented stimuli in rhesus monkeys: I. Orientation. *Exp. Brain Res.* **32**, 445–58.

Dean, P. (1979). Visual cortex ablation and thresholds for successively presented stimuli in rhesus monkeys: II Hue. *Exp. Brain Res.* **35**, 69–83.

Dean, P. (1982). Visual behavior in monkeys with inferotemporal lesions. In *Analysis of visual behavior* (ed. D.J. Ingle, M.A. Goodale, and R.J.W. Mansfield), pp. 587–628. MIT Press, Cambridge, Massachusetts.

Desimone, R. and Duncan, J. (1995). Neural mechanisms of selective attention. *Ann. Rev. Neurosci.* **18**, 193–222.

Desimone, R., Albright, T.D., Gross, C.G., and Bruce, C. (1984). Stimulus selective properties of inferior temporal neurons in the macaque. *J. Neurosci.* **4**, 2051–62.

Desimone, R., Schein, S.J., Moran, J., and Ungerleider, L.G. (1985). Contour, color and shape analysis beyond the striate cortex. *Vision Res.* **25**, 441–52.

DeWeerd, P., Desimone, R., and Ungerleider, L.G. (1996). Cue-dependent deficits in grating orientation discrimination after V4 lesions in macaques. *Vis. Neurosci.* **13**, 529–38.

De Weerd, P., Peralta, M.R., Desimone, R., and Underleider, L. (1999). Loss of attentional stimulus selection after extrastriate cortical lesions in macaques. *Nat. Neurosci.* 2, 753–8.

Deyoe, E.A., Hockfield, S., Garren, H., and Van Essen, D.C. (1990). Antibody labeling of functional subdivisions in visual cortex: Cat-301 immunoreactivity in striate and extrastriate cortex of the macaque monkey. *Vis. Neurosci.* 5, 67–81.

Deyoe, E.A., Felleman, D.J., Vanessen, D.C., and McClendon, E. (1994). Multiple processing streams in occipitotemporal visual cortex, *Nature* 371, 151–4.

Dias, E.C. and Segraves, M.A. (1999). Muscimol-induced inactivation of monkey frontal eye field: effects on visually and memory-guided saccades. *J. Neurophysiol.* 81, 2191–214.

Dineen, J. and Keating, E.G. (1981). The primate visual system after bilateral removal or striate cortex. Survival of complex pattern vision. *Exp. Brain Res.* 41, 338–45.

Dobkins, K.R. and Albright, T.D. (1994). What happens if it changes color when it moves? The nature of chromatic input to macaque visual area MT. *J. Neurosci.* 14, 4854–70.

Duffy, C.J. and Wurtz, R.H. (1991). Sensitivity of MST neurons to optic flow stimuli. I. A continuum of response selectivity to large-field stimuli. *J. Neurophysiol.* 65, 1329–45.

Dursteler, M.R. and Wurtz, R.H. (1988). Pursuit and optokinetic deficits following chemical lesions of cortical areas MT and MST. *J. Neurophysiol.* 60, 940–65.

Dursteler, M.R., Wurtz, R.H., and Newsome, W.T. (1987). Directional pursuit deficits following lesions of the foveal representation within the superior temporal sulcus of the macaque monkey. *J. Neurophysiol.* 57, 1262–87.

Eysel, U.T. and Schweigart, G. (1999). Increased receptive field size in the surround of chronic lesions in the adult cat visual cortex. *Cereb. Cortex* 9, 101–9.

Felleman, D.J. and Van Essen, D.C. (1987). Receptive field properties of neurons in area V3 of macaque monkey extrastriate cortex. *J. Neurophysiol.* 57, 889–920.

Felleman, D.J. and Van Essen, D.C. (1991). Distributed hierarchical processing in the primate cerebral cortex. *Cereb. Cortex* 1, 1–47.

Felleman, D.J., Xiao, Y.P., and McClendon, E. (1997). Modular organization of occipito-temporal pathways—cortical connections between visual area 4 and visual area 2 and posterior inferotemporal ventral area in macaque monkeys. *J. Neurosci.* 17, 3185–200.

Ferrera, V.P., Nealey, T.A., and Maunsell, J.H.R. (1994a). Responses in macaque visual area V4 following inactivation of the parvocellular and magnocellular lgn pathways. *J. Neurosci.* 14, 2080–8.

Ferrera, V.P., Rudolph, K.K., and Maunsell, J.H. (1994b). Responses of neurons in the parietal and temporal visual pathways during a motion task. *J. Neurosci.* 14, 6171–86.

Ffytche, D.H., Guy, C.N., and Zeki, S. (1996). Motion specific responses from a blind hemifield. *Brain* 119, 1971–82.

Fiorentini, A. and Berardi, N. (1980). Perceptual learning specific for orientation and spatial frequency. *Nature* 287, 43–4.

Florence, S.L. and Kaas, J.H. (1995). Large-scale reorganization at multiple levels of the somatosensory pathway follows therapeutic amputation of the hand in monkeys. *J. Neurosci.* 15, 8083–95.

Fuster, J.M., Bauer, R.H., and Jervey, J.P. (1981). Effects of cooling inferotemporal cortex on performance of visual memory tasks. *Exp. Neurol.* 71, 398–409.

Gaffan, E.A., Harrison, S., and Gaffan, D. (1986). Single and concurrent discrimination learning by monkeys after lesions of inferotemporal cortex. *Quart. J. Exp. Psychol. B, Comp. Physiol. Psychol.* 38, 31–51.

Gallant, J.L., Connor, C.E., Rakshit, S., Lewis, J.W., and Van Essen, D.C. (1996). Neural responses to polar, hyperbolic, and Cartesian gratings in area V4 of the macaque monkey. *J. Neurophysiol.* 76, 2718–39.

Gegenfurtner, K.R., Kiper, D.C., Beusmans, J.M., Carandini M., Zaidi, Q., and Movshon, J.A. (1994). Chromatic properties of neurons in macaque MT. *Vis. Neurosci.* 11, 455–66.

Gegenfurtner, K.R., Kiper, D.C., and Levitt, J.B. (1997). Functional properties of neurons in macaque area V3. *J. Neurophysiol.* 77, 1906–23.

Gilbert, C.D., Das, A., Ito, M., Kapadia, M., and Westheimer, G. (1996). Spatial integration and cortical dynamics. *Proc. Natl Acad. Sci., USA* 93, 615–22.

Girard, P., Salin, P.A., and Bullier, J. (1991). Visual activity in areas V3a and V3 during reversible inactivation of area V1 in the macaque monkey. *J. Neurophysiol.* 66, 1493–503.

Glickstein, M. (1988). The discovery of the visual cortex. *Sci. Am.* 259, 118–27.

Glickstein, M. and Fahle, M. (2000). Visual disturbances following gunshot woulds of the cortical visual area. *Brain* 123 (special suppl.), 1–101.

Gold, J., Bennett, P.J., and Sekuler, A.B. (1999). Signal but not noise changes with perceptual learning. *Nature* 402, 176–8.

Goodale, M.A. and Milner, A.D. (1992). Separate visual pathways for perception and action. *Trends Neurosci.* 15, 20–5.

Graziano, M.S., Yap, G.S., and Gross, C.G. (1994). Coding of visual space by premotor neurons. *Science* 266, 1054–7.

Gregory, R.L. (1961). The brain as an engineering problem. In *Current problems in animal behavior* (ed. W.H. Thorpe and O.L. Zangwill), pp. 547–65. Cambridge University Press, Cambridge.

Gross, C.G. (1973). Visual functions of inferotemporal cortex. In *Handbook of sensory physiology* (ed. R. Jung), pp. 451–82. Springer, Berlin.

Gross, C.G., Bender, D.B., and Rocha-Miranda, C.E. (1969). Visual receptive fields of neurons in inferotemporal cortex of the monkey. *Science* 166, 1303–6.

Gross, C.G., Bender, D.B., and Gerstein, G.L. (1979). Activity of inferior temporal neurons in bahaving monkeys. *Neuropsychologia* 17, 215–29.

Grusser, O.J. and Landis, T. (1991). *Visual agnosias and other disturbances of visual perception and cognition.* CRC Press, Boca Raton, Florida.

Hawken, M.J., Parker, A.J., and Lund, J.S. (1988). Laminar organization and contrast sensitivity of direction-selective cells in the striate cortex of the Old World monkey. *J. Neurosci.* 8, 3541–8.

Heywood, C.A. and Cowey, A. (1987). On the role of cortical area V4 in the discrimination of hue and pattern in macaque monkeys. *J. Neurosci.* 7, 2601–17.

Heywood, C.A., Shields, C., and Cowey, A. (1988). The involvement of the temporal lobes in colour discrimination. *Exp. Brain Res.* 71, 437–41.

Heywood, C.A., Gadotti, A., and Cowey, A. (1992). Cortical area V4 and its role in the perception of color. *J. Neurosci.* 12, 4056–65.

Heywood, C.A., Gaffan, D., and Cowey, A. (1995). Cerebral achromatopsia in monkeys. *Eur. J. Neurosci.* 7, 1064–73.

Holmes, E.J. and Gross, C.G. (1984). Effects of inferior temporal lesions on discrimination of stimuli differing in orientation. *J. Neurosci.* 4, 3063–8.

Horel, J.A., Voytko, M.L., and Salsbury, K.G. (1984). Visual learning suppressed by cooling the temporal pole. *Behav. Neurosci.* 98, 310–24.

Horgan, N.F. and Finn, A.M. (1997). Motor recovery following stroke: a basis for evaluation. *Disabil. Rehabil.* 19, 64–70.

Hubel, D.H. and Wiesel, T.N. (1968). Receptive fields and functional architecture of monkey striate cortex. *J. Physiol.* 195, 215–43.

Hubel, D.H., Wiesel, T.N., and LeVay, S. (1976). Functional architecture of area 17 in normal and monocularly deprived macaque monkeys. *Cold Spring Harb. Sympos. Quant. Biol.* 40, 581–9.

Humphrey, N.K. and Weiskrantz, L. (1967). Vision in monkeys after removal of the striate cortex. *Nature* 215, 595–7.

Hupé, J.M., Chouvet, G., and Bullier, J. (1999). Spatial and temporal parameters of cortical inactivation by GABA. *J. Neurosci. Methods* 86, 129–43.

Huxlin, K.R. and Pasternak, T. (1999). Mechanisms of training-induced improvements in complex motion perception after PMLS lesions in the cat. *J. Neurosci. Abstr.* 25, 501.

Huxlin, K.R. and Pasternak, T. (2001). Long-term neurochemical changes after visual cortical lesions in the adult cat. *J. Comp. Neurol.* 429, 221–41.

Huxlin, K.R., Price, T., and Pasternak, T. (2000a). Cellular changes associated with visual recovery after cortical lesions in adult cats. *Soc. Neurosci. Abstr.* 26, 1063.

Huxlin, K.R., Saunders, R.C., Marchionini, D., Pham, H.A., and Merigan, W.H. (2000b). Perceptual deficits after lesions of inferotemporal cortex in macaques. *Cereb. Cortex* 10, 671–83.

Keating, E.G. (1979). Rudimentary color vision in the monkey after removal of striate and preoccipital cortex. *Brain Res.* 179, 379–84.

Keating, E.G. and Horel, J.A. (1976). Cortical blindness after overlapping retinal-striate lesions: a limit to plasticity in the central visual system. *Brain Res.* 101, 327–39.

Kluver, H. and Bucy, P.C. (1997). Preliminary analysis of functions of the temporal lobes in monkey. *J. Neuropsychiatry Clin. Neurosci.* 9, 606–20.

Kobatake, E. and Tanaka, K. (1994). Neuronal selectivities to complex object features in the ventral visual pathway of the macaque cerebral cortex. *J. Neurophysiol.* 71, 856–67.

Komatsu, H., Ideura, Y., Kaji, S., and Yamane, S. (1992). Color selectivity of neurons in the inferior temporal cortex of the awake macaque monkey. *J. Neurosci.* 12, 408–24.

Kulikowski, J.J., Walsh, V., McKeefry, D., Butler, S.R., and Carden, D. (1994). The electrophysiological basis of colour processing in macaques with V4 lesions. *Behav. Brain Res.* 60, 73–8.

Latto, R. (1986). The role of inferior parietal cortex and the frontal eye-fields in visuospatial, discriminations in the macaque monkey. *Behav. Brain Res.* 22, 41–52.

Lennie, P. (1998). Single units and visual cortical organization. *Perception* 27, 889–935.

Levitt, J.B., Yoshioka, T., and Lund, J.S. (1995). Connections between the pulvinar complex and cytochrome oxidase-defined compartments in visual area V2 of macaque monkey. *Exp. Brain Res.* 104, 419–30.

Li, C.S., Mazzoni, P., and Andersen, R.A. (1999). Effect of reversible inactivation of macaque lateral intraparietal area on visual and memory saccades. *J. Neurophysiol.* 81, 1827–38.

Logothetis, N.K., Guggenberger, H., Peled, S., and Pauls, J. (1999). Functional imaging of the monkey brain [see comments]. *Nat. Neurosci.* 2, 555–62.

Lund, J.S. (1988). Anatomical organization of macaque monkey striate visual cortex. *Ann. Rev. Neurosci.* 11, 253–88.

Malpeli, J.G. (1999). Reversible inactivation of subcortical sites by drug injection. *J. Neurosci. Methods* 86, 119–28.

Malpeli, J.G., Schiller, P.H., and Colby, C.L. (1981). Response properties of single cells in monkey striate cortex during reversible inactivation of individual lateral geniculate laminae. *J. Neurophysiol.* 46, 1102–19.

Manning, F.J. (1971). Punishment for errors and visual-discrimination learning by monkeys with inferotemporal cortex lesions. *J. Comp. Physiol. Phychol.* 75, 146–52.

Martin, J.H. and Ghez, C. (1999). Pharmacological inactivation in the analysis of the central control of movement. *J. Neurosci. Methods* 86, 145–59.

Maunsell, J.H. and Newsome, W.T. (1987). Visual processing in monkey extrastriate cortex. *Ann. Rev. Neurosci.* 10, 363–401.

Maunsell, J.H.R. and Van Essen, D.C. (1983). Functional properties of neurons in the middle temporal area or the macaque monkey. I. Selectivity for stimulus direction, speed and orientations. *J. Neurophysiol.* **49**, 1148–67.

Maunsell, J.H.R., Sclar, G., Nealy, T.A., and DePriest, D.D. (1992). Extraretinal representations in area V4 in the macaque monkey. *Vis. Neurosci.* **7**, 561–73.

Merigan, W.H. (1996). Basic visual capacities and shape discrimination after lesions of extrastriate area V4 in macaques. *Vis. Neurosci.* **13**, 51–60.

Merigan, W.H. (2000). Cortical area V4 is critical for certain texture discriminations, but this effect is not dependent on attention. *Vis. Neurosci.* **17**, 1–10.

Merigan, W.H. and Maunsell, J.H. (1993). How parallel are the primate visual pathways? *Ann. Rev. Neurosci.* **16**, 369–402.

Merigan, W. and Pham, H.A. (1998). V4 lesions in macaques affect both single- and multiple-viewpoint shape discriminations. *Vis. Neurosci.* **15**, 359–67.

Merigan, W.H., Katz, L.M., and Maunsell, J.H.R. (1991). The effects of parvocellular lateral geniculate lesions on the acuity and contrast sensitivity of macaque monkeys. *J. Neurosci.* **11**, 994–1001.

Merigan, W.H., Nealey, T.A., and Maunsell, J.H. (1993). Visual effects of lesions of cortical area V2 in macaques. *J. Neurosci.* **13**, 3180–91.

Merzenich, M.M., Kaas, J.H., Wall, J., Nelson, R.J., Sur, M., and Felleman, D. (1983). Topographic reorganization of somatosensory cortical areas 3b and 1 in adult monkeys following restricted deafferentation. *Neuroscience* **8**, 33–55.

Meunier, M., Bachevalier, J., Murray, E.A., Malkova, L., and Mishkin, M. (1999). Effects of aspiration versus neurotoxic lesions of the amygdala on emotional responses in monkeys. *Eur. J. Neurosci.* **11**, 4403–18.

Miller, M., Pasik, P., and Pasik, T. (1980). Extrageniculostriate vision in the monkey. VII. Contrast sensitivity functions. *J. Neurophysiol.* **43**, 1510–26.

Motter, B.C. (1993). Focal attention produces spatially selective processing in visual cortical areas V1, V2, and V4 in the presence of competing stimuli. *J. Neurophysiol.* **70**, 909–19.

Nakamura, H., Gattass, R., Desimone, R., and Ungerleider, L.G. (1993a). The modular organization of projections from area-V1 and area-V2 to area-V4 and TEO in macaques. *J. Neurosci.* **13**, 3681–91.

Nakamura, H., Gattass, R., Desimone, R., and Ungerleider, L.G. (1993b). The modular organization of projections from areas V1 and V2 to areas V4 and TEO in macaques. *J. Neurosci.* **13**, 3681–91.

Newsome, W.T. and Paré, E.B. (1988). A selective impairment of motion perception following lesions or the miadle temporal visual area (MT). *J. Neurosci.* **8**, 2201–11.

Newsome, W.T., Wurtz, R.H., Dursteler, M.R., and Mikami, A. (1985). Deficits in visual motion processing following ibotenic acid lesions of the middle temporal visual area of the macaque monkey. *J. Neurosci.* **5**, 825–40.

Olavarria, J.F. and Van Essen, D.C. (1997). The global pattern of cytochrome oxidase stripes in visual area V2 of the macaque monkey. *Cereb. Cortex* **7**, 395–404.

Orban, G.A., Saunders, R.C., and Vandenbussche, E. (1995). Lesions of the superior temporal cortical motion areas impair speed discrimination in the macaque monkey. *Eur. J. Neurosci.* **7**, 2261–76.

Pasik, P. and Pasik, T. (1973). Extrageniculostriate vision in the monkey. V. Role of accessory optic system. *J. Neurophysiol.* **36**, 450–7.

Passingham, R.E. (1972). Visual discrimination learning after selective prefrontal ablations in monkeys (*Macaca mulatta*). *Neuropsychologia* **10**, 27–39.

Pasternak, T. (1987). Discrimination of differences in speed and flicker rate depends on directionally selective mechanisms. *Vision Res.* **27**, 1881–90.

Pasternak, T. and Merigan, W.H. (1994). Motion perception following lesions of the superior temporal sulcus in the monkey. *Cereb. Cortex* 4, 247–59.

Pasternak, T., Horn, K.M., and Maunsell, J.H.R. (1989). Deficits in speed discrimination following lesions of the lateral suprasylvian cortex in the cat. *Vis. Neurosci.* 3, 365–75.

Pasupathy, A. and Connor, C.E. (1999). Responses to contour features in macaque area V4. *J. Nerophysiol.* 82, 2490–502.

Phinney, R.E. and Siegel, R.M. (2000). Speed selectivity for optic flow in area 7a of the behaving macaque. *Cereb. Cortex* 10, 413–21.

Poppel, E., Held, R., and Frost, D. (1973). Residual visual function after brain wounds involving the central visual pathways in man. *Nature* 243, 295–6.

Quintana, J. and Fuster, J.M. (1993). Spatial and temporal factors in the role of prefrontal and parietal cortex in visuomotor integration. *Cereb. Cortex* 3, 122–32.

Quintana, J., Fuster, J.M., and Yajeya, J. (1989). Effects of cooling parietal cortex on prefrontal units in delay tasks. *Brain Res.* 503, 100–10.

Rainer, G. and Miller, E.K. (2000). Effects of visual experience on the representation of objects in the prefrontal cortex [see comments]. *Neuron* 27, 179–89.

Ratcliff, G., Ridley, R.M., and Ettlinger, G. (1977). Spatial disorientation in the monkey. *Cortex* 13, 62–5.

Read, H.L. and Siegel, R.M. (1997). Modulation of responses to optic flow in area 7a by retinotopic and oculomotor cues in monkey. *Cereb. Cortex* 7, 647–61.

Reynolds, J.H., Pasternak, T., and Desimone, R. (2000). Attention increases sensitivity of V4 neurons [see comments]. *Neuron* 26, 703–14.

Ridley, R.M. and Ettlinger, G. (1975). Tactile and visuo-spatial discrimination performance in the monkey: the effects of total and partial posterior parietal removals. *Neuropsychologia* 13, 191–206.

Rockland, K.S. and Van Hoesen, G.W. (1994). Direct temporal-occipital feedback connections to striate cortex (V1) in the macaque monkey. *Cereb. Cortex* 4, 300–13.

Rodman, H.R., Gross, C.G., and Albright, T.D. (1989). Afferent basis of visual response properties in area MT of the macaque. I. Effects of striate cortex removal. *J. Neurosci.* 9, 2033–50.

Roe, A.W. and Tso, D. (1997). The functional architecture of area V2 in the macaque monkey. Physiology, topography, and connectivity. *Cereb. Cortex* 12, 295–333.

Rolls, E.T., Treves, A., Tovee, M.J., and Panzeri, S. (1997). Information in the neuronal representation of individual stimuli in the primate temporal visual cortex. *J. Comput. Neurosci.* 4, 309–33.

Rudolph, K.K. (1997). Motion and form perception after lesions of cortical areas MT/MST and V4 in the macaque. Doctoral dissertation. Department of Brain and Cognitive Science. Rochester, NY: University of Rochester.

Rudolph, K.K. and Pasternak, T. (1996). Motion and form perception after lesions of areas MT/MST and V4 in the macaque. *Invest. Ophthalmol. Vis. Sci.* 37 (suppl.), 5486.

Rudolph, K. and Pasternak, T. (1999). Transient and permanent deficits in motion perception after lesions of cortical areas MT and MST in the macaque monkey. *Cereb. Cortex* 9, 90–100.

Rushworth, M.E.S., Nixon, P.D., and Passingham, R.E. (1997). Parietal cortex and movement. 2. Spatial representation. *Exp. Brain Res.* 117, 311–23.

Sakata, H., Shibutani, H., Ito, Y., Tsurugai, K., Mine, S., and Kusunoki, M. (1994). Functional properties of rotation-sensitive neurons in the posterior parietal association cortex of the monkey. *Exp. Brain Res.* 101, 183–202.

Schein, S.J. and Desimone, R. (1990). Spectral properties of V4 neurons in the macaque. *J. Neurosci.* 10, 3369–89.

Schilder, P., Pasik, P., and Pasik, T. (1972). Extrageniculostriate vision in the monkey. 3. Circle VS triangle and 'red VS green' discrimination. *Exp. Brain Res.* 14, 436–48.

Schiller, P.H. (1993). The effects of V4 and middle temporal (MT) area lesions on visual performance in the rhesus monkey. *Vis. Neurosci.* 10, 717–46.

Schiller, P.H. (1995). Effect of lesions in visual cortical area V4 on the recognition of transformed objects. *Nature* 376, 342–4.

Schiller, P.H. and Lee, K. (1991). The role of the primate extrastriate area V4 in vision. *Science* 251, 1251–3.

Schiller, P.H. and Lee, K. (1994). The effects of lateral geniculate nucleus, area V4, and middle temporal (MT) lesions on visually guided eye movements. *Vis. Neurosci.* 11, 229–41.

Schiller, P.H., True, S.D., and Conway, J.L. (1980). Deficits in eye movements following frontal eye-field and superior colliculus ablations. *J. Neurophysiol.* 44, 1175–89.

Schoups, A.A., Vogels, R., and Orban, G.A. (1995). Human perceptual learning in identifying the oblique orientation: retinotopy, orientation specificity and monocularity. *J. Physiol.* 483, 797–810.

Schwarcz, R., Hökfelt, T., Fuxe, K., Jonsson, G., Goldstein, M., and Terenius, L. (1979). Ibotenic acid-induced neuronal degeneration: a morphological and neurochemical study. *Exp. Brain Res.* 37, 199–216.

Seidemann, E., Poirson, A.B., Wandell, B.A., and Newsome, W.T. (1999). Color signals in area MT of the macaque monkey. *Neuron* 24, 911–17.

Sereno, M.I., Dale, A.M., Reppas, J.B., Kwong, K.K., Belliveau, J.W., Brady, T.J., Rosen, B.R., and Tootell, R.B. (1995). Borders of multiple visual areas in humans revealed by functional magnetic resonance imaging [see comments]. *Science* 268, 889–93.

Shadlen, M.N., Britten, K.H., Newsome, W.T., and Movshon, J.A. (1996). A computational analysis of the relationship between neuronal and behavioral responses to visual motion. *J. Neurosci.* 16, 1486–510.

Shipp, S. and Zeki, S. (1985). Segregation of pathways leading from area V2 to areas V4 and V5 of macaque monkey visual cortex. *Nature* 315, 322–5.

Siegel, R.M. and Read, H.L. (1997). Analysis of optic flow in the monkey parietal area 7a. *Cereb. Cortex* 7, 327–46.

Snyder, L.H., Batista, A.P., and Anderson, R.A. (1997). Coding of intention in the posterior parietal cortex. *Nature* 386, 167–70.

Snyder, L.H., Batista, A.P., and Anderson, R.A. (1998). Change in motor plan, without a change in the spatial locus of attention, modulates activity in posterior parietal cortex. *J. Neurophysiol.* 79, 2814–19.

Stoerig, P. and Cowey, A. (1992). Wavelength discrimination in blindsight. *Brain* 115, 425–44.

Taira, M., Tsutsui, K.-I., Jiang, M., Yara, K., and Sakata, H. (2000). Parietal neurons represent surface orientation from the gradient of binocular disparity. *J. Neurophysiol.* 83, 3140–6.

Tanaka, K. (1992). Inferotemporal cortex and higher visual functions. *Curr. Opin. Neurobiol.* 2, 502–5.

Tanaka, M., Lindsley, E., Lausmann, S., and Creutzfeldt, O.D. (1990). Afferent connections of the prelunate visual association cortex (areas V4 and DP). *Anat. Embryol.* 181, 19–30.

Ungerleider, L.G. and Brody, B.A. (1977). Extrapersonal spatial orientation: the role of posterior parietal, anterior frontal, and inferotemporal cortex. *Exp. Neurol.* 56, 265–80.

Ungerleider, L.G. and Mishkin, M. (1982). Two cortical visual systems. In *The analysis of visual behavior* (ed. D.J. Ingle, R.J.W. Mansfield) and M.S. Goodale, pp. 549–86. MIT press, Cambridge, Massachusetts.

Vogels, R., Saunders, R.C., and Orban, G.A. (1997). Effects of inferior temporal lesions on two types of orientation discrimination in the macaque monkey. *Eur. J. Neurosci.* 9, 229–45.

von der Heydt, R. and Peterhans, E. (1989). Mechanisms of contour perception in monkey visual cortex. I. Lines of pattern discontinuity. *J. Neurosci.* 9, 1731–48.

Walker, M.F., Fitzgibbon, E.J., and Goldberg, M.E. (1995). Neurons in the monkey superior colliculus predict the visual result of impending saccadic eye movements. *J. Neurophysiol.* **73**, 1988–2003.

Walsh, V., Butler, S.R., Carden, D., and Kulikowski, J.J. (1992*a*). The effects of V4 lesions on the visual abilities of macaques: shape discrimination. *Behav. Brain Res.* **50**, 115–26.

Walsh, V., Kulikowski, J.J., Butler, S.R., and Carden, D. (1992*b*). The effects of lesions of area V4 on the visual abilities of macaques: colour categorization. *Behavi. Brain Res.* **52**, 81–9.

Walsh, V., Carden, D., Butler, S.R., and Kulikowski, J.J. (1993). The effects of V4 lesions on the visual abilities of macaques: hue discrimination and colour constancy. *Behav. Brain Res.* **53**, 51–62.

Walsh, V., Le Mare, C., Blaimire, A., and Cowey, A. (2000). Normal discrimination performance accompanied by priming deficits in monkeys with V4 or TEO lesions. *Neuroreport* **11**, 1459–62.

Wandell, B.A., Poirson, A.B., Newsome, W.T., Baseler, H.A., Boynton, G.M., Huk, A., Gandhi, S., and Sharpe, L.T. (1999). Color signals in human motion-selective cortex. *Neuron* **24**, 901–9.

Watamaniuk, S.N.J., Sekuler, R., and Williams, D.W. (1989). Direction perception in complex dynamic displays: the integration of direction information. *Vision Res.* **29**, 47–60.

Weiskrantz, L. (1986). *Blindsight: a case study and implications.* Oxford University Press, Oxford.

Weiskrantz, L. and Cowey, A. (1967). Comparison of the effects of striate cortex and retinal lesions on visual acuity in the monkey. *Science* **155**, 104–6.

Weiskrantz, L. and Saunders, R.C. (1984). Impairments of visual object transforms in monkeys. *Brain* **107**, 1033–72.

Wild, H.M., Butler, S.R., Carden, D., and Kulikowski, J.J. (1985). Primate cortical area V4 is important for colour constancy but not wavelength discrimination. *Nature* **313**, 133–5.

Williams, D.W. and Sekuler, R. (1984). Coherent global motion percepts from stochastic local motions. *Vision Res.* **24**, 55–62.

Xiao, Y., Zych, A., and Felleman, D.J. (1999). Segregation and convergence of functionally defined V2 thin stripe and interstripe compartment projections to area V4 of macaques. *Cereb. Cortex* **9**, 792–804.

Yamasaki, D.S. and Wurtz, R.H. (1991). Recovery of function after lesions in the superior temporal sulcus in the monkey. *J. Neurophysiol.* **66**, 651–73.

Zeki, S. (1983*a*). Colour coding in the cerebral cortex: the reaction of cells in monkey visual cortex to wavelengths and colours. *Neuroscience* **9**, 741–65.

Zeki, S. (1983*b*). The distribution of wavelength and orientation selective cells in different areas of monkey visual cortex. *Proc. R. Soc. Lond. B, Biol. Sci.* **217**, 449–70.

Chapter 6

Magnetic stimulation in studies of vision and attention

Amanda Ellison, Lauren Stewart, Alan Cowey, and Vincent Walsh

Introduction

Neuropsychology attempts to draw inferences about normal brain function from the behaviour of patients with brain lesions. The contribution of this approach to what we know about brain function today cannot be overstated. Even so, the approach is not without its limitations—brain lesions are often quite diffuse and may result in functional reorganization within the brain. Furthermore, the lesions are enduring; we are never afforded the opportunity to see how a patient would perform a given task in the absence of their lesion. Transcranial magnetic stimulation (TMS) offers a 'virtual lesion' method of investigating the effects of cortical dysfunction that is free of the limitations mentioned above. It can disrupt cognitive functions with a spatial resolution of approximately 1 cm on the scalp and its effects are transient, lasting a few tens of milliseconds, so that any effects observed are not masked by reorganization, which occurs over much longer time scales. Moreover, the temporal resolution allows one to asks questions about the timing of cortical processing.

TMS involves applying a brief magnetic pulse, or a train of pulses, to the scalp to induce a local electrical field, which, in turn, alters the local electrical field in the underlying surface of the brain. The modern age of magnetic stimulation began as recently as 1985 when Barker *et al.* first stimulated the human motor cortex with a 2 Tesla pulse. The sequence of events in delivery of a single pulse begins with an electrical current of up to 8 kA, generated by a capacitor and discharged into a circular or figure-of-eight-shaped coil that, in turn, produces a magnetic pulse of up to 2 Tesla. The pulse has a rise time of approximately 200 μs and a duration of 1 ms and, due to its intensity and brevity, changes at a rapid rate. The changing magnetic field generates an electric field resulting in neural activity. The net change in charge density in the cortex is zero. In addition to single-pulse stimulation, some stimulators can deliver trains of pulses up to a rate of 50 Hz. Rapid rate stimulation carries a small risk of inducing seizures so stimulation parameters, e.g. intensity and rate of repetition, must be kept within the recommended safety limits (Wassermann 1998).

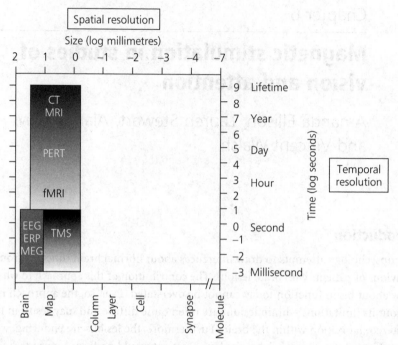

Fig. 6.1 TMS has spatial and temporal resolutions that allow it to occupy an interaction area, time, and space not accessible to other techniques.

The specificity of TMS is remarkable in both space and time. Figure 6.1 shows the resolution of TMS and some of the other techniques used in studying brain function in human subjects and it is clear that there is often a trade-off between space and time. Event-related potentials (ERPs) have good temporal but poor spatial resolution, whereas positron emission tomography (PET) and functional magnetic resonance imaging (fMRI) have the reverse—good resolution in the spatial but less in the temporal domain. TMS, like magnetoencephalography (MEG), combines good spatial and temporal resolution. Good spatial and temporal resolution are impressive, but the question to be asked of any technique is, 'what new *functional* resolution does it offer?' Can TMS be used to explore functions that could not be studied by other means? Can it offer a more elegant, quicker, or less invasive solution to some of the problems that can be addressed through other techniques?

Techniques such as PET, fMRI, ERPs, and MEG can provide a correlation of neural activity with a dependent variable, e.g. recorded muscle activity at a distal site, subjective self-report of the subject, behavioural measures such as reaction time or errors on a task. However, since TMS acts as a virtual lesion technique, rather than asking whether activity in a given area is correlated with some dependent variable, TMS asks whether or not it is *necessary* for a given function.

TMS studies of visual cortex

Amassian *et al.* (1989) were the first to demonstrate the power of TMS in psychological studies of vision. They delivered single-pulse TMS over the occipital cortex of subjects while they performed a letter-identification task. Performance was impaired when TMS was applied between 60 and 140 ms after the onset of the presentation of the stimuli and, when it was applied between 80 and 100 ms after stimulus onset, subjects were incapable of detecting any of the letters. This result was soon replicated and correlated with visual evoked potential (VEP) latencies in clinically normal and abnormal subject groups. Amassian and colleagues also took their experiment a significant stage further by showing that TMS could unmask a visual mask (like disinhibition) and thus improve performance. In the latter experiment subjects were presented with the same letter-identification arrays followed, 100 ms later, by a high contrast visual mask and single-pulse TMS was applied at various intervals after the presentation of the mask. The effect of TMS was to prevent the presentation of the second stimulus (the mask) from impeding identification of the first stimulus, as was the case without TMS. Fig. 6.2 shows the reciprocal effects of TMS in the two experiments. In these two experiments lies the foundation for all subsequent studies of visual cognition using TMS. One can either impair visual performance by interfering with the transmission of relevant visual signals or one can improve performance by interfering with the transmission of irrelevant or competing stimuli.

In a recent study, Cowey and Walsh (2001*a,b*) have shown that TMS can be used to probe the neural substrates of awareness. Phosphenes were induced by TMS to

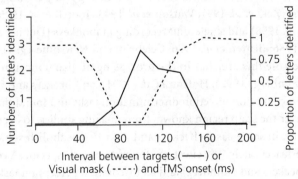

Fig. 6.2 Amassian's experiments. The solid line (left ordinate) represents the number of letters correctly identified in trigrams when single-pulse TMS was applied at the time after stimulus onset shown on the abscissa. When TMS was applied at 0 to 40 ms after the onset of the letters there was virtually no effect of TMS on recognition. But TMS applied between 60 and 140 ms after stimulus onset impaired performance and reduced recognition to zero between 80 and 100 ms. The dashed line (right ordinate) shows the proportion of letters correctly identified in the presence of a visual mask when TMS was applied after the mask. This function resembles the inverse of the recognition paradigm.

examine the integrity of visual cortex in a peripherally blind subject who had suffered optic nerve damage and to compare the results with those obtained by stimulating the same regions in normally sighted individuals and in a hemianopic subject who possesses blindsight in the impaired field. The TMS-induced phosphenes obeyed Emmert's law of size scaling in blindsighted and sighted subjects irrespective of whether the stimulation was applied over the midline of the occipital cortex (Fig. 6.3 left panel) to produce stationary phosphenes or over visual area V5 (Fig. 6.3 right panel) to produce moving phosphenes. The farther away was the surface on to which the phosphenes were 'projected', the larger they were perceived to be. However, extensive and intensive stimulation of the damaged left hemisphere in the blindsight subject did not yield phosphenes, even when applied to V5 on that side. The phosphenes reported by the peripherally blind subject (Fig. 6.3(b)) were as easily elicited and as reproducible as those seen by other subjects but their spatial distribution suggests that retinotopic mapping in this subject's V1 is degraded. Despite the coarser spatial mapping the blind subject showed otherwise normal phosphenes including the perception of movement when V5 was stimulated (Fig. 6.3 right panel). These findings are strongly supportive of the view that visual awareness requires the presence of an intact V1.

The location of extrastriate area V5, just posterior to the meeting point of the ascending limb of the inferior temporal sulcus and the lateral occipital sulcus (Watson *et al.* 1993), makes it particularly accessible to stimulation with TMS and, to date, there have been several studies that have stimulated V5 with the aim of investigating the involvement of this area in visual motion processing (Hotson *et al.* 1994; Beckers and Zeki 1995; Walsh *et al.* 1998*b*; Stewart *et al.* 1999; Pascual-Leone and Walsh 2001). The results of these studies have added to already existing evidence from imaging studies (Zeki *et al.* 1991; Watson *et al.* 1993; Tootell *et al.* 1995; Reppas *et al.* 1997; Smith *et al.* 1998) and single-unit recording in monkeys (Dubner and Zeki 1971; Mikami *et al.* 1986; Britten *et al.* 1996; Celebrini and Newsome 1994) in reinforcing the specialized role this area has in the processing of visual motion information. Beckers and Homberg (1992), Hotson *et al.* (1994), and Beckers and Zeki (1995) all used forced-choice motion direction discrimination tasks and found that single-pulse TMS applied over the scalp region known, from imaging studies, to overlie cortical V5 could disrupt or, in some cases (Beckers and Zeki 1995), abolish subjects' ability to perform this task accurately. The effect was found to be task-specific. A colour discrimination task (Beckers and Homberg) and an orientation perception task (Beckers and Zeki) were both unaffected and site-specific. The finding that TMS over V5 can abolish motion direction discrimination builds on results from imaging studies but, whilst these have shown a correlation between motion direction perception and activity in V5, the TMS studies demonstrate the necessity of this area for accurate performance on this task.

A recent study by Stewart *et al.* (1999) demonstrates that TMS delivered over V5 can elicit moving phosphenes. Stimulation was delivered over points within a 3 cm × 3 cm

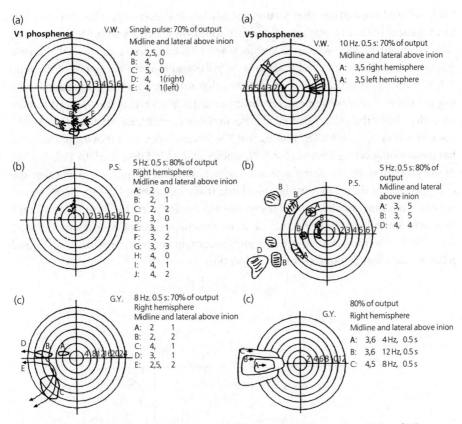

Fig. 6.3 Examples of retinotopic mapping of TMS-induced phosphenes over VI and V5 (moving phosphenes): (a) in a normally sighted observer V.W.; (b) in a retinally blind subject P.S.; and (c) in a hemianopic patient G.Y. The coordinates give the site of stimulation in dorsal–lateral order. For example, 3, 5 indicates that the coil was centred 3 cm above the inion and 5 cm lateral. In the case of V1 stimulation, as the coil is moved dorsally and forward, away from the inion, the phosphenes migrate inferiorly (cf. A and C part (c)), and, as the coil is moved laterally from the midline, the phosphenes migrate further from the vertical meridian, in the contralateral visual field (cf. A and B part (c)). In the retinally blind subject P.S. (b), the phosphenes were clustered in the central 3° of the visual field despite stimulation being delivered between 2 and 4 cm above the inion and up to 3 cm lateral. Where phosphenes were elicited beyond the central 2°, they are in the opposite direction to that predicted by normal retinotopic mapping, i.e. stimulating more dorsally yielded more superior rather than inferior phosphenes. P.S. drew all his phosphenes as small smudges about 1° across. As they overlapped extensively, only their centres are marked. The arrowheads on the medial outlines of phosphenes D and E in (c) indicate that the phosphene extended much further into the periphery to a border that could be indicated only vaguely by the subject. In V5 stimulation all three subjects reported moving phosphenes. In G.Y. the centripedal direction was particularly strong, as indicated by the arrows. In P.S. at the same scalp position a few seconds apart yielded phosphenes with different positions. Such extensive variability was not seen in six sighted subjects.

grid, centred on a point that structural MRI scans have suggested overlies V5. Stimulation intensity was 30–100% of maximum output and both single- and repetitive-pulse TMS were used. Subjects were asked to indicate when they saw a phosphene, to describe it, and to draw it on polar graph paper. Seven out of the nine subjects tested reported seeing phosphenes that moved. Some subjects described a vague impression of movement, e.g. 'as if the edges of a vertical line seemed to bow inwards', while others described vivid, directional movement, e.g. 'drifting rightwards, not continuous' (Fig. 6.4). The finding that TMS over V5 can elicit moving phosphenes has methodological significance for TMS studies of the kind described. In TMS studies of the visual system, the absence of any easily measurable output has meant that the coil position on the scalp must be calculated from anatomical MRI scans. However, anatomy and functionality do not always overlap precisely and the location of V5 may vary between individuals by up to 2 cm in its anterior–posterior coordinates (Watson *et al.* 1993). The induction of moving phosphenes, in contrast, provides a quick and reliable functional demonstration of V5 location.

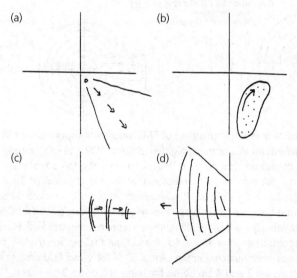

Fig. 6.4 Moving phosphenes. Four examples of moving phosphenes drawn by subjects following stimulation over V5. (a) The subject described this as 'a movement of a single point in a static field': TMS was applied 2 cm dorsal to inion and 6 cm left of the midline at 1.4 T, 5 Hz for 500 ms. (b) Described as 'similar to a random dot array; black dots on a white background; appears to move upwards and rightwards'. Stimulation site, left hemisphere, 2 cm dorsal and 6 cm lateral to inion; stimulation rate, 5 Hz at 1.8 T for 0.5 s. (c) Described as 'drifing right, not continuous'. Stimulation site, right hemisphere 2 cm dorsal and 5 cm lateral to inion; stimulation rate, 10 Hz at 1.4 T for 1 s. (d) Described as 'a block of visual noise that jumps to the left'. Stimulation site, right hemisphere, 2 cm dorsal and 4 cm lateral to inion; stimulation rate, single pulse at 1.4 T.

The results of both the direction discrimination experiments and the moving phosphene experiment also reveal something about the organization of area V5. In Beckers and Homberg's study, TMS over V5 disrupted direction discrimination only when the moving stimulus was in the hemifield contralateral to the site of stimulation, suggesting that, in man as in monkey, it is the contralateral hemifield that is mapped in each V5. In the moving phosphene experiment, the pattern of phosphenes elicited corresponded to a strictly retinotopically organized system, i.e. stimulation of left V5 produced moving phosphenes in the right visual hemifield and vice versa and moving the coil up and down caused the location of the phosphenes to move down and up respectively. Results from both these studies also suggest a relative lateralization of motion processing to the left hemisphere. Beckers and Homberg found a much more marked reduction in performance when TMS was applied over left compared to right V5 and moving phosphenes elicited by TMS over V5 were more easily produced with left V5 stimulation than right. A left lateralization of motion processing is in line with PET scanning results (Zeki et al. 1991; Lueck et al. 1989), but neuropsychological evidence would not seem to support such a lateralization. A possible reason for the disparity between TMS and neuropsychological findings may be the nature of the disruption produced in each instance. The damage sustained by neuropsychological patients is obviously enduring and patients learn to perform tasks using alternative strategies. TMS, in contrast, produces a transient disruption that is too short for any such changes to occur.

The characteristic properties of V5 neurons have also been highlighted using TMS. Beckers and Homberg report that TMS-induced deficits in direction discrimination were most marked for movement away from the fovea rather than towards it. Similarly, the moving phosphenes elicited by Stewart et al. were most often reported to be moving away from the fovea. These results are consistent with findings by Albright (1989) that V5 possesses more neurons tuned for motion away from the fovea than towards it. Hence, stimulation over V5 will affect a greater proportion of centrifugally tuned compared to centripetally tuned neurons.

Aside from revealing some of the properties of V5, TMS has been used to affect V5 function. Stewart et al. (1999) designed an analogue of a motor learning experiment in which TMS had been found to affect learning in a frequency-specific manner such that a low rate of stimulation impeded learning whilst a high rate enhanced it (Pascual-Leone et al. 1999). The study was designed to assess whether TMS could also affect learning in a non-motor modality such as vision. In addition, if TMS applied over V5 could affect the degree to which learning occurred, V5 itself could be considered to be a neural substrate of learning. TMS was applied over V5 while subjects learned a visual motion task that required detection of a target defined by the conjunction of shape and direction. Three subject groups participated. One group received no TMS; the other two received TMS at 3 and 10 HZ, respectively during learning occurred over 4 days (1.5 hours/day). While all subjects learned the task significantly, the 3 Hz stimulation group learned significantly less than either the no TMS group or the 10 Hz stimulation

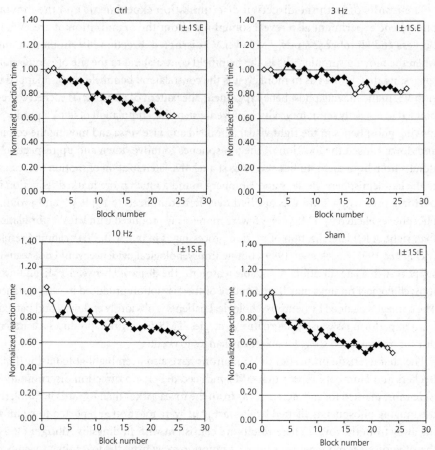

Fig. 6.5 The effects of different rates of TMS on perceptual learning of visual motion. Subjects practised for over 100 trials on a motion detection task. The control group did not receive TMS; the sham group received TMS with the coil directed away from the cortex. The two TMS groups received either 3 HZ or 10 Hz TMS on each trial. At 3 Hz the reaction times improved less than in any of the other groups. It is important to note that the 3 Hz group received fewer TMS pulses than the 10 Hz group (from Stewart *et al.* 1999).

group (Fig. 6.5). This frequency-specific effect of TMS on learning suggests that TMS effects on learning may generalize across modalities and that learning visual motion detection may arise from activity within V5 rather than from some 'higher centre' outside sensory cortex.

Studies of attention

The role of the parietal cortex in visual attention is a question of central concern. Several imaging and neuropsychological studies point to a particular role for this area in orienting attention while others emphasize its role in visual binding. Frequently, the same tasks are used to address the two different issues. Ashbridge *et al.* (1997) applied TMS over the parietal visual cortex of subjects while they were performing 'pop-out' or conjunction visual search tasks in arrays containing eight distractors. Magnetic stimulation had no detrimental effect on the performance of pop-out search but did significantly increase reaction times on conjunction search when stimulation was applied over the right parietal cortex 100 ms after the onset of the visual display. Stimulation had no effect on the number of errors made. The results suggest that a subregion of the right parietal lobe is important for conjunction search but not for pre-attentive pop-out. This is consistent with timing data from studies of single cells in monkeys and the hypothesis that parietal areas generate a signal that projects back to extrastriate visual areas to enhance the processing of features in a restricted part of the visual field (see Chapter 2, this volume for the underlying anatomical and functional connections). The timing of the effect indicates that TMS disrupts the mechanisms underlying the focal attention necessary for feature binding in conjunction search. The results also highlight the efficacy of TMS as a complement to other spatial and temporal mapping techniques.

The role of the parietal cortex, like that of any other area, may change with experience and Walsh *et al.* (1998*a*) extended the paradigm used by Ashbridge *et al.* to study the effects of learning. Performance on a wide range of perceptual tasks improves with practice. Most accounts of perceptual learning are concerned with changes in neuronal sensitivity or changes in the way a stimulus is represented. Another possibility is that different areas of the brain are involved in performing a task during, as opposed to after, learning it. Walsh *et al.* observed that single-pulse TMS to the right parietal cortex impaired visual conjunction search when the stimuli were novel and required a serial search strategy, but not once the particular search task had been learned (Fig. 6.6). Hence, the right parietal cortex has a role in novel but not learned visual conjunction search. The effect of TMS returns when a different, novel, serial search task is presented.

Following damage to the right parietal cortex, patients often exhibit neglect of the left side of space or the left side of objects (see Chapter 7, this volume). One possible explanation for this is that, because the two hemispheres operate in a mutually inhibitory manner, damage to the right cortical hemisphere not only leads to a reduced capacity to orient to information in the left-world, but also to disinhibition of the left parietal cortex and thus an exaggerated tendency to attend to the right-world. By applying single-pulse TMS to the parietal cortex 50 ms before subjects were required to detect a small electrical stimulus delivered to the fingers, Seyal *et al.* (1995) were able to demonstrate that sensitivity to tactile stimuli was *increased* in the hand ipsilateral to stimulation. Using repetitive-pulse TMS, Pascual-Leone *et al.* (1994) modelled visual extinction, another feature of parietal cortex damage. Subjects were presented with either one or two asterisks to detect on a computer monitor and received trains of pulses contralateral to the stimulated hemisphere only when targets were presented in both hemifields simultaneously. Subjects were significantly impaired by unilateral TMS over the parietal cortex when visual stimuli were presented in both visual fields simultaneously.

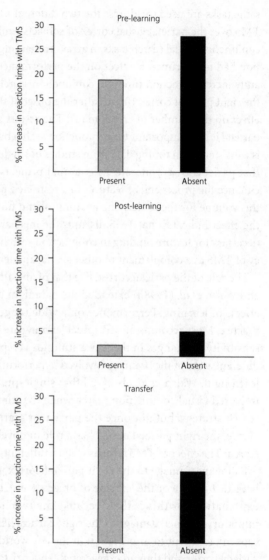

Fig. 6.6 TMS can be used to assess the role of cortical areas at different stages of learning and expertise. Walsh *et al.* (1998*a*) applied TMS over posterior parietal cortex during the performance of visual search tasks. (Top) When subjects are presented with a previously unseen visual search task there are large costs in reaction times for both target present and target absent trials. (Middle) After subjects have trained to become efficient on the search task the deficits are no longer induced by TMS. (Bottom) When the same subjects are again presented with a new visual search task, the effects of TMS are reinstated.

TMS may also be able to model visual neglect. Neglect is widely studied in neuropsychological patients but there are many differences between patients and the tendency is for the phenomenon to be transient. In a study by Fierro *et al.* (2000) subjects were briefly presented (50 ms) with bisected lines and required to judge whether the left, right, or neither side was longer. In control trials there was a pseudoneglect tendency, consistent with right hemisphere bias, to report the left as longer. On TMS trials, pulses were delivered at 115% of motor threshold at 25 Hz for 400 ms over left or right parietal cortex at the time of stimulus onset. Right parietal stimulation corrected the pseudoneglect but left parietal and sham TMS did not change the subjects' behaviour.

Stimulation to the parietal cortex reduced the ability to detect stimuli. Being able to reproduce neglect is an important step in modelling the phenomenon and one wonders whether a reaction time approach might increase the sensitivity of this particular assay. At the other end of the clinical scale, Olivieri *et al.* (1999) have reversed rather than reproduced a neuropsychological phenomenon. They studied patients with right or left hemisphere brain lesions and gave TMS to frontal or parietal cortex of the intact hemisphere 40 ms after the subjects were presented with unilateral or bilateral tactile stimuli to be detected. Those patients with right hemisphere lesions showed a reduction in extinction when TMS was given over the left frontal region, thus supporting the interpretation of Kinsbourne (1977) and Seyal *et al.* (1995).

Looking forward

The use of TMS has many applications in the vision sciences that await the attentions of researchers. The effects of learning and plasticity are good paradigms for investigating cortical change and the potential for combining TMS with other neuroimaging techniques will widen the scope of its utility in the study of vision.

Acknowledgements

The authors' works are supported by the Medical Research Council, the Dr Hadwen Humane Research Trust, and the Royal Society.

References

Albright, T.D. (1989). Centrifugal directional bias in the middle temporal visual area (MT) of the macaque. *Vis. Neurosci.* 2 (2), 177–88.

Amassian, V.E., Cracco, R.Q., Maccabee, P.J., Cracco, J.B., Rudell, A.P., and Eberle, L. (1989). Suppression of visual perception by magnetic coil stimulation of human occipital cortex. *Electroencephalogr. Clini. Neurophysiol.* 74, 458–62.

Amassian, V.E., Cracco, R.Q., Maccabee, P.J., Cracco, J.B., Rudell, A.P., and Eberle, L. (1993). Unmasking human visual perception with the magnetic coil and its relationship to hemispheric asymmetry. *Brain Res.* 605, 312–16.

Ashbridge, E., Walsh, V., and Cowey, A. (1997). Temporal apsects of visual search studied by transranial magnetic stimulation. *Neuropsychologia* 35, 1121–31.

Barker, A.T., Jalinous, R., and Freeston, I.L. (1985). Non-invasive magnetic stimulation of human motor cortex. *Lancet* i, 1106–7.

Beckers, G. and Homberg, V. (1992). Cerebral visual motion blindness: transitory akinetopsia induced by transcranial magnetic stimulation of human area V5. *Proc. R. Soc. Lond.* B 249, 173–8.

Beckers, G. and Zeki, S. (1995). The consequences of inactivating areas V1 and V5 on visual motion perception. *Brain* 118, 49–60.

Britten, K.H., Newsome, W.T., Shadlen, N.M., Celebrini, S., and Movshon, J.A. (1996). A relationship between behavioural choice and the visual responses of neurons in macaque MT. *Vis. Neurosci.* 13 (1), 87–100.

Celebrini, S. and Newsome, W.T. (1994). Neuronal and psychophysical sensitivity to motion signals in extrastriate area MST of the Macaque monkey. *J. Neurosci.* 14 (7), 4109–24.

Corbetta, M., Miezin, F.M., Shulman, G.L., and Petersen, S.E. (1991). Selective attention modulates extrastriate visual regions in humans during visual feature discrimination and recognition. *Ciba Found. Sympo.* 163, 165–75.

Corbetta, M., Shulman, G.L., Miezin, F.M., and Petersen, S.E. (1995). Superior parietal cortex activation during spatial attention shifts and visual feature conjunction. *Science* 270, 802–5.

Coslett, H.B. and Monsul, N. (1994). Reading with the right hemisphere: evidence from transcranial magnetic stimulation. *Brain and Lang.* 46, 98–211.

Cowey, A. and Walsh, V. (2001a). Tickling the brain: studies of visual sensation, perception and cognition by transcranial magnetic stimulation. *Prog. Brain Res.*, 134, 129–43.

Cowey, A. and Walsh, V. (2001b). Magnetically induced phosphenes in sighted, blind and blindsighted observers. *NeuroReport* 11, 3269–73.

Day, B.L., Dressler, D., Maertens de Noordhoot, A., Marsden, C.D., Nakashima, K., Rothwell, J.C., and Thompson, P.D. (1989). Electric and magnetic stimulation of the human motor cortex: surface EMG and single motor unit responses. *J. Physiol.* 412, 449–73.

Dubner, R. and Zeki, S.M. (1971). Response properties and receptive fields of cells in an anatomically defined region of the superior temporal sulcus in the monkey. *Brain Res.* 35, 528–32.

Epstein, C.M., Meador, K.J., Loring, D.W., Wright, R.J., Wiseman, J.D., Shgeppard, S., Lah, J.J., Puhlavich, F., Gaitan, L., and Davey, K.R. (1999). Localization of speech arrest with transcranial magnetic brain stimulation. *J. Clin. Neurophysiol.* 110 (6), 1073–9.

Eyre, J.A., Miller, S., and Ramesh, V. (1991). Constancy of central conduction delays during development in man: investigation of motor and somatosensory pathways. *J. Physiol.* 434, 441–52.

Fierro, B., Brighina, F., Oliveri, M., Piazza, A., La Bua, V., Buffa, D., and Bisiach, E. (2000). Contralateral neglect induced by right posterior parietal rTMS in healthy subjects. *Neuroreport* 11, 1519–21.

Flament, D., Hall, E.J., and Lemon, R.J. (1992). The development of corticomotorneuronal projections investigated using magnetic brain stimulation in the infant macaque. *J. Physiol.* 447, 755–68.

Flitman, S.S., Grafman, J., Wassermann, E.M., Cooper, V., O'Grady, J., Pascual-Leone, A., and Hallett, M. (1998). *Neurology* 50, 175–81.

Friedman-Hill, S.R., Robertson, L.C., and Treisman, A. (1995). Parietal contributions to visual feature binding: evidence from a patient with bilateral lesions. *Science* 269, 853–5.

Gomez-Tortosa, E., Pascual-Leone, A., Grafman, J., Alway, D., Nichelli, P., and Hallett, M. (1993). Induction of transient hemiattention to visual stimuli by rapid-rate transcranial magnetic stimulation (rTMS) of parietal areas. *Neurology* 43, A345.

Hotson, J.R. and Anand, S. (1999). The selectivity and timing of motion processing in human temporo-parieto-occipital cortex: a transcranial magnetic stimulation study. *Neuropsychologia* 37 (2), 169–80.

Hotson, M., Braun, D., Herzberg, W., and Boman, D. (1994). Transcranial magnetic stimulation of extrastriate cortex degrades human motion direction discrimination. *Vision Res.* 34, 2115–23.

Ilmoniemi, R.J., Virtanen, J., Ruohonen, J., Karhu, J., Aronen, H.J., Naatanen, R., and Katila, T. (1997). Neuronal responses to magnetic stimulation reveal cortical reactivity and connectivity. *NeuroReport* 8, 3537–40.

Jalinous, R. (1991). Technical and practical aspects of magnetic nerve stimulation. *J. Clin. Neurophysiol.* 8, 10–25.

Jennum P., Friberg, L., Fuglsang-Frederiksen, A., and Dam, M. (1994). Speech localization using repetitive transcranial magnetic stimulation. *Neurology* 44, 269–73.

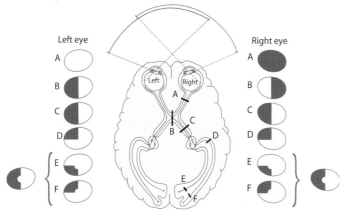

Plate 1 Visual field defects (scotomata) caused by lesions at different levels of the visual system. Retinal lesions produce unilateral, incongruent scotomata in the affected eyes (and hemifields), and so do optic nerve defects (A). Lesions of the chiasm (B), optic tract, lateral geniculate nucleus (LGN), and optic radiation (D, E, F) produce lesions only in the contralesional hemifield that are roughly congruent, i.e. cover the same area when tested monocularly. The same is true for the primary, or striate, visual cortex, area 17. Lesions of extrastriate cortical areas often create blindness in one quadrant while the other one is spared, due to the fact that the representations of the upper and lower visual field are separated in extrastriate cortical areas (cf. Fig. 7.7). From Fahle (2003b). (See Fig. 7.1.)

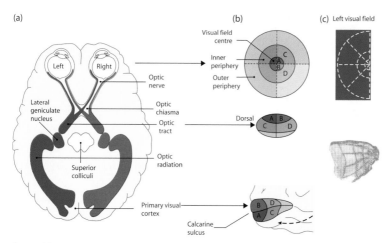

Plate 2 (a) Projection from both halves of both retinae to the LGN and primary visual cortex. (b, c) Topography of the projection of the visual world on to the primary visual cortex. The centre of gaze, corresponding to the fovea, is represented at the occipital pole; the horizontal meridian, i.e. the horizontal line running through the centre of gaze, is represented in the depth of the calcarine fissure that runs almost horizontally on the medial side of the occipital cortex (cf. Plate 3). The vertical meridian, the vertical line running through the centre of gaze, separates the projection to the right hemisphere from that to the left hemisphere. It is represented *parallel* both above and below the horizontal meridian. This is to say that each primary visual cortex contains a map of the visual world resembling a (spherical) Mercator's projection, with the fovea corresponding to one of the poles, and the vertical and horizontal meridians corresponding to, say, the 0° (horizontal) and the 90° and 270° deg meridians (vertical); ((c), lower part). Visualization of the projection to the primary visual cortex. The stimulus displayed in the upper part of the graph produces the cortical activation displayed in the lower part (compare also Fig. 7.4). (After Fahle 2003b; (c) after Tootell et al. (1982).) (See Fig. 7.2.)

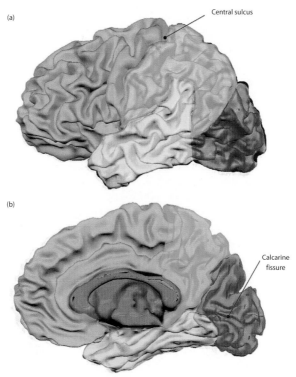

Plate 3 (a) Lateral view of a human brain (that of the author) representing the surface between cortical grey and underlying white matter. Blue, frontal lobe; green, parietal lobe; yellow, temporal lobe; red, occipital lobe, (b) Medial view of the same brain. (See Fig. 7.3.)

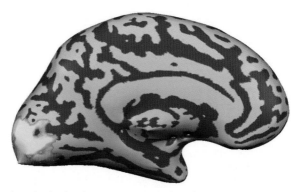

Plate 4 Representation of a simulated scotoma as it appears in functional magnetic imaging during stimulation through the right eye. Visual cortex is stimulated by means of a contrast-reversing checkerboard extending in the right half of the visual field from the fovea to about 25 deg. eccentricity, with a blank area without flicker. This artificial scotoma was located at 15 deg. eccentricity and had a diameter around 5 deg., roughly corresponding to the blind spot. For details regarding the method of functional magnetic resonance imaging, see Chapter 4, this volume. (See Fig. 7.8.)

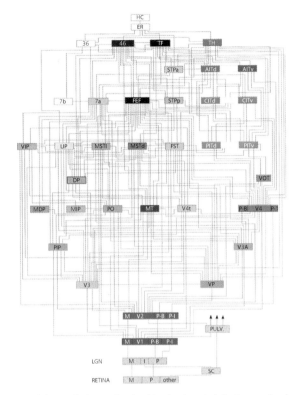

Plate 5 Schematic view of the cortical areas involved in visual analysis in the monkey brain, based on the pattern of axonal connections between areas, as well as on differences in cytoarchitectonic and electrophysiological properties of single neurons. (From van Essen *et al.* (1992).) (See Fig. 7.9.)

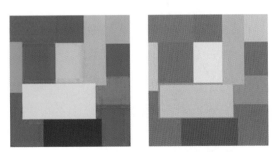

Plate 6 To the left is a chromatic Mondrian pattern and, to the right, its achromatic counterpart. (See Fig. 8.2.)

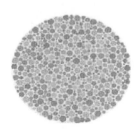

Plate 7 An Ishihara plate is composed of small circles with random luminance variation. The numeral is defined by colour difference. (See Fig. 8.3.)

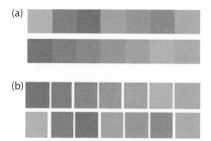

(a)

(b)

Plate 8 (a) The lower figure is a row of abutting equiluminant patches ordered in chromaticity. Above, the identical patches are presented as a jumbled array. Although M.S. was unable to discriminate between any of the constituent patches, he was able to discriminate between the ordered and jumbled arrays. In (b) the patches no longer abut and M.S. can no longer tell the arrays apart. (See Fig. 8.4.)

Plate 9 The figure is composed of an achromatic checker-board (draught board) in which a green cross is embedded. When the luminance of each square is rapidly varied from moment to moment, M.S. effortlessly detects the location of the green cross. The rapid fluctuation in luminance, to which the M-channel is sensitive, would render it ineffective in detecting the chromatic contour. Detection must presumably be mediated by a preserved P- or K-channel. (See Fig. 8.5.)

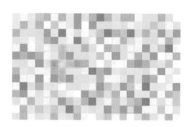

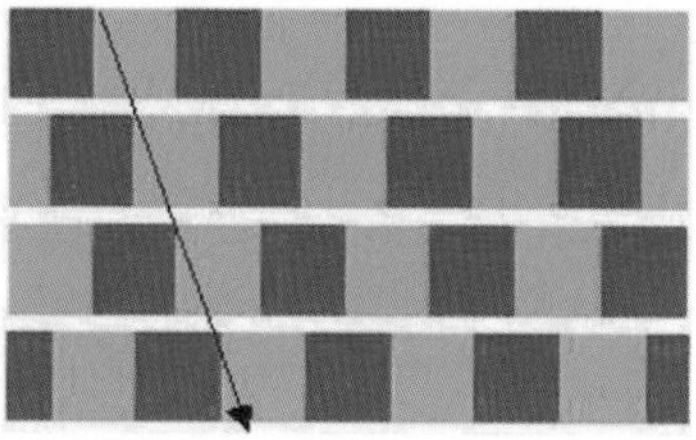

Plate 10 The figure shows four successively presented frames of an equiluminant display where the phase of the pattern is shifted a quarter of a cycle. The direction of motion (left-to-right) can only be ascertained by matching successive green/red borders. If red/green and green/red borders cannot be distinguished, the direction of motion will be ambiguous. (See Fig. 8.7.)

Plate 11 (c) shows an equiluminant chromatic grating constructed by sinusoidally modulating red and green in spatial antiphase, as shown in (a). Where red and green are mixed in equal proportion, creating yellow, the grating will appear dimmer because of brightness subadditivity. (d) and (e) show two examples of gratings where luminance had been added as shown in (a) to compensate for the effects of subadditivity. A drifting equiluminant grating will appear to move considerably more slowly than a luminance grating (f) drifting at the same speed. By adding an appropriate amount of luminance compensation, the grating is perceived as moving even *more* slowly by both M.S. and normal observers. Since subadditivity is the result of P-channel colour-opponency, this implies that M.S. retains intact colour input into the motion system. (See Fig. 8.8.)

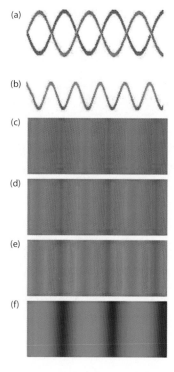

(a)

(b)

(c)

(d)

(e)

(f)

Kinsbourne, M. (1977). Hemi-neglect and hemisphere rivalry. *Advan. Neurol.* 18, 41–9.

Luck, S.J. and Hillyard, S.A. (1994). Electrophysiological correlates of feature analysis during visual search. *Psychophysiology* 31, 291–308.

Lueck, C.J., Zeki, S., Friston, K.J., Deiber, M.P., Cope, P., Cunningham, V.J., Lammertsma, A.A., Kennard, C., and Frackowiak, R.S. (1989). The colour centre in the cerebral cortex of man. *Nature* 340, 386–9.

Maccabee, P.J., Eberle, L., Amassian, V.E., Cracco, R.Q., Rudell, A., and Jayachandra, M. (1990). Spatial distribution of the electric field induced in volume by round and Figure 8 magnetic coils: relevance to activation of sensory nerve fibres. *Electroencephalogr. Clin. Neurophysiol.* 76, 131–41.

Michelucci, R., Valzania, F., Passarelli, D., Santangelo, M., Rizzi, R., Buzzi, A.M., Tempestini, A., and Tassinari, C.A. (1994). Rapid-rate transcranial magnetic stimulation and hemispheric language dominance: usefulness and safety in epilepsy. *Neurology* 44, 1697–700.

Mikami, A., Newsome ,W.T., and Wurtz, R.H. (1986). Motion selectivity in macaque visual cortex. I. Mechanisms of direction and speed selectivity in extrastriate area MT. *J. Neurophysiol.* 55 (6), 1308–27.

Mottaghy, F.M., Hungs, M., Brugmann, M., Sparing, R., Boroojerdi, B., Foltys, H., Huber, W., and Topper, R. (1999). Facilitation of picture naming after repetitive transcranial magnetic stimulation. *Neurology* 53, 1806–12.

Oliveri, M., Rossinin, P.M., Traversa, R., Cicinella, P., Filippi, M.M., Pasqualetti, P., Tomaiulo, F., and Caltagirone, C. (1999). Left frontal transcranial magnetic stimulation reduces contralateral extinction in patients with unilateral right brain damage. *Brain* 122, 1731–9.

Pascual-Leone, A. and Torres, F. (1993). Plasticity of the sensorimotor cortex representation of the reading finger in Braille readers. *Brain* 116, 39–52.

Pascual-Leone, A. and Walsh, V. (2001). Fast backprojections from the motion to the primary visual area necessary for visual awareness. *Science* 292, 510–12.

Pascual-Leone, A., Houser, C.M., Reese, K., Shotland, L.I., Grafman, J., Sato, S., Valls-Sole, J., Brasil-Neto, J.P., Wasserman, E.M., and Cohen, L.G. *et al.* (1993). Safety of rapid-rate transcranial magnetic stimulation in normal volunteers. *J. Electroencephalogr. Clin. Neurophysiol.* 89, 120–30.

Pascual Leone, A., Gomez Tortosa, E., Grafman, J., Alway, D., Nichelli, P., and Hallett, M. (1994). Induction of visual extinction by rapid-rate transcranial magnetic stimulation of parietal lobe. *Neurology* 44, 494–8.

Pascual-Leone, A., Tarazona, F., and Keenan, J. (1999). Transcranial magnetic stimulation and neuroplasticity. *Neuropsychologia* 37 (2), 207–17.

Paus, T., Jech, R., Thompson, C J., Comceau, R., Peters, T., and Evans, A.C. (1997). Transcranial magnetic stimulation during positron emission tomography: a new method for studying connectivity of the human cerebral cortex. *J. Neurosci.* 17, 3178–84.

Penfield, W. and Rasmussen, T. (1949). Vocalization and arrest of speech. *Arch. Neurol. Psychiatry* 61, 21–7.

Reppas, J.B., Niyogi, S., Dale, S.M., Sereno, M.I., and Tootell, R.B.H. (1997). Representation of motion boundaries in retinotopic human visual cortical areas. *Nature* 388, 175.

Seyal, M., Ro, T., and Rafal, R. (1995). Increased sensitivity to ipsilateral cutaneous stimuli following transcranial magnetic stimulation of the parietal lobe. *Ann. Neurol.* 38, 264–7.

Smith, A.T., Greenlee, M.W., Singh, K.D., Kraemer, F.M., and Hennig, J. (1998). The processing of first- and second-order motion in human visual cortex assessed by, functional magnetic resonance imaging (fMRI). *J. Neurosci.* 18 (10), 3816–30.

Stewart, L.M, Battelli, L., Walsh, V., and Cowey, A. (1999). Motion perception and perceptual learning: a magnetic stimulation study. *J. Electroencephalogr. Clin. Neurophysiol.* 51, 34–50.

Tootell, R.B.H., Reppas, J.B., Dale, A.M., Look, R.B., Sereno, M.I., Malach, R., Brady, T.J., and Rosen, B.R. (1995). Visual motion after effect in human cortical area MT revealed by functional magnetic resonance imaging. *Nature* 375, 139–41.

Topper, R., Mottaghy, F., Brugmann, M., Noth, J., and Huber, W. (1998). Facilitation of picture naming by focal transcranial magnetic stimulation of Wernicke's area. *Exp. Brain Res.* 121, 371–8.

Walsh, V. (2000). Reverse engineering the human brain. *Phil. Trans. R. Soc. A* 358, 497–511.

Walsh, V. and Cowey, A. (1998). Magnetic stimulation studies of visual cognition. *Trends Cogn. Sci.* 2, 103–10.

Walsh, V. and Rushworth, M. (1999). A primer of magnetic stimulation as a tool for neuropsychology. *Neuropsychologia* 37 (2), 125–36.

Walsh, V., Ashbridge, E., and Cowey, A. (1998a). Cortical plasticity in perceptual learning demonstrated by transcranial magnetic stimulation. *Neuropsychologia* 36, 45–9.

Walsh, V., Ellison, A., Battelli, L., and Cowey, A. (1998b). Task-specific impairments and enhancements induced by magnetic stimulation of human visual area V5. *Proc. R. Soc. Lond. B* 265, 537–43.

Wassermann, E.M. (1998). Risk and safety of repetitive transcranial magnetic stimulation: report and suggested guidelines from the International Workshop on the Safety of Repetitive Transcranial Magnetic Stimulation. *Electroencephaolgr. Clin. Neurophysiol.* 108 (1), 1–16.

Wassermann, E.M., Blaxton, T.A., Hoffman, E.A., Berry, C.D., Oletsky, H., Pascual-Leone, A., and Theodore, W.H. (1999). Repetitive transcranial magnetic stimulation of the dominant hemisphere can disrupt visual naming in temporal lobe epilepsy patients. *Neuropsychologia* 37, 537–44.

Watson, J.D, Myers, R., Frackowiak, R.S., Hajnal, J.V., Woods, R.P., Mazziotta, J.C., Shipp, S., and Zeki, S. (1993). Area V5 of the human brain: evidence from a combined study using positron emission tomography and magnetic resonance imaging. *Cereb. Cortex* 3 (2), 79–94.

Zeki, S., Watson, J.D.G., Lueck, C.J., Friston, K.J., Kennard, C., and Frackowiak, R.S.J. (1991). A direct demonstration of functional specialization in human visual cortex. *J. Neurosci.* 11, 641–9.

Part 5

Psychophysics: patient studies

Chapter 7

Failures of visual analysis: scotoma, agnosia, and neglect

Manfred Fahle

Introduction

This chapter covers different types of failure to analyse the visual world, starting with the complete loss of vision, *blindness*, as well as blindness for circumscribed parts of the visual field, *scotomata*. These disturbances of visual perception can be adequately assessed by different perimetric methods. But vision is disturbed in some patients even though they are able to detect bright points—the method used to assess the visual field in clinical tests (perimetry). These patients will show normal results in perimetry in spite of severe problems of visual perception.

'Vision' is not just one single unified capacity, but has many components, partly sub-served by different cortical areas. The number of separate and functionally distinct visual cortical areas may be above 40 or even 50. Defects of different areas may lead to specific symptoms characterized by relatively distinct deficits of visual perception, e.g. difficulties in discriminating colours, perceiving motion, seeing depth, or discriminating retinal image motion due to eye movements from motion due to object movements.

The second part of the chapter presents some syndromes characterized by difficulties in perceiving of and discriminating between different domains or submodalities of vision, while leaving most others intact, such as acquired inability to assess visual motion, or acquired colour blindness caused by cerebral damage (achromatopsia, see also Chapter 8, this volume).

On a more complex level of image analysis, the features detected in the different sub-modalities have to be bound together to segregate figures from their surround and to create object representations. I will argue that this process of object synthesis is heavily influenced by prior learning and experience and involves not only button-up processing governed by the sensory input but also top–down influences from 'higher' processing levels, making it difficult to find intact low-level analysis even if exclusively higher-level centres have been damaged.

Finally, the visual object representations formed in the cortex have to be matched with stored representations of objects in order to identify the class and possibly the identity of the object perceived. Problems in object formation are traditionally called agnosias, and a short survey of the different types will be given in the third part (see also Chapter 10, this volume). The individual steps of visual analysis may not be separated from each other as clearly as outlined above, due to the reflexive nature of cortical pattern analysis, with strong feedback from higher stages of analysis on earlier stages, but the deficits are still sufficiently different to justify—and to require—a distinction between these syndromes.

The chapter ends with an overview of the most astonishing examples—in my view—of failed visual perception: simultanagnosia; neglect; and Balint's syndrome. These syndromes share the phenomenon that conscious perception of objects in (parts of) the peripheral visual field is absent in spite of intact stimulation of the primary visual cortex by these objects.

It would be a great advantage if precise knowledge about the normal function of the visual system and about visual perception could supply us with a sound framework to classify all the different symptoms encountered in patients and to precisely infer structural brain defects from behavioural symptoms, and vice versa. As it stands, such a detailed knowledge of the exact operations taking place during analysis of visual scenes is still fragmentary in spite of recent advances in neurobiological research. These advances, many of which are outlined in the first part of this book (see especially Chapters 1, 2, and 5), indeed help to understand the sometimes puzzling symptoms encountered in neuropsychological patients. I will try to fill in some gaps of knowledge by means of speculation in the following section to produce a consistent taxonomy of symptoms encountered in visual neuropsychology. Hopefully, the resulting picture will be at least consistent and plausible to some readers. Overall, the chapter will combine the theoretical background with clinical findings and with a description of at least some of the methods used to diagnose patients suffering from failures of visual analysis.

Blindness, scotomata, and visual information processing

Complete failure to see: blindness and scotomata

Certainly the most severe and fundamental disturbance of visual perception is blindness, the complete lack of subjective perception and of responsiveness to visual stimulation—hence an apparent failure of visual analysis. Blindness may occur not only for the entire visual field, but also parts of the field may become blind while others still elicit a perception. Hence, testing visual acuity, the resolution limit at the centre of the visual field, is not at all sufficient to assess visual function in patients suffering from lesions of the visual system. The entire visual field has to be tested. Circumscribed areas of 'blindness' are called scotomata. They can be the result of lesions on the level of the retina, optic nerve, lateral geniculate nucleus (LGN), optic radiation, or visual cortex.

On the retinal level radiation coming from visual objects is transformed to activate neurons and some early image processing is achieved such as enhancement of luminance- and hue-contrasts. Lesions on this level result in scotomata of just the affected eye. Defects in the right and left retinae usually subtend over noncorresponding visual field

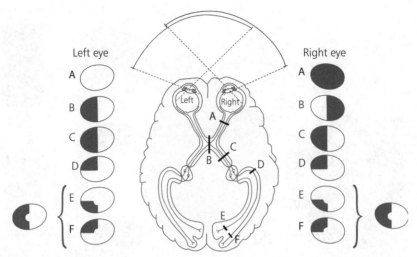

Fig. 7.1 Visual field defects (scotomata) caused by lesions at different levels of the visual system. Retinal lesions produce unilateral, incongruent scotomata in the affected eyes (and hemifields), and so do optic nerve defects (A). Lesions of the chiasm (B), optic tract, lateral geniculate nucleus (LGN), and optic radiation (D, E, F) produce lesions only in the contralesional hemifield that are roughly congruent, i.e. cover the same area when tested monocularly. The same is true for the primary, or striate, visual cortex, area 17. Lesions of extrastriate cortical areas often create blindness in one quadrant while the other one is spared, due to the fact that the representations of the upper and lower visual field are separated in extrastriate cortical areas (cf. Fig. 7.7). From Fahle (2003b). (See Plate 1, colour plate section.)

portions of both eyes. These scotomata, for example, result from increased intraocular pressure (glaucoma) or from deficits in blood supply to the retina or optic nerve.

Lesions of the optic nerve peripheral to the partial crossing-over of fibres at the optic chiasm (Fig. 7.1) usually cause visual field defects for only one eye, while those beyond the chiasm, i.e. in the optic tract, lead to corresponding, or congruent scotomata in both eyes. The same is true for lesions located in the LGN, the optic radiation, and the visual cortex. Figure 7.1 summarizes the effects of lesions of the visual system on the visual fields of the patients. It should be noted that lesions of the optic tract and optic radiation generally produce scotomata less congruent in the two eyes than lesions of (primary) visual cortex do, since fibres from the two eyes seem to finally converge to form a retinotopic map only in the cortex (Walsh and Hoyt, 1969; see, however, Teuber *et al.* 1960). Hence fibres from corresponding locations of both retinae may not necessarily run very close to each other in the optic radiation.

The cortical representation of the fovea is located at the posterior pole of the brain, i.e. in the occipital cortex. The representation of the horizontal meridian, i.e. the horizontal line in the visual field through the fixation point, is represented in the depth of the calcarine fissure (Fig. 7.2) which runs through the medial bank of the occipital

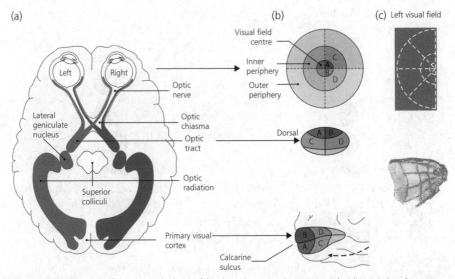

Fig 7.2 (a) Projection from both halves of both retinae to the LGN and primary visual cortex. (b, c) Topography of the projection of the visual world on to the primary visual cortex. The centre of gaze, corresponding to the fovea, is represented at the occipital pole; the horizontal meridian, i.e. the horizontal line running through the centre, is represented in the depth of the calcarine fissure that runs almost horizontally on the medial side of the occipital cortex (cf. Fig. 7.3). The vertical meridian, the vertical line running through the centre of gaze, separates the projection to the right hemisphere from that to the left hemisphere. It is represented *parallel* above and below the horizontal meridian. This is to say that each primary visual cortex contains a map of the visual world resembling a (spherical) Mercator's projection, with the fovea corresponding to one of the poles, and the vertical and horizontal meridians corresponding to, say, the 0° (horizontal) and the 90° and 270° deg meridians (vertical); ((c), lower part). Visualization of the projection to the primary visual cortex. The stimulus displayed in the upper part of the graph produces the cortical activation displayed in the lower part (compare also Fig. 7.4). (After Fahle 2003b; (c) after Tootell *et al.* (1982).) (See Plate 2, colour plate section.)

cortex, close to the midsagittal plane of the brain (cf. Fig. 7.3). In the early nineteenth century, neuropsychological investigations by a Japanese ophthalmologist, Tatsuji Inouye (translation: Glickstein and Fahle 2000; see also Wilbrand 1887, 1890; Wilbrand and Sänger 1904, 1917; Henschen 1896; Kleist 1923; Mingazzini 1908; Munk 1878; Foerster 1890), on patients suffering from circumscribed gun-shot wounds of the occipital cortex revealed this representation. Inouye's investigation, moreover, showed that: (1) the central visual field (1–3°) is overrepresented in the primary visual cortex: its representation occupies almost one-quarter of this cortex (Fig. 7.4 is overly conservative in this respect); (2) the upper part of the visual cortex, on the upper lip of the calcarine fissure, represents the lower half of the visual field, while the lower part represents the upper part of the visual field; and (3) the representation of the vertical meridian, the vertical line through the fixation point separating the left from the right visual

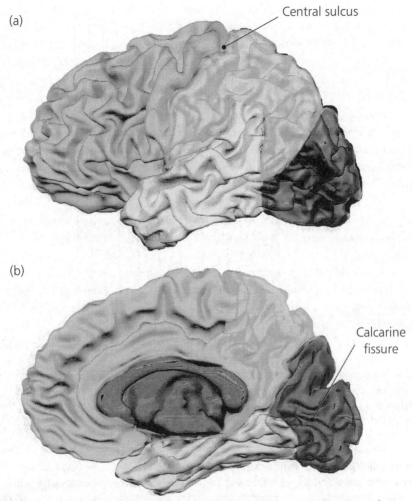

(a)

Central sulcus

(b)

Calcarine
fissure

Fig. 7.3 (a) Lateral view of a human brain (that of the author) representing the surface between cortical grey and underlying white matter. Blue, frontal lobe; green, parietal lobe; yellow, temporal lobe; red, occipital lobe, (b) Medial view of the same brain. (See Plate 3, colour plate section for colour coding.)

field, runs *parallel* to the horizontal meridian and separates the primary visual cortex, Brodmann area BA17 (Fig. 7.5) from the secondary projection, BA18 (Fig. 7.4; Glickstein and Fahle 2000). In many patients, a foveal sparing with a diameter of 0.5–2° is found in blindness of one-half of the visual field, i.e. hemianopia. The underlying cause may be a bilateral cortical representation of the fovea or else a double blood supply for the foveal representation in the primary visual cortex.

Injuries of all structures up to the optic radiation lead to a deficient *transmission* of information towards the visual cortex, while injuries of the visual cortex lead to a

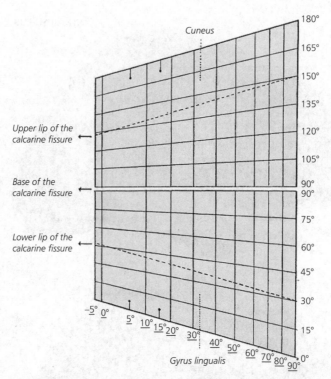

Fig. 7.4 Visual field representation on the human primary visual cortex as deduced from investigations on gunshot wounds by nineteenth century ophthalmologist Inouye (from Glickstein and Fahle 2000). The upper part of the visual scene (0°–90°) is represented in the lower part of the calcarine fissure while the lower part of the visual surround (90°–180°) is represented in the upper part of the primary visual cortex. Hence, the lower part of the vertical meridian separates the primary visual cortex from the dorsal (upper) part of area 18, while the upper part of the vertical meridian is represented on the border between the primary visual cortex and the ventral (lower) portion of area 18, the first extrastriate visual area. As a consequence, only the primary visual cortex contains a continuous representation of the contralateral visual field while the extrastriate areas above and below the calcarine fissure each only represent one quadrant of the visual field. (0° indicates fovea; 90° outer border of visual field.)

deficient cortical *representation* of parts of the visual field. This distinction is important for rehabilitation (see Chapter 11, this volume). In the case of, say, a retinal defect, the information regarding the corresponding part of the visual field does not even enter the visual system, and there is no possibility of retrieving it by *adaptive* processes in the brain. (Recovery of function in partially damaged fibres will, of course, improve performance in all types of patients.) On the other hand, defects of representation due to an injury of circumscribed portions of the (primary) visual cortex can, in principle, be overcome by other cortical neurons taking over the analysis of the information from the defective cortical representation areas (cf. Eysel 2002; Gilbert and Wiesel 1992;

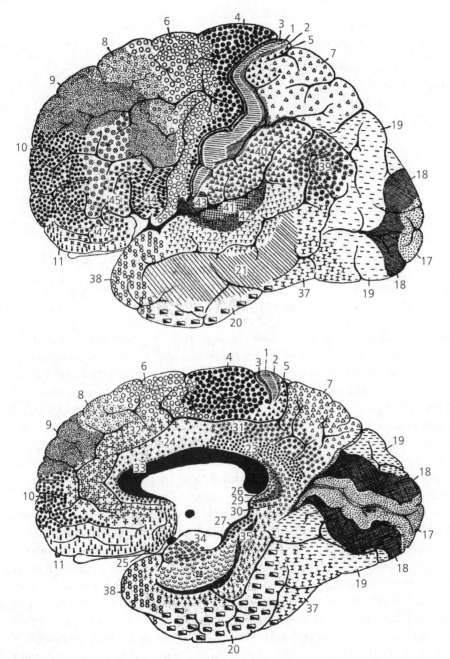

Fig. 7.5 Segmentation of the human cortex on the basis of cytoarchitecture (from Brodmann (1909)).

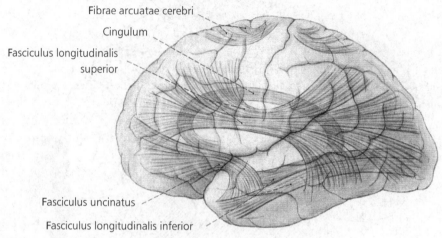

Fibrae arcuatae cerebri

Cingulum

Fasciculus longitudinalis superior

Fasciculus uncinatus

Fasciculus longitudinalis inferior

Fig. 7.6 Main fibre tracts in the human brain.

Fahle and Poggio 2002). Hence, there can be hope for improvement through active restructuring of cortical connectivity after cerebral lesions, while this is not the case for lesions of the retina and optic nerve. Only little hope exists for lesions of LGN and optic radiation since most (90%) of retinal fibres project through these structures, and it is unclear how much visual information is conveyed through other pathways, including the superior colliculus (see Chapters 2, 5, and 9 this volume, and Fig. 7.6). For deficits in reception (retina) or transmission of visual information (optic nerve, tract, radiation, LGN), the only hope presently seems to lie in compensatory behaviours that enable the patients to better cope with their deficits. In the future, neural prostheses and/or transplantations may provide further help.

As mentioned above, optic nerve fibres partly cross at the chiasm, and the crossing fibres stem from the nasal retina representing the temporal half of the visual field. As a consequence, the primary visual cortex of each hemisphere represents the contralateral half of the visual field, and a complete loss of one hemisphere leads to complete blindness in the corresponding half of the visual field, the so-called homonymous hemianopia. Hemianopias often—but not always—are associated with problems of space exploration, with increased latencies for eye movements towards the blind hemifield, and an almost random rather than systematic visual search of the space contralateral to the lesion. Smaller lesions of visual cortex often lead to homonymous quadrantanopia, the loss of vision in one quadrant of the visual field. The reason is that the representations of the upper and lower quadrants are relatively well segregated: there are at least three representations of the upper quadrant bellow the calcarine fissure in cortical areas 17, 18, and 19 (see Fig. 7.7(a)), while the three or more representations of the lower visual field quadrant are represented above the calcarine fissure in separate parts of areas 17, 18, and 19 (Fig. 7.7(b), cf. also Fig. 7.4).

As a rule, the size of scotomata is unrelated to visual acuity, as long as the fovea is spared (Lenz 1909; Wilbrand and Sänger 1917). Not surprisingly, patients are most debilitated by lesions in the centre of the visual field where resolution is best in healthy observers. The acuity loss caused by foveal lesions will, e.g. make reading difficult or even impossible and hinder object discrimination in general.

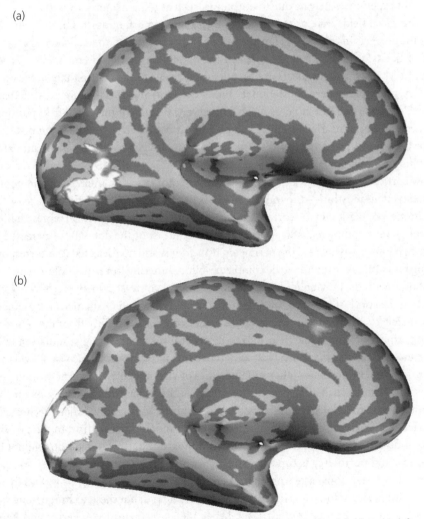

(a)

(b)

Fig. 7.7 Representation of the upper right quadrant of the author's visual field on his left cortical hemisphere as revealed by functional magnetic resonance imaging. (a) The cortical surface has been partly flattened to visualize the cortical areas buried in the sulci, too (Brain Voyager Software), (b) Representation of the lower visual field quadrant in the same observer.

Visual field testing: perimetry

To assess visual function, testing visual acuity is not sufficient, as mentioned above. While acuity is a very sensitive indicator of the quality of the eye's optical system and of foveal function at the centre of the retina, it only tests a small portion of the visual field and hence of the visual system. Patients are often not aware of defects in their visual fields, similar to our unawareness of the physiological blind spot in the temporal field of view. Hence, testing of the entire visual field is important in patients suffering from symptoms in the field of visual neuropsychology. At least part of the problems the patient experiences may be due to a scotoma, such as in hemianopic dyslexia.

The visual fields were originally tested by bringing in bright objects of different size from the periphery, and by marking at what distance from the centre, i.e. at what eccentricity, they were first detected by the patient (Aubert and Foerster 1857; von Graefe 1856). Smaller objects are first detected closer to the centre than larger ones. Today, many perimeters use stationary rather than moving dots that are presented at a contrast just above threshold of normal observers for each of the visual field positions tested (Aulhorn and Harms 1972). If a patient cannot detect a dot at a given position, this failure indicates a relative damage in the ability to detect differences in luminance at this visual field position and, hence to detect luminance contrast there. (Why and how cortical lesions can lead to diffuse relative scotomata is an interesting and poorly investigated question—one must assume destruction of a (large) percentage of the neuronal population in the corresponding afferent fibre tracts or cortical representation rather than a complete eradication.) Next, the contrast of the dot will be increased to the maximum possible for the perimeter. If the dot is still not detected, the corresponding retinal area is assumed to be completely blind, suffering from an absolute scotoma.

Both methods, moving in dots of defined size and contrast (kinetic perimetry) and testing the contrast required for detection at a given position (static perimetry), make it possible to quantitatively assess the decline of contrast sensitivity from the centre to the periphery of the visual field, and to detect regions where visual stimulation fails. Perimetry is a standard clinical test and, if patients pass this test, their visual fields are considered to be normal—other submodalities of vision such as colour or motion perception are not usually tested in the periphery of the visual field. The reasons for this limitation are manifold. Testing for motion detection is much more difficult technically, patients suffering from isolated defects of, say, motion perception in part of the visual field are rare (and, since this is not a standard test, the few who do will not be found), and perimetry is time-consuming and not popular with patients anyway. There have been some attempts to measure flicker fusion frequency as well as form, orientation, and colour discrimination in the visual field, but these techniques are not used in clinical practice (Aubert 1857; Leber 1869; Wertheim 1894; Ferree and Rand 1920; Aulhorn and Harms 1972; Teuber et al. 1960). Today, it is possible to test the visual field in addition by means of more objective methods, e.g. in patients unable to cooperate. The methods employed are monitoring the pupil response to presentation

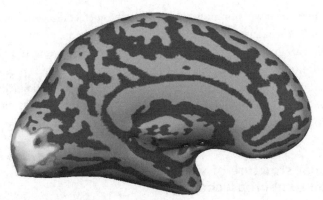

Fig. 7.8 Representation of a simulated scotoma as it appears in functional magnetic imaging of the author's right hemisphere during stimulation through the right eye. Visual cortex is stimulated by means of a contrast-reversing checkerboard extending, in the right half of the visual field, from the fovea to about 25 deg. eccentricity, with a blank area, without flicker. This artificial scotoma was located at 15 deg. eccentricity and had a diameter around 5 deg., corresponding to the blind spot. For details regarding the method of functional magnetic resonance imaging, see Chapter 4, this volume. (See Plate 4, colour plate section.)

of either luminance- or pattern-defined stimuli (Barbur 1995) or testing the cortical response to visual stimuli by sum potential recordings that may even differentiate between the contributions of different parts of the visual field (Slotnick *et al.* 2001; see also Chapter 3, this volume) or by functional magnetic resonance imaging (fMRI; see Fig. 7.8 for an example of a scotoma, see also Chapter 4, this volume).

The patients' task during perimetry is to gaze steadily at a central fixation point and not to move their eyes while a bright dot is presented sequentially often at a hundred or more different positions in the visual field. Whenever the dot appears, the patient is required to press a button, while not being allowed to look at the newly appeared dot, as would be the 'natural' reaction. If there are one or several scotomata, the dots within these regions will not be perceived and are presented not just once, but several times, to discriminate between absolute and relative scotomata, further increasing examination time to 15 minutes and more per eye. Recent advances trying to make perimetry more 'physiological' include the use of eye-tracking. In this method, the eye of the patient is tracked by a camera and its position measured by a computer. The patient looks at points appearing on a monitor, i.e. he or she performs a saccadic eye movement towards the point (Repnow *et al.* 1995). If the computer detects a correct direction and amplitude of this saccade, the new dot is considered to be located in an intact portion of the visual field—an assumption not necessarily true as is evident from the phenomenon of blindsight (see Chapter 9, this volume). However, the number of patients showing blindsight spontaneously and with sufficient spatial resolution is low enough not to pose a practical problem. Moreover, even patients suffering from visual field defects with blindsight will not move their eyes in the correct direction unless forced to make a saccade in whatever direction but will wait for the next dot they consciously perceive. This 'gaze'-perimetry is: (1) somewhat faster than the conventional perimetry based on button-pressing; (2) less exhausting for the patient; and (3) uses a monitor to present the stimuli so that the method can, in principle, test the visual field not just for contrast detection. The stimulus serving as the target can be defined by motion among stationary dots, by a (slightly) differing colour, by stereoscopic depth, or a multitude of other features.

The modular structure of visual cortices and its relation to neuropsychology

A failure of visual stimulus analysis can follow not just from blindness for the part of the visual field where the stimulus is presented, as is the case with a scotoma. The failure can also be due to a failure to discriminate the stimulus, i.e. the figure, from its surround. For example, a stimulus that differs from its surround not by its luminance but by a different stimulus attribute such as colour can only be detected by a colour-sensitive mechanism. This type of patient would not be blind at any position of the visual field, and perimetry might yield normal results since it only tests the patient's ability to discriminate between two luminances and, hence, his or her sensitivity for luminance contrast. Still, colour, or motion, or stereodetection might be defective, leading to a circumscribed defect of the corresponding submodality in part of the visual field. These types of defects will be discussed in detail at the beginning of the section on 'Visual indiscriminations'. Here I will give a short overview of the neuronal basis and some explanations why these defects are still incompletely understood.

During the last decades, electrophysiological investigations in animals (see Chapters 1, 2, and 5, this volume) and later functional Magnetic Resonance Imaging, fMRI (see Chapter 4, this volume) have greatly refined the cytoarchitectonic map initially developed by Brodmann (1909; see Fig. 7.5). We now discriminate between about 40 different areas in the monkey cortex that are all involved in the analysis of the visual world and might represent different modules of processing (see Fig. 7.9). Many of these areas contain a complete topographically ordered representation of the (contralateral half of the) visual field, i.e. their own ordered map of the outer world. Why so many representations and not just one? Comparing the cortex of man with the cortices of less 'brainy' animals such as the cat shows that the primary projection cortices for visual, auditory, and somatosensory information constitute a much larger proportion of the brain in these (and other) animals than they do in man. Obviously, the primary sensory cortices are necessary to process the sensory information while the additional cortical areas, often called 'association' areas, add additional capabilities to (wo)man not available to simpler animals. It seems that, during evolution, some additional capabilities were built into the cortex—at least partly by duplicating existing areas and devoting them to new tasks. I would like to hypothesize that different cortical areas as

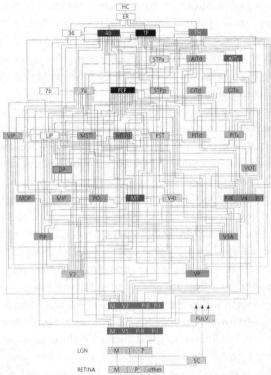

Fig. 7.9 Schematic view of the cortical areas involved in visual analysis in the monkey brain, based on the pattern of axonal connections between areas, as well as on differences in cytoarchitectonic and electrophysiological properties of single neurons. (From van Essen *et al.* (1992).) (See Plate 5, colour plate section.)

shown in Fig. 7.9 fulfil at least slightly different tasks during the analysis of the visual world—certainly not a very audacious hypothesis.

Destruction of each one of these areas should lead to a deficit in at least one aspect of visual perception (see the beginning of the section 'Visual indiscriminations' for a detailed analysis). These deficits might be quite subtle indeed since, beyond the primary visual cortex, at least some areas receive input from both hemispheres, and defects in one area of one hemisphere can be partly compensated for by the corresponding contralateral area. Moreover, the ensemble of areas works together and, as the results of fMRI investigations demonstrate very convincingly, most stimuli activate quite a number of different areas. So we cannot expect the same clear symptoms from destruction of any of these 'downstream' (i.e. 'higher'!) areas as we get from defects of the primary visual cortex, especially since the system has a fair amount of plasticity even in adults to (partly) compensate for lost functions, perhaps through other areas taking over part of the task. But we can expect that defects of these 'higher' cortical areas will nevertheless lead to partial failures of visual analysis for certain stimuli, and examples will be given below. These results clearly demonstrate that the view that introspection gives us on visual perception as being one unified entity is incorrect. Even though seeing the world appears to be a simple unitary process, this process has separable elements that may be damaged individually, leaving a view of the world that more or less selectively lacks one or several specific dimension(s).

Unfortunately, however, our knowledge about the exact contributions of almost all of these cortical areas is sparse, for a number of reasons. To start with, earlier researchers in neuropsychology quite often did not know the exact location of lesions in their patients, and only in relatively few patients could this localization be clarified after the patients' deaths. Today, this problem has been overcome by the improvements of imaging techniques that make possible to localize most cortical defects by recording the sum potentials reflecting brain activity (see Chapter 3, this volume), by computed tomography (CT), and especially by magnetic resonance imaging (MRI; see Figs 7.7 and 7.8, and Chapter 4, this volume). A second, still virulent problem is that we do not know exactly what and where the individual cortical areas lie that are homologous to the monkey's areas shown in Fig. 7.9. After all, our brains differ substantially from those of monkeys (thank goodness!) not only regarding the size and number of folds, but also regarding the arrangement of areas. (For example, the foveal representation in man is far more medial than in monkey, where it is situated on the lateral occipital cortex.) A third problem is that lesions in humans usually destroy more than one area, even if some of them only partially, and that fibres of passage between neighbouring areas might be destroyed, too. Hence, it is not surprising that patients seldom present 'pure' symptoms and that the exact relationships between the structure and function of visual cortical areas are still largely unknown.

Visual information-processing in the cortex: parallel processing and feedback

Given the rich and extended pattern of cortical areas analysing the visual world, strokes and other cortical injuries quite often involve parts of the 'visual' cortex that makes up, according to some estimates, around one-third of the human cortex. As we just saw, different parts of this system subserve different aspects of visual analysis and on different levels of abstraction. Over the last century, a solid body of descriptions has accumulated describing the resulting symptoms, and several systems to categorize them and to associate symptoms to different levels of (failed) analysis have emerged. The one used in this chapter is firmly based on these earlier systems, with a few modifications.

A failure of adequate response to visual stimulation in the absence of absolute scotomata—and usually intact colour-, motion-, and stereovision, i.e. failure of object analysis without severe loss in contour detection—is usually called an agnosia. An often-used distinction is between apperceptive and associative agnosias (Lissauer 1890 'Seelen blindheit'; cf. Chapter 10, this volume). In short, apperceptive agnosias describe problems on a more fundamental level of perception: patients are unable to form visual objects and to reliably segregate figure from ground (Benton and Tranel 1993). Patients suffering from associative agnosia, on the other hand, are able to perform this early step of pattern analysis, but fail to categorize the figure they segregated from its surround and hence fail to recognize the objects in spite of the fact that they are able to bind together the isolated features. These clinical syndromes will be described in detail in the section 'Apperceptive and associative agnosias', while some neuronal aspects are presented here.

Understanding neuropsychological symptoms in vision in full would require the understanding of the normal structure and function of the neuronal machinery that subserves visual perception. From the knowledge about this function outlined in Chapters 1, 2, and 5 in this volume, we now have a concept of cortical function quite different from that of a couple of decades ago. Cortical processing is no longer considered to be a one-way sequence of hierarchical levels of (increasingly complex and symbolic) information-processing, but rather a highly complex entity of feedforward and feedback projections (see especially Chapter 2). With such a view, which emphasizes the effects of top–down influences from 'higher' cortical areas to 'lower' ones, factors such as attention and expectation gain importance even for the very first steps of visual pattern analysis (e.g. Ullman 1995). A second important insight is the distributed and parallel processing of visual information in the cortex. Different aspects of stimuli are analysed in parallel processing streams (e.g. colour, motion; see Chapter 5, this volume), and we have good evidence for a partial separation between processing of contours versus (homogeneous) areas (see the next subsection and the later subsection 'Neuronal mechanisms for contour and position detection'; Welpe *et al.* 1980; Grossberg 1991; Paradiso and Nakayama 1991).

On the other hand, the brain uses not *maximally* distributed processing—if it would, as Lashley thought (see Bach *et al.* 1960), there would not exist any specific losses for specific functions such as colour or form perception, and neither would agnosias exist. The brain obviously processes similar features, or objects in nearby locations, so we find (visual) retinotopy, (auditory) tonotopy, and (somatosensory) somatotopy in primary sensory areas, as well as some type of 'object-topy' in higher areas, e.g. all faces seem to be processed in adjacent parts of the cortex, enabling the syndrome of (isolated) prosopagnosia (failure to recognize faces; see the eponymous section). As a consequence of the feedback nature of the system, the identification of an object seems to occur usually in an iterative way. First, in a very fast process, a preliminary hypothesis is produced about what type of object might be present. Thorpe *et al.* (1996) demonstrated that cortical potentials evoked by presentation of natural scenes containing animals versus those not containing animals start to differ from each other as early as 150 ms after the start of stimulus presentation. This is to say that, after such short time, the brain has already made a hypothetical decision about a rather complex dichotomy, namely, between animate and inanimate scenes. However, the pattern recognition task is by no means finished by that time, but higher security and precision of analysis require extensive additional computation.

Given these facts, it is not surprising that the electrical activities evoked by a visual stimulus in 'early' and 'higher' visual areas overlap over quite a substantial time, as is evident from Fig. 2.9 in Chapter 2, and it has been argued that the failure of agnosic patients to correctly identify objects may be due to the fact that they stop too early during the iterative process of object synthesis in the visual brain (Zihl and von Cramon 1986). Both theoretical (e.g. Hinton 1981) and empirical findings (e.g. Fahle and Poggio 2002) indicate moreover that processing and storage of information are not strictly separated in the brain: changing perceptual memory is associated with changing perception.

To sum up, anatomical, electrophysiological, and computational evidence all support a view of cortical pattern analysis as an iterative process involving the simultaneous activity of many cortical areas that deal with visual information-processing on different levels of complexity. This new view poses some problems for a clear-cut discrimination between the effects of associative disturbances on one hand and apperceptive ones on the other, since not only do disturbances on the level of perception hinder association, but also the other way round! This view of cortical processing immediately explains why it may be difficult to discriminate between apperceptive and associative agnosias in patients (see the section 'Apperceptive and associative agnosias'). Even if these defects involve different levels of information processing, the lower level will not function normally if the higher one is defective. Still, it seems fair to discriminate, not only computationally but also in the cortex, between different levels of processing in feature analysis and hence between different levels of defect. But we should always be aware that even lesions on 'high' levels of processing can have effects on performance on the 'low' levels, especially for difficult perceptual stimuli requiring iterative processing.

Different levels and separate channels of visual information-processing

In the following, I would like to propose an operational distinction between the different levels of visual analysis, loosely based on the modular structure of visual cortex as out-lined in the subsection on 'The modular structure of visual cortices' and the parallel pro-cessing as outlined in the preceding subsection. The first level achieves predominantly the *detection of contours*, or boundaries between areas, supplying information about the type of edge, its position, orientation, sharpness, and contrast—similar to the primal sketch of visual scenes proposed by Marr (1982). The perceived quality of areas defined by these boundaries is to a large extent determined by the information collected at these contour boundaries. An example for a feature extracted at this level is a difference in luminance (hence a luminance contrast), the feature tested in conven-tional perimetry. But a large number of features can contribute to contour definition, such as differences in colour, stereo-depth, motion direction, or velocity, and many more, often based on differences in texture (see the beginning of the section on 'Visual indiscriminations').

Two parallel systems seem to exist—one detecting boundaries (e.g. by means of spatial bandpass–filtering) and the other one representing (larger) areas (spatial

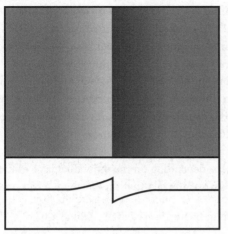

Fig. 7.10 Craik-O'Brian-Cornsweet illusion. While the areas on both far ends of the divide have exactly the same luminance (cover the middle part of the figure and you will see for yourself), they appear at different brightness. The reason is the sharp transition between high and low intensity which is clearly perceived by the visual system. The information on intensity collected at this border is extrapolated towards the adjacent area, while the slow gradient of luminosity that brings both areas back to identical intensity levels is largely ignored by the early stages of the visual system and is eventually eliminated. (From Fahle (2003a).)

lowpass-filter). Features such as colour, luminance, and texture, represented partly by an area-system, seem to be filled in into the areas delineated by the contours, and starting from the contours (Welpe *et al.* 1980; Paradiso and Nakayama 1991; Grossberg 1991). One striking demonstration is the Craik-O'Brien-Cornsweet illusion, where two fields of identical luminance appear in quite different brightness due to the fact that the areas close to the borders between the two fields have different contrast polarity (Fig. 7.10).

Another forceful argument for the pre-eminent importance of borders is the so-called stabilized image. Our eyes constantly perform irregular high-frequency, low-amplitude motions that move the retinal image of the outer world over short distances on the retina. If the image of the outer world is stabilized on the retina (say by immobilizing the eye), the world fades within a few dozens of seconds. Note that the stabilization will have no influence on those photoreceptors illuminated by homogeneous areas—their input stays constant anyway. The only receptors that will experience a difference between a stabilized and an unstabilized image are the ones at boundaries. While the moving contour prevents local adaptation of the underlying photoreceptors, this changes as soon as the boundaries are stabilized and local adaptation takes its toll.

While the boundary system is certainly the most important channel for visual information-processing, a second independent system probably exists which conveys information about areas (cf. the subsection 'Neuronal mechanisms for contour and position detection'; Welpe *et al.* 1980). Moreover, a second categorization is important: between a system analysing primarily colour and fine detail (P-system) and another one dealing primarily with motion signals and important for action (M-system; see

Ungerleider and Mishkin 1982; Milner and Goodale 1995; Westwood *et al.* 2002; Patla and Goodale 1996; Goodale *et al.* 1991; cf. also Ettlinger 1990; Vaina 1994).

The results of single-cell recordings in animals, mostly macaque monkeys, indicate that the striate cortex as well as early extrastriate areas subserve fundamental visual operations such as detection of contours, as well as analysis of orientation and spatial frequency (plus some forms of grouping and figure-ground segmentation, see below; Peterhans and von der Heydt 1991). Disturbances on this level of image processing, i.e. failures to detect and identify contours and borders, and to fill in the adjacent areas, are not usually called agnosias, but rather scotomata or visual field defects, or cerebral achromatopsia, or motion blindness, depending on the individual type of defect. As a general name for this class, and to stress the fact that they share a defect on the same

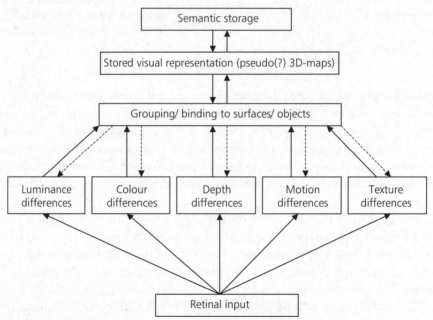

Fig. 7.11 Schematic overview of the levels of cortical information-processing and the symptoms arising from disturbances on the different levels. On the first level, boundaries are detected based on transitions in luminance, hue, (stereoscopic) depth, motion direction or speed, texture, or other cues, e.g. second-order features in these submodalities. Defects on this level lead to symptoms that are called indiscriminations. On the next level, contours, or boundaries are combined and bound together to form objects. Defects on this level lead to apperceptive agnosias. On a third level, the objects are compared with stored representations of objects encountered earlier, i.e. the present object is categorized and hence recognized. Defects on this level lead to associative agnosias, e.g. to prosopagnosia if only recognition of faces is defective, or alexia if the defect concerns words. The recognized object is usually linked to a noun (semantic storage). Missing of this link leads to optic aphasia.

level of processing—between complete blindness on one side and the intact detection of contours and areas without the ability to form objects on the other side (apperceptive agnosia; see the beginning of the section 'Apperceptive and associative agnosias')—I would propose the term 'indiscriminations' (see Fig. 7.11). These indiscriminations will be dealt with in detail in the first two subsections of 'Visual indiscriminations', while the third subsection presents methods to test these functions.

The second level is the *binding together* of individual contour elements to coherent objects. This is by no means an easy task in natural environments due to partial overlap between objects, shadows adding contours that do not represent object borders, and motion blur, to name a few problems. Disturbances on this level usually receive the label 'apperceptive agnosias'. The third level then would be *recognition* of the objects formed on the second level, mainly on the basis of the contour information collected on the first level. Disorders on this level are generally called associative agnosias (see the last two subsections of 'Apperceptive and associative agnosias'), since the association between the visual image and its stored representation has been lost. One may or may not continue to discriminate a fourth level that connects the recognized object with the appropriate noun, but this level may not be specific for *visual* neuropsychology. Disturbances on this fourth level are called optic aphasias (see the eponymous subsection), reflecting the fact that the object can be identified, but the connection to its name is lost (while the person still knows the correct noun; compare Mendola *et al.* 1999). As mentioned above, these levels cannot be separated during normal operation. They do not work sequentially but at least partly in synchrony, so defects on each of the levels will necessarily influence the operation of the other levels, even the 'lower' ones, at least when extremely difficult perceptual tasks have to be solved.

The above distinction of levels will serve as a useful way to categorize the symptoms of patients in visual neuropsychology, even if the levels cannot be separated from each other as precisely as one would like. Deficits on the level of binding together of contours, i.e. of object formation and object identification, will be discussed in the section 'Apperceptive and associative agnosias'.

Visual indiscriminations and failures of space representation

Visual indiscriminations: failures to extract (object) boundaries in visual scenes

Defects of detecting luminance and colour contrasts

There appears to be no unique role for *luminance contrast* in the detection of contours. Contours between objects can be defined by differences in hue, saturation, reflectance, stereoscopic depth, texture, motion velocity or motion direction of elements, time of appearance of elements, and quite a number of other, more complex features, such as the amount of variation in any of these domains over space and/or time (so-called second-order features; e.g. Zanker *et al.* 1998; Chapter 4, this book). But *luminance* contrast is the only feature contributing to contour detection that is routinely tested in clinical practice, mostly due to the fact that this test is technically easy to perform and that virtually all contours in natural environments have a contrast component—hence patients suffering from defects in detecting luminance contrast are most severely handicapped. Defects anywhere in the retina and along the visual pathways up to the primary visual cortex will produce defects in contrast detection as well as in all other submodalities that can contribute to contour detection. Hence, testing one dimension is sufficient to assess the damage. After all, detecting a luminance (or colour) contrast is a prerequisite for most other processes of feature analysis such as stereovision and orientation discrimination. But just testing patients' ability to detect luminance contrast is not sufficient for lesions that involve cortical areas beyond the primary visual cortex. Injuries of cortical areas beyond V1, the primary visual area receiving the bulk of the afferent fibres from the retina via the lateral geniculate nucleus, often do not result in absolute scotomata as detected by conventional perimetry.

An example of such an incomplete defect is a condition called 'cerebral amblyopia' where the perceptions of form and of colour are defective in the contralesional hemifield while luminance detection is preserved (see below; Mauthner 1881; Gelpke 1899; Poppelreuter 1917; Teuber *et al.* 1960; Zihl and von Cramon 1986). A number of patients have been described as suffering from relatively isolated defects of abilities such as detecting motion or colour. Examples for defects of *colour* processing caused by cortical injury are discussed in detail in Chapter 8, this volume (see also Samelsohn 1881; Scotti and Spinnler 1970; Tzavaras *et al.* 1971; Assal *et al.* 1969; Damasio *et al.* 1980a; Green and Lesell 1977; Lewandowsky 1908; Lhermitte *et al.* 1969; Pearlman *et al.* 1975; Mendola and Corkin 1999; Cronin-Golomb *et al.* 1993; Troscianko *et al.* 1996). In short, bilateral destruction of several cortical areas, including Area V4, can lead to the so-called cortical achromatopsia. Patients suffering from this type of 'indiscrimination' lose the ability to discriminate between colours on the basis of hue or saturation. They only perceive shades of grey, in spite of intact retinal ganglion cells of all three types and in spite of the fact that they can still faintly perceive borders between directly adjoining coloured patches if the differences are sufficiently large. Object colour can no longer be 'filled in' from the borders, and the patients are unable to find an object on the basis of its colour. Moreover, patients may be unable to name the colour that is characteristic of an object (Zihl and von Cramon 1986) or to correctly sort colours (de Renzi *et al.* 1972; cf. also de Renzi and Spinnler 1967). The defect of colour perception may be present in only a part of the visual field—most often, one of the upper quadrants—and often is associated with problems in identifying faces (prosopagnosia; see the eponymous subsection). Lesions usually are located in the medial and lateral occipitotemporal gyri.

Defects of detecting and discriminating motion- or time-defined boundaries

Another submodality of visual perception that has been reported as being defective in patients without distinct scotomata as revealed by perimetry is *motion detection*.

Already the gestalt psychologists knew that an object could be defined by 'common fate', e.g. common direction of motion. We must first clarify how motion information can contribute to the detection of boundaries between areas and hence define an object before dealing with deficits of this ability.

The case is similar to that of visual perception in general, which to introspection appears as a unitary entity while it consists of many partly independent submodalities (see the subsection on 'The modular structure of visual cortices'). Similarly, introspection tends to create the wrong impression regarding the sequence of events when it comes to analysing moving objects. I expect that most people not familiar with neurophysiology would suppose that our brains first detect objects and subsequently analyse their movements. A number of experiments show that this is not the case, at least not always. On the lowest level of motion analysis, the elementary motion detector signals that a contrast edge has moved, usually from one position in space to a nearby position. The detector is so simple (Fig. 7.12) that it cannot discriminate between moving versus appropriately flickering targets. It just differentiates between dynamic versus stationary stimuli as well as between different directions of motion.

The local motion signals from many motion detectors, each with a spatially restricted receptive visual field, are combined with each other. They thus create an object, defined, e.g. by common motion relative to a stationary background, by a difference in the speed of element motion, or else by a difference in the direction of element motion. In this way, motion information can contribute to the detection of borders in the visual field, and can by itself define an object. Low-level motion information, such as differences in the speed of moving dots (one special case being stationary dots) can serve as input for the contour detection system, thus defining an object that would otherwise be invisible. (The same is true for stereoscopic depth perception: an object may be defined purely by disparity differences between the object and its surround, the principle underlying the so-called random-dot stereograms (Julesz 1971; see the next subsection), and even differences in the presentation times of identical elements in different areas of the visual field can lead to the perception of contours between these areas (Fahle 1993).)

It seems that there are only very few reports in the literature on patients suffering from relatively isolated but severe disturbances of motion perception. In all cases, the patient's detection or discrimination of moving stimuli had deteriorated rather selectively (Pötzl and Redlich 1911; Goldstein and Gelb 1918; Zihl et al. 1983; Greenlee and Smith 1997; cf. also Smith et al. 1998; Vaina et al. 1999; Braun et al. 1998; Vaina et al. 1990, 2000, 2001a; Cowey and Vaina 2000; Vaina and Rushton 2000; Clifford and Vaina 1999; Vaina 1989, 1998; Vaina and Cowey 1996; and Vaina et al. 2001b for fMRI-correlates of different levels of motion processing in humans). Patients with severe symptoms typically see the object both at the start and the end of its trajectory, but not in-between, and some who had been tested for the perception of apparent motion did not experience any motion impression. A number of additional patients described in the literature suffered from disturbances of motion perception that were either due to the so-called cerebral amblyopia which is not specific for motion perception (cf. Zihl and

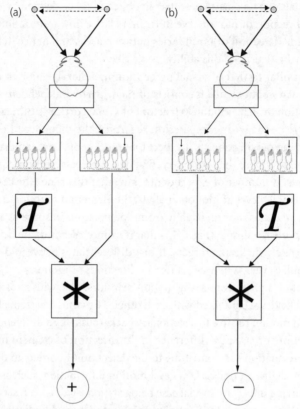

Fig. 7.12 The elementary motion detector. A stimulus moving from left to right (solid horizontal line) will first activate the left receptor and, after a delay depending on the speed of motion, will subsequently activate the right receptor. (a) During that interval, the activation of the left receptor has passed through the delay line and arrived at the multiplication unit where it meets the activation from the right receptor which does not have to cross a delay line. Hence, the multiplication unit produces an output. Leftward motion (interrupted horizontal line), on the other hand, will first activate the right receptor and subsequently, after a delay, the left detector. When the activation from the right detector arrives at the multiplication unit, the other factor, coming from the left detector, is zero, and thus will be the result of the multiplication. The same is true when the activation from the left receptor finally arrives at the multiplication unit. By that time, the activation from the right receptor has long decayed, one of the factors is zero, and the multiplication unit signals 'no movement'. (b) A delay line at the output of the other i.e. right receptor, creates a motion detector for the opposite direction, i.e. leftwards. Both detectors can be activated by repetitive, i.e. flicker stimulation.

von Cramon 1986), or due to loss of perception of motion-in-depth associated with a loss of depth perception (see the next subsection).

The best-studied and most pronounced case of 'motion-blindness' is that of a 43-year-old patient who had suffered from a bilateral occlusion of the parieto-occipital superior cerebral veins. Her visual fields were intact on both sides. The patient experienced all moving objects as jumping from one position to the next, rather than as in smooth motion, and had problems even in judging the speed at which a cup filled with coffee or in perceiving the mimics of her conversational counterpart. Crossing the street was dangerous for her since she could not estimate the speed of approaching cars, and she had problems navigating in crowded places due to an inability to anticipate the paths of other pedestrians. Interestingly, her ability to perform visually guided pursuit eye movements was also defective. The most probable cause for the defects was a bilateral injury to the medial temporal as well as the occipital gyri (cf. Fig. 7.3). In addition, a disconnection between striate cortex and some prestriate cortical areas may have played an important role (Zihl *et al.* 1983).

Defects to detect or discriminate contours defined by depth, by orientation differences, and 'cerebral amblyopia'

A defect of *stereoscopic depth* perception, and hence the ability to detect boundaries based on depth differences, that is not linked to oculomotor abnormalities occurs in a relatively low proportion of patients after head trauma (Hart 1969). Usually, loss of fusion, i.e. of the ability to direct both eyes to exactly the same direction and to superimpose both retinal images, will lead to loss of stereoscopic vision in these trauma patients (Danta *et al.* 1978). The small phorias that almost all of us have and that lead to a small squint in the dark when a fusional impulse is missing might express themselves if fusion is defective. Relatively isolated defects of stereoscopic depth perception have been described as well as those combined with scotomata (Anton 1899; Pick 1901; Poppelreuter 1917; Holmes 1918*a*,*b*; Birkmayer 1951; Benton and Hécaen 1970; Hamsher 1978; Lehmann and Walchi 1975; Rizzo and Damasio 1985; Rizzo 1989; Rothstein and Sacks 1972; cf. also Servos *et al.* 1995).

Depth perception not only relies on binocular disparities between the two retinal images, but also on several distinct cues (e.g. Fahle and Troscianko 1991). It seems that the ability to make use of at least several of these cues can be disrupted independently, usually after bilateral injuries (Danta *et al.* 1978; Birkmayer 1951; Kramer 1907; Holmes and Horax 1919; Gloning 1965). Complete loss of (not only stereoscopic) depth perception is often associated with the patient's inability to appreciate the third dimension of perception: the world appears like the image on a monitor-screen (Riddoch 1917; Holmes and Horrax 1919; Faust 1947; Gloning 1965; cf. also Vaina 1989). This complete loss of the third dimension, at least in some patients, disrupts one of the important constancies, namely size constancy (see the subsection 'Failures to achieve object constancy'). Retinal signals contain information about location of objects (direction, distance), their size, and speed that have to be converted from retinal space into egocentric space that is independent of eye- and head-movements in order for subjects to be able to navigate through their visual world.

There have been only a few reports on an isolated inability to perform figure–ground discrimination—and hence to detect boundaries—on the basis of *orientation differences*, or, more generally, on the basis of differences in texture, or spatial frequency (Kartsounis and Warrington 1991; Riddoch and Humphreys 1986; cf. also Davidoff and Warrington 1993; Humphrey *et al.* 1996; cf. also Warrington and Rabin 1970; Humphrey *et al.* 1995; Hamsher *et al.* 1992). (Spatial frequency is, to a first approximation, a measure of the coarseness versus fineness of a pattern, e.g. a grating: a fine sinewave grating has a high spatial frequency, a coarse grating a low spatial frequency.)

We will not deal in detail with further features that can serve to detect borders and hence serve as a prerequisite for figure–ground segregation. Suffice it to say that gradients in the amount of variation over space or time in most of the features outlined above (e.g. differences in luminance contrast) will lead to the perception of borders between the areas differing in regard to this feature. But these features are not tested in neuropsychological patients and, while we plan to extend the range of tests applied in the future, no results are available as yet.

The indiscriminations described here may be related to the so-called cerebral amblyopias that are defined by a loss of clearly defined visual perception without complete loss of vision (see above and Ferrier 1881; Mauthner 1881; Bender and Bodis-Wollner 1978; Riddoch 1917). Patients experience a stimulus presented within the amblyopic region as 'foggy' and blunt, and they are unable to detect its form, colour, or motion direction—while they can still discriminate between stationary and moving objects. These are symptoms not unlike those for some patients suffering from blindsight (see Chapter 9, this volume). In some patients, the size of the residual visual field changes and fluctuates over time with occasional 'obscurations' (Bender and Teuber 1946, Wilbrand and Sänger 1892; Poppelreuter 1917; Gelb and Goldstein 1922). These fluctuations have a correlate in the visual evoked cortical responses (Zihl and Schmid 1989), and both dark- and bright-adaptation may be decreased (Aulhorn and Harms 1972).

Mislocation of objects in space

Mislocalization of objects in the visual field is not uncommon, leading to a perception of objects as closer to the centre of gaze in some but not all patients suffering from scotomata in the peripheral visual field (e.g. Poppelreuter 1917; Riddoch 1935; Ratcliff and Davies-Jones 1972; Beyer 1895). Poppelreuter (1917) found a mislocalization of object positions towards the fovea in patients suffering from peripheral scotomata caused by lesions in the occipital or parietal lobe (cf. also Holmes 1918*b*; Hannay *et al.* 1976; Lenz 1944; Massironi *et al.* 1990). In hemianopic patients, the subjective 'straight ahead' is often shifted and the vertical meridian is rotated (Lenz 1909; Gelb 1926; Zihl and von Cramon 1986). Patients with left-sided lesions, especially of parietal or temporal occipital cortex, experience as 'vertical' a line tilted clockwise (up to 20°). These patients, surprisingly, experience a horizontal line as tilted counterclockwise, and the subjective straight-ahead seems to be shifted to the right (i.e. towards the scotoma; Axenfeld 1894; Liepmann and Kalmus 1900; Bender and Jung 1948; Zihl and von Cramon 1986). These changes were sometimes present (but less pronounced) even without accompanying visual field defects (cf. also bisection tasks in neglect patients in the subsection 'Tests for detecting spatial neglect in patients').

Neuronal mechanisms for contour and position detection

A highly speculative explanation is that antagonistically organized receptive fields might code visual field position, similarly to the coding of motion direction. Decreasing the influence of one type of input, e.g. of one motion direction, by looking for a while at a waterfall, will result in the perception of the opposite motion direction when subsequently looking at a stationary object. The same neuronal mechanism of adaptation or selective gain change might cause a displacement or sideward shift of the subjective 'straight-ahead', coupled with a displacement of the subjective positions of the horizontal and vertical meridians. Patients suffering from these symptoms often suffer from uni- or bilateral lesions of the occipitoparietal cortex, especially the supramarginal and angular gyri (Lenz 1909, 1944; Gelb 1926; Teuber and Mishkin 1954; de Renzi et al. 1971; Benton et al. 1975; Zihl and von Cramon 1986; cf. also the phenomenon of 'past pointing' after lesions of the brainstem and a possible role of eye position control). Another line of explanation is presented in the context of simultanagnosia (see the subsection 'Visual disorientation in simultagnosia').

The luminance and colour perceptions of homogeneous *areas* between the contours are created probably partly by extrapolation, or filling in, from these contours, and partly from a separate area system (see the subsection 'Different levels and separate channels of visual information-processing'; Welpe et al. 1980; Grossberg 1991). The same may be true for stereoscopic depth, where depth differences seem to be computed only relative to the next contour (see e.g. Fahle and Westheimer 1995).

In texture- and motion-defined contours, even the homogeneous areas contain (luminance-defined) contour elements. There, orientation, or distribution of elements, or else motion-speed or -direction are the important parameters to discriminate between figure and ground. This differentiation can be achieved only by mechanisms that group together different visual field positions according to the exact type of feature within a given feature domain, i.e. that discriminate not only between stationary and moving, but between different directions of motion and create an object consisting of (all) elements showing this feature. We can still assume that boundaries are the important feature extracted from the image, but with texture-defined stimuli, boundaries are detected in a more indirect way, or on a *second level* that compares, e.g. the velocities from motion detectors on the first level, and groups those with similar outputs, thus creating boundaries between areas (second-order processing, see e.g. Zanker et al. 1998; Chapter 4, this volume). An analogue in the domain of luminance contrast would be an area defined by a difference in contrast, rather than in luminance: this would be a contrast in contrast, while the two areas would not differ in mean luminance, so there would not be a luminance contrast at the border between the two areas. This reminds us that, within each of the levels, there may be several steps or sublevels of processing.

Searching for indiscriminations in the visual field: component perimetry

Due to a process called filling-in, most neuropsychological patients suffering from scotomata in their visual field are not aware of these 'dark holes' in their fields. This phenomenon is loosely related to the fact that we are not aware of the blind spot in our temporal visual field caused by the exit of the optic nerve from the eye—in both cases, there is no representation in the (primary) visual cortex of a restricted part of the visual field. Even fewer patients are aware of regions in their visual fields where they do not experience colour, or motion. Given the resulting relative rarity of reports in the literature on patients suffering from relatively isolated defects in detecting, e.g. stimulus motion, with (largely) preserved discrimination of luminance contrasts, we developed a new screening method for visual field defects that should be able to detect such deficits in patients. It is based on a method proposed by Aulhorn and Köst (1988) that was initially developed to diagnose defects in contrast detection.

For this screening method, observers sit close to a monitor screen that displays different types of dynamic stimuli so that a large part of the visual field is stimulated simultaneously. The original method employed visual noise consisting of randomly moving black and white dots presented in the central 30° of the visual field. Virtually all patients suffering from scotomata caused by lesions on the level of retina, optic nerve, optic tract, and optic radiation were able to detect their visual field defects when looking at this stimulus, while only about half of the patients with scotomata due to cortical lesions detected their defects when gazing at the stimulus of the original method (Aulhorn and Köst 1988). We extended the method by adding test stimuli defined purely by differences in hue (colour) without any luminance contrast, i.e. stimuli that were isoluminant and would appear as homogeneous to any colour-blind system (Bachmann and Fahle 2000). A second extension was the use of figures, more precisely checkerboards (or draught boards) defined purely by stereoscopic depth, direction of motion, or time of element appearance—dots were flickered in these latter displays, always appearing a couple of frames later in one type of checks than in the other type. Schematic displays of some sample stimuli of this new method, component perimetry, are shown in Fig. 7.13.

In two studies, we tested around 100 patients suffering from infarctions of either the posterior or medial cerebral arteries with a monitor subtending eccentricities up to around 40°, larger than in the previous studies (Bachmann and Fahle 1998, 2000; Spang *et al.* 2001). In contrast to the earlier studies that used a smaller monitor, around 90% of these patients were able to subjectively experience their scotomata when looking steadily at these stimuli, often only in the far periphery of the monitor (Bachmann and Fahle 2000). Patients usually experienced their scotomata as regions where the stimulus was not as dynamic as in the rest of the visual field, or was completely stationary, or else as moving more slowly, being less colourful, or missing the checkerboard structure. By and large, the positions of the scotomata the patients drew by felt-tip on

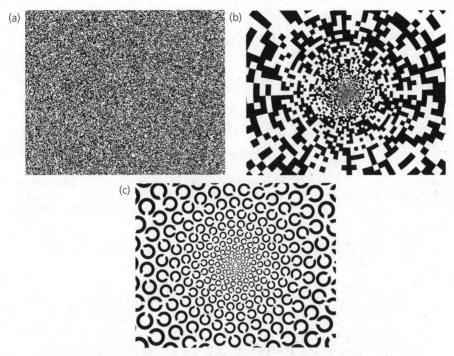

Fig. 7.13 Some examples of the stimuli used for component perimetry testing. These are individual stationary frames from a sequence of dynamic stimuli presented to a large part of the visual field of the patients (diameter between about 60 and more than 80 degrees of visual angle). (a)-(c) The stimuli consist either of dynamic noise defined by luminance or hue, by differences in motion direction, depth, or by rotating stimuli.

the monitor were similar to the defects revealed by automated perimetry that was performed on all patients immediately after the tests of component perimetry. Hence the method, requiring about 10 minutes per patient for five different submodalities, is a relatively sensitive screening tool for visual field defects. However, the subjective defects tended to be smaller than the more objective size revealed by conventional perimetry, probably due to filling-in mechanisms.

In the context of visual neuropsychology, the main interest is in patients with discrepancies between the results of conventional contrast perimetry on one hand and those of component perimetry on the other hand. If contrast perimetry yields normal visual fields, while the more subjective component perimetry shows defects, the patient may either be 'false-positive', i.e. imagining the defect, or else contrast detection might be relatively normal while some other visual function, such as colour, motion, or depth perception is defective. Figure 7.14 presents the results of one of almost a dozen patients with distinct differences between the results of contrast versus component perimetry that we have found so far. While the visual field for contrast perimetry is almost normal (Fig. 7.14(a)),

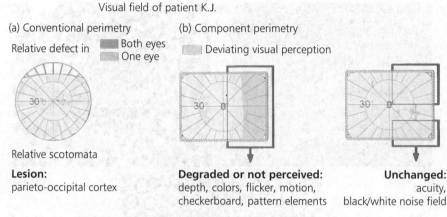

Visual field of patient K.J.

(a) Conventional perimetry

Relative defect in
■ Both eyes
■ One eye

(b) Component perimetry

■ Deviating visual perception

Relative scotomata

Lesion:
parieto-occipital cortex

Degraded or not perceived:
depth, colors, flicker, motion,
checkerboard, pattern elements

Unchanged:
acuity,
black/white noise field

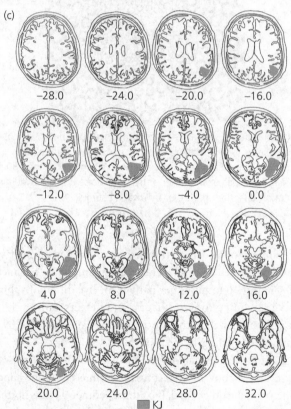

(c)

−28.0   −24.0   −20.0   −16.0

−12.0   −8.0   −4.0   0.0

4.0   8.0   12.0   16.0

20.0   24.0   28.0   32.0

■ KJ

Fig. 7.14 Test results of (a) conventional and (b) component perimetry in a patient suffering from an indiscrimination in the domain of colour and motion processing with largely intact luminance detection. (c) schematic representation of the cortical lesion of the patient whose results are shown in (a) and (b), as revealed by magnetic resonance imaging (as seen from below; after Bachmann and Fahle, unpublished).

the patient perceives strong differences between his right and left visual hemifields when looking at those patterns of component perimetry that test colour or motion perception (Fig. 7.14(b)). The brain lesion as revealed by MRI is shown schematically in Fig. 7.14(c), showing defects in the left hemisphere that spare the optic radiation and primary visual cortex while involving parts of the temporal and parietal cortex.

Obviously, these rather subjective screening tests have to be complemented by more quantitative measurements such as colour-, motion-, and stereo-perimetry. We are presently developing these methods, partly making use of gaze perimetry (see the sub-section 'Visual field testing: perimetry'). The results of the screening tests strongly suggest that a certain proportion of patients after infarctions of posterior cerebral cortex suffer from circumscribed scotomata of the indiscrimination-type with intact contrast detection, hence largely normal visual fields as tested by conventional perimetry.

Failures to achieve object constancy

In natural environments, objects tend to appear under different circumstances, at different distances, in different orientations, with different illuminations, and at different positions in the visual field. Usually, this variance of appearance does not pose a noticeable problem for visual object recognition in humans. Again, the problem may appear trivial at first glimpse but it is far from trivial, in spite of the ease with which humans usually solve the task. The retinal area covered by a cup at a viewing distance of 5 metres is about one-hundredth of the area covered by that same cup at a distance of 0.5 metres. Nevertheless, the cup appears to have the same size at both distances, due to a neuronal mechanism of size constancy that takes into account the distance of objects when their size is assessed. Disturbances of this mechanism, e.g. in patients suffering from a loss of depth perception (see above), lead to changes in the apparent size of objects presented at different distances: objects perceived as nearer than they actually are appear too small (micropsia), while those perceived as further away than they are appear too big (macropsia) (cf. Holmes 1918*a*).

Similarly, we recognize objects that are rotated or shifted in the visual field, producing quite different retinal images. This constancy is probably achieved through extensive learning and storage of many typical (or canonical) views of the object, and not primarily by producing a three-dimensional model that is subsequently translated and rotated until it fits the actual position and view of the object in the outer world (Bülthoff *et al.* 1995; Dill and Fahle 1999) while the final construction of a 'true' three-dimensional representation in Marr's (1982) sense cannot be excluded. Patients have been described who experience profound difficulties in matching views of three-dimensional objects after *rotation* or across shifts of perspective (e.g. de Renzi *et al.* 1969; Warrington and Taylor 1973, 1978; Humphreys and Riddoch 1984, 1985; Levine 1978), usually after lesions in the right posterior hemisphere, especially the inferior parietal lobe (Warrington and Taylor 1973; Warrington 1982). This deficit was called 'perceptual categorization deficit' by Warrington and colleagues. These patients have relatively few problems in everyday life, probably due to the redundancy present in most visual scenes of everyday life.

The capability to perceive objects in the same colour (colour constancy), irrespective of the illuminant, may suffer an isolated defect. The wavelength sent out by objects depends on their surface properties and on the light source illuminating them. While the surface property is relatively constant and helps in identifying the object, the illuminant is not constant, but varies greatly between light bulbs, neon tubes, and sunlight—and even strongly between the sunlight at midday versus sunrise or sunset. Photographic film correctly mirrors these variations of wavelength composition originating from identical surfaces under different illuminants, leading to clearly different object colours on film. To the human observer, quite to the contrary, the object's colour stays constant—due to the mechanism of *colour constancy*. Two studies proved that the ability of colour constancy might be lost in patients while colour vision as such is spared (Rüttiger *et al.* 1999; see Chapter 8, this volume). Changes of luminance, on the other hand, seem to be automatically compensated for by the fact that cortical neurons are primarily concerned with contrasts rather than with absolute intensities, since object contrasts are independent of the intensity of the illuminant.

Failures to achieve a stable representation of extrapersonal space

Even the discrimination between the effects of ego-motion (self-motion) versus object motion in vision may become defective. There are two possible reasons for the perception of object motion on the retina, namely, motion of the object in the outer world, or else motion of the eye. To discriminate between these two possibilities, and to prevent the brain from misinterpreting retinal image motion as object motion during eye movements, an efference copy is relayed from the oculomotor centres to the visual cortex, containing information on the velocity and direction of the intended motion (Fig. 7.15; von Holst and Mittelstaedt 1950). When an injury of the brain involves the centre mediating this efference copy, the patient is impaired in discriminating between motion of objects versus eye movements—and, consequently, strong subjective object movements will be experienced during each (smooth) eye movement. Indeed, a patient suffering from such symptoms has been described in the literature (Haarmeier *et al.* 1997), and many more will have not been diagnosed for lack of adequate testing.

The problem of discriminating between motion of the retinal image due to object motion versus eye- or body-motion leads to the more general question of how humans achieve a stable representation of *extrapersonal space*. Due to the extreme specialization of our central retina, we steadily perform a saccadic scanning of the outer world by eye movements and obviously synthesize from this sequential scanning a relatively stable representation of the visual world. This representation cannot be achieved in the primary or secondary visual cortices, areas 17 through 19, since these areas are *retinotopically*

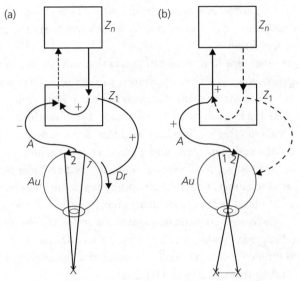

Fig 7.15 The principle of the 'efference-copy'. Whenever we move the eyes (e.g. from 1 to 2), the centres planning the movements of the eyes (Z_n) send a copy of the signal aimed at the eye muscles to a control instance (Z_1) that subtracts this signal from a signal caused by retinal motion. (a) If the retinal motion is caused by eye movements, the two signals cancel each other out. (b) If the retinal motion is caused by object motion, Z_1 does not receive an efference copy and the retinal motion signal (A) is not cancelled. The brain is able, on the basis of this signal, to discriminate between retinal motion caused by object motion versus retinal motion caused by eye motion. A defect of this system leads to the subjective impression of a moving world during each eye movement. (After von Holst and Mittelstaedt (1950).)

organized. Hence, the part of the outer world they represent is determined by the actual eye position. Subsequent cortical areas, especially in the parietal lobe, no longer code the outer world in *precise or exclusively* retinotopic coordinates. Some of the cells in these areas in the frontal eye fields and in the superior colliculus increase their firing rate if a saccadic movement is intended towards the target (Wurtz *et al.* 1986) or even shift their receptive fields, i.e. the part of the world they represent, to the target position of an intended saccade prior to the start of the saccade. Neurons in these areas of parietal cortex represent space partly in *egocentric* rather than retinotopic co-ordinates, but in a complex way that is described as 'gain field' (Andersen 1995). These neurons receive signals from vestibular and proprioceptive sources as well as information about eye position to create a coordinate system relative to the (whole) body, representing objects relative, e.g. to the head or trunk. This type of representation is highly useful for all motor activities, whether performed by the hand (grasping) or eye (saccading to a target). This level of egocentric representation roughly corresponds to Marr's (1982) '$2\frac{1}{2}$'-dimensional sketch of the world. Failure to achieve this level, e.g. due to a failure of the efference copy of eye movements, will lead to the instability of the visual world experienced by the patient as described above (Haarmeier *et al.* 1997) and probably plays a major role in Balint's syndrome and simultanagnosia (see eponymous subsection).

There is still another type of representation and that will become important for the understanding of neglect (see the eponymous subsection). That is the allocentric representation related to Marr's three-dimensional sketch. (But while Marr believed in a real three-dimensional reconstruction of object representations, recent evidence indicates that often a number of different two-dimensional views are stored instead of the computation of a complete three-dimensional reconstruction; see Bülthoff *et al.* 1995 and cf. Hinton 1981.) The *allocentric* coordinate system codes objects primarily through the spatial relations between their components. This type of representation allows constancy of object recognition during object rotation. If a watch is rotated by 90°, its retinal image changes considerably, and this is certainly even more true for, say, a human being. Failure in creating an allocentric representation of objects will lead to strong problems for identification of objects presented in unusual orientations, or perhaps even when tilting the head or when lying down.

In summary, constancy mechanisms exist for a number of aspects of visual object perception, such as illuminant, size, object position, and extrapersonal space, and their failure, while probably most often not correctly diagnosed, leads to distinct disturbances in the perception of the outer world (e.g. Riddoch 1935). This ends the description of defects on a relatively early level of visual information-processing, where contours are detected in the visual input and their positions in space are computed. Next, we will deal with the formation of objects from contours, and with the failures of this process.

Apperceptive and associative agnosias

Contour binding, object formation, and their failures: illusory conjunctions and apperceptive agnosias

Following border, or contour extraction, the next level of visual information-processing is the binding or grouping (these words will be used as synonyms) together of those borders belonging to the same region or surface and hence to the same object. Binding of contours to a coherent representation of a surface and finally to an object leads to the formation of a gestalt that is distinct from its surround such as in figure – ground segregation. This seems to be an easy feat since humans do it all the time quite effortlessly. But, when researchers in artificial intelligence started to teach vision to their computers, they soon realized the complexities inherent in natural scenes. Objects are not usually presented in isolation but close to other objects. They may be partly occluded by other objects. They are not homogeneous but textured and hence not all contours represent borders, especially if there are shadows cast on to the object. In short, it is not an easy task to combine contours extracted from an image into object representations. Even the intact human visual system sometimes fails in this task. For example, when a (reasonable) number of different forms such as different digits are

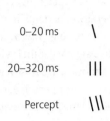

0–20 ms

20–320 ms

Percept

Fig. 7.16 The feature-inheritance effect. A single vernier stimulus is presented for a very short time (20 ms), followed by a grating consisting of five straight lines, presented for a much longer time (e.g. 300 ms). Observers will not perceive the single vernier, but all of the elements of the subsequent grating will be perceived as offset in the direction of the leading vernier in spite of not being offset. This is to say that the vernier target presented first bequeaths its offset to the subsequent grating. (After Herzog and Fahle (2002).)

presented shortly and in different colours and with a subsequent mask, observers are usually able to correctly identify all the digits and all the colours, but, relatively often, they err in the assignment between digits and colours when asked to describe what they have just seen. So they will perceive one digit in the colour of another digit (Treisman and Schmidt 1982).

Another demonstration of incorrect binding of features is the so-called feature-inheritance effect (Herzog *et al.* 2001). A line slanted to, say, the right is presented for some hundredths of a second. A grating of five vertical lines follows immediately afterwards, displayed for a much longer time (see Fig. 7.16). Observers do not consciously perceive the single line, but just the grating, and they perceive all the grating elements as slanted to the right (cf. Herzog and Fahle 2002 for a similar effect). Obviously, the earlier stimulus has bequeathed one of its features, slant, to the following grating by means of feature binding. This is another indication that, in the visual system, features from different positions and sometimes from different points in time are combined in order to form objects, and that this process may fail even in healthy observers. The presentation time of the first stimulus required for this phenomenon to occur is significantly increased in unmedicated schizophrenic patients (Brand *et al.* 2001), indicating the complex nature of the binding process that ultimately leads to illusory conjunctions.

Different theories try to explain how the binding process might be achieved in the human brain. They postulate to employ spatial neighbourhood of representations or else synchronous firing of neurons coding the same object (Singer 1999). Grouping had been thought to be driven exclusively by bottom–up processes (Farah 1990, p. 149), while more recently, the importance of top–down influences is becoming clearer (see the subsection 'Visual information-processing in the contex' and Chapters 2,10, this volume). The ability to bind together the contours detected on the first level of feature analysis in order to create object representations in the brain is impaired in some patients. For these patients, the world appears as a jumble of lines, colours, and movements, mostly without circumscribed and defined objects, probably not unlike some contemporary abstract paintings.

Agnosic patients ('agnosia' was given its name by Freud in 1891) fail to recognize objects in spite of sufficiently preserved visual fields, preserved elementary visual functions such as luminance, colour and motion perception, and sufficient general intellectual and language capabilities. The deficit of recognition is not limited to the naming of objects but is equally obvious in nonverbal testing, such as matching, copying, or discriminating between even simple visual stimuli. (Therefore, patients having problems with comparing the size of simple geometrical objects (e.g. Taylor and Warrington, 1973) can be considered as borderline to apperceptive agnosia, if their visual fields are intact.) These patients, suffering from *apperceptive* agnosias, are so severely handicapped that they often appear as blind to a casual observer. They perceive local colours and lines, but these do not constitute surfaces and objects (may be not unlike the situation in patients who achieve vision late in life by remedy of an inborn optical problem of the eyes; see Gregory and Wallace 1963; Fine *et al.* 2002). Hence they cannot bind together contours across breaks, e.g. caused by small occluding objects (see Grüsser and Landis 1991; Farah 1990), trace dotted lines, or avoid being distracted by scratches on a painting. Straight lines are better recognized than curved ones, while interrupted lines are worst (e.g. Goldstein and Gelb 1918; cf. also Corkin 1979; Mooney 1957; Russo and Vignolo 1967), indicating that the problem of binding together isolated contours can arise on different levels of processing. Real objects yield better results than photographs or line drawings, possibly due to the fact that patients rely partly on noncontour information such as colour or texture, hence on the 'area'-system. Usually, the patients recognize objects based on haptic or auditory sensory information while not recognizing the same objects based on visual signals (Goldstein and Gelb 1918; Brown 1975; Rubens 1979; Adler 1944; Alexander and Albert 1983; Efron 1968; Benson and Greenberg 1969; Campion and Latto 1985; Campion 1987; Landis *et al.* 1982) and visual imagery seems to be preserved (Servos and Goodale 1995). Patients may develop a strategy of tracing contours by hand- or eye-movements and to recognize shapes from these trajectories.

Some patients seem to suffer from apperceptive agnosia only for stationary images, another indication for partly separated processing of motion information (see Chapter 5, this volume). It is no wonder that the patients suffering from an apperceptive agnosia in Lissauer's (1890) terminology are unable to copy even simple drawings, as is described in detail in Chapter 10, this volume. This failure indicates that conscious perception does not have direct access to the neuronal representation of the outer world in the primary visual cortex since there a retinotopically ordered representation of the image exists, the copying of which should result in an acceptable copy of the 'real' object—at least during steady fixation.

The cause underlying these deficits is damage to the occipital and parietal cortex (sparing primary visual cortex), usually diffuse rather than focal, possibly affecting the white matter more than the grey matter of the brain (Landis *et al.* 1982).

Failure of object identification in associative agnosias: theory

Once the contours are grouped together to form surfaces and object-representations, the next step is to *recognize* these object representations. In patients suffering from associative agnosias, this step of analysis is selectively impaired. Konorski (1967) discriminated nine different object categories that together cover the entire field of object recognition and that have been described as being selectively impaired in neuropsychological patients: (1) small, manipulable objects; (2) large objects (e.g. furniture); (3) non-manipulable objects (e.g. houses); (4) facial identity; (5) emotional facial expression; (6) animals and animated objects; (7) letters and signs; (8) handwriting; (9) limb-positions. For all of these visual objects, isolating individual objects and discriminating them from the background, i.e. achieving figure–ground discrimination, is only a first step of object identification. The ultimate goal is not just to know that there are three separate objects, but also to know *what* these objects are.

Let's assume the first two steps of visual analysis have been successfully solved: all relevant boundaries between objects have been identified, and those corresponding to different objects have been bound together, forming stable object- or at least surface-representations. (As mentioned above, this is a very difficult task without top-down information about possible ways of grouping, i.e. without stored templates of objects, so it may fail even though the neuronal mechanisms at the lower level are still intact.) But let's assume that we have never before seen the object. It follows that we would not know what it is used for, what material it is made from, whether or not it is fragile, and so on—and, of course, we would not know its name. Familiar things are quite another matter: we have all this information stored in our brain. When looking at familiar objects the task is to find, on the basis of the current representation of an object we are looking at, the corresponding stored representation containing all this information. This may be easy for everyday objects, but is difficult for others that we know less well (what exact type of bird or of flower is it we are looking at?) as well as for objects seen from an unfamiliar perspective (cf. Warrington 1985).

For objects we have never seen before, we somewhat resemble patients suffering from associative agnosia: we can copy the object's image well enough, contour by contour, as shown in Chapter 10, this volume, but we do not know what we are copying here. (Admittedly, we may have an idea due to similar objects we saw in the past.) In reality, the task is even more difficult for the patient since we still have the neuronal machinery in place that guides the search for relevant contours in the image and that steers the binding of elements, e.g. in analogy to other, similar objects we have encountered before. The patient, on the other hand, having lost the ability to store representations of visual objects or to access this storage, may not have a single blueprint of a visual object at hand and hence lacks the concept of a visual object. All image analysis in this patient and hence both contour detection and binding has to be driven in a strictly 'bottom–up' way, i.e. entirely on the basis of sensory information. That type of analysis is much more difficult and prone to error than a process guided by top–down influence, i.e. by a concept of what the object looks like.

I would propose that associative agnosias are failures of a patient's ability to find a stored representation matching the representation of the visual object at hand (cf. Hécaen and Angelergues 1963; Critchley 1964; Gloning *et al.* 1968; Damasio 1985; Damasio *et al.* 1990a). As mentioned in the introduction to this chapter, we still do not know exactly how visual information is analysed in the healthy brain. But a growing body of evidence suggests the use of distributed processing in neuronal networks with strong feedback connections (e.g. Palm 1982; Chapter 2, this volume; the subsection 'Visual information-processing in the cortex'). These types of networks are relatively tolerant to defects of single elements, as well as of noise in the input, and can complete stimuli that are incomplete. Feeding the raw primal contour information into this network would lead to an output corresponding to the most similar object representation stored so far—the processes of object formation and object recognition would not be separated but take place simultaneously, in the same network, and would moreover incorporate visual memory.

One may wonder why this type of associative neuronal network still needs the stage of contour extraction and binding of features and does not analyse the 'raw' retinal image on a point-by-point basis, as supplied by the optic nerve. A plausible answer evolved from research in artificial intelligence. The network only works reliably if similar objects produce similar inputs to the network. This requirement is not met by a pixel-by-pixel input directly representing the retinal activation. Processes such as contour extraction and contour binding are a necessary prerequisite for object formation and identification. The excitation of individual photoreceptors signalling an object depends strongly on the level of illuminance, on wavelength composition of the illuminant, on the distance of the object, its position in the visual field, and its orientation to name just some parameters. All these accidental features that are irrelevant for object recognition have to be eliminated as completely as possible. To concentrate on the *form* of the object, by extracting its outer borders, is obviously a good way to achieve the goal of constancy: coding the object in similar ways irrespective of the above-mentioned accidental parameters.

In summary, associative agnosias are characterized by a failure to associate the representation of a presently displayed object with a stored representation of this object, and by a lack of top–down control in pattern analysis. Will this view be consistent with the results of patient studies? The next subsection will bring the answer!

Associative agnosias: patient studies

Associative agnosias in a strict sense are characterized by four criteria: (1) no (absolute) scotomata—or else, as is the case in most agnosic patients, scotomata that will not, by themselves, prevent object recognition. (The extended lesions required for agnosias, unfortunately, are most often associated with visual field defects.); (2) difficulty or inability to recognize visually presented objects as evidenced not only in naming, but also in nonverbal tests; (3) preserved ability to separate figure and ground (hence no pronounced problems in navigating through the environment) and preserved ability to copy and match stimuli. This feature is in strong contrast with apperceptive agnosias; (4) Preserved ability to recognize and name objects or people through other sense modalities such as audition, touch, or smell, and intact intelligence (Rubens and Benson 1971; Albert *et al.* 1975; Bauer 1982; Hécaen and de Ajuriaguerra 1956; Levine 1978; Levine and Calvanio 1989; Mack and Boller 1977; Macrae and Trolle 1956;

McCarthy and Warrington 1986; Pillon *et al.* 1981; Ratcliff and Newcombe 1982; Riddoch and Humphreys 1987*a,b*; Wapner *et al.* 1978; Lissauer 1890; Bender and Feldman 1972; de Renzi 1986*b*; Heidenhain 1927; Hécaen *et al.* 1974; Kertesz 1979; Humphreys and Riddoch 1987*a, b*; cf. also Davidoff and Wilson 1985).

Even though matching of objects as well as copying is intact, this does not mean that perception as such is normal, as is implied by Teuber's (1968) famous definition of 'a normal percept, stripped of its meaning'. This definition mirrors the view, of this time, of perception as a strictly feedforward hierarchical system. In a feedback system, however, where recognition is achieved through an interactive process involving different levels of processing, one would indeed expect simple 'perception' to be disturbed even if 'only' the process of object *recognition* is defective. Indeed, associative agnosics *do* suffer from serious impairments also of object perception (not just of object identification) such as impairments when copying or comparing drawings (Humphreys and Riddoch 1987*a,b*; cf. Levine and Calvanio 1989; Mendez 1988; Ratcliff and Newcombe 1982). Hence, the slavish line-by-line copying of associative agnostics is no surprise. The same is true for the fact that their speed of copying is far slower than that of normal observers, but differs little between 'possible' and 'impossible' (and hence unfamiliar) objects, while normal observers copy familiar objects much faster than unfamiliar ones. The performance of agnosic patients decreases markedly for tachistoscopic stimulus presentations as well as for photographs (compared to real objects) and especially for line drawings (probably due to lack of information from the 'area' system, for example about the colour and shading of objects; see subsections 'Different levels and separate channels of visual information processing' and 'Neuronal mechanisms for contour and position detection'). They also experience great problems with binding together objects that are partly occluded or that are symbolized by (strongly) interrupted lines as in the Gollin-figures (Gollin 1960; we all probably use top–down information to solve this task) or in hidden figures (Corkin 1979). Additional— rather than incomplete—information, on the other hand, improves performance in some patients, e.g. aiding categorization by supplying (auditory) information about the context in which the objects normally occur (e.g. Duensing 1952, 1953; Rubens and Benson 1971; cf. also Taylor and Warrington 1971). Finally, at least some of the patients suffering from associative agnosia experience severe difficulties in reading since they have to analyse words in a letter-by-letter way (see the subsection 'Alexia and optic aphasia').

Farah (1990) differentiates between two types of agnosia: (1) agnosia for objects that have to be decomposed into parts and hence require fast serial processing while representation is easy since the parts are simple (e.g. words) and (2) agnosia for objects represented as complex entities, where representation is more difficult while no fast serial processing is required.

There has been some controversy about which type of cortical damage causes associative agnosias. Some authors favour as an explanation left-sided lesions of occipital/temporal cortex (Warrington 1985; Boudouresques *et al.* 1972; Feinberg *et al.* 1986; Pillon *et al.* 1981; Hécaen and de Ajuriaguerra 1956; McCarthy and Warrington

1986 cf. also Bisiach *et al.* 1979*b*), while others postulate bilateral damage of the inferior or temporo-occipital junction (Alexander and Albert 1983), or else of the right side (Boudouresques *et al.* 1979; Levine 1978), or find associative agnosias as the result of diffuse brain damage (Taylor and Warrington 1971).

Specific associative agnosias: prosopagnosia

Associative agnosias may relate to all types of objects, or else to certain types of objects only and to the discrimination between classes of objects or else between individuals. The best-known example for associative agnosia for a (more or less!) limited class of objects certainly is *prosopagnosia* (Bodamer 1947), the failure to recognize faces (e.g. Pallis 1955; Assal *et al.* 1984; Bornstein and Kidron 1959; Cole and Perez-Cruet 1964; De Renzi 1986*a,c*; Kay and Levin 1982; Lhermitte and Pillon 1975; Nardelli *et al.* 1982; Shuttleworth *et al.* 1982; Beyn and Knyazeva 1962; Bornstein *et al.* 1969; Cohn *et al.* 1977; Warrington and James 1967; Newcombe 1979; Whiteley and Warrington 1977; Levine 1978; Kertesz 1979; Hécaen and Angelergues 1962, 1963; Benton and van Allen 1972; Benson *et al.* 1974; Benton 1980; Damasio *et al.* 1990*b*; Gloning *et al.* 1966; Hamsher *et al.* 1979; Landis *et al.* 1986, 1988; Mazzucchi and Biber 1983; Pevzner *et al.* 1962; Tranel *et al.* 1988; Sergent and Villemure 1989; Rondot *et al.* 1967). It seems not to be caused by the fact that faces are more complex and similar to each other than most other visual objects, i.e. just the most difficult to discriminate.

This deficit corresponds well to the fact that many neurons in inferotemporal cortex respond best to defined views of different faces (see Chapter 1, this volume). Face recognition may involve several, partially separable processes that could be disturbed independently—such as identification of a face as distinct from other object categories versus identification of the facial *expression* of a person. Hence, even within prosopagnosia, there may be different subtypes: patients experiencing difficulties in recognizing either the identity of faces (Bruyer *et al.* 1983; Shuttleworth *et al.* 1982), or else the emotional expression (Kurucz and Feldmar 1979), or both (Etcoff 1984). Some patients lose the ability to discriminate individual animals (Newcombe 1979; Bornstein *et al.* 1969; Assal *et al.* 1984; Young 1988), or animal species (Bornstein 1963; Boudouresques *et al.* 1979; Damasio *et al.* 1982; Gomori and Hawryluk 1984; Lhermitte *et al.* 1972; Lhermitte and Pillon 1975; Pallis 1955), plants (Boudouresques *et al.* 1979; Gomori and Hawryluk 1984; Whiteley and Warrington 1977), or even to judge food (Damasio *et al.* 1982; Michel *et al.* 1986; Whiteley and Warrington 1977), clothing (Damasio *et al.* 1982; Shuttleworth *et al.* 1982), or discriminate makes of cars (Boudouresques *et al.* 1979; Damasio *et al.* 1982; Gomori and Hawryluk 1984; Lhermitte *et al.* 1972; Lhermitte and Pillon 1975; Newcombe 1979; Shuttleworth *et al.* 1982; cf. also Benton and van Allen 1968).

Objective measures such as event-related brain potentials (ERPs; see Chapter 3, this volume), the psychogalvanic skin response, or reaction times demonstrated better preservation of face recognition on the basis of matching tasks in some patients than would have to be expected (Bauer 1984; Tranel and Damasio 1985, 1988; Renault *et al.* 1989; Bauer and Verfaellie 1988; de Haan *et al.* 1987*a, b*; Bruyer *et al.* 1983; cf., however, Newcombe *et al.* 1989; and see also the discussion on discrimination without awareness in Chapter 9, this volume). Hence, similarly to neglect (see subsection 'Evidence for preserved processing of visual input'), some object formation may take place unnoticed by the 'owner' of the brain in one form (memory-impaired) of prosopagnosia).

The defects underlying prosopagnosia always include the right hemisphere, and generally an additional left-sided defect of the parieto-occipital area, most often with a left superior quadrantanopia. (cf. Meadows 1974*a,b*; Torii and Tamai 1985; de Renzi *et al.* 1986.)

Alexia and optic aphasia

Alexia (or dyslexia), the inability to read other than in a letter-by-letter way with preserved writing and comprehension of spoken language, might be considered to be an agnosia for words—at least if it is not caused by visual field defects (e.g. Mesulam 1985; Damasio and Damasio 1983; Warrington and Shallice 1979; 1980). In patients, alexia is caused most often by concentric narrowing of the visual field, with a remaining central field diameter of less than approximately 3°, or else a reduction of visual acuity, rather than by defects of higher cortical areas. Therefore, perimetric testing (see the subsection 'Visual field testing: perimetry') is essential in all patients suffering from alexia. Even hemianopia, i.e. blindness in one visual hemifield (see the subsection 'Complete failure to see: blindness and scotomata'), will produce strong disturbances of reading (see Zihl 1995).

More pertinent to the topic of agnosias is the 'pure' alexia caused by certain lesions of the left posterior cortex, as are most cases of object agnosia without prosopagnosia. Latency to decipher individual words increases linearly with word length in these patients (Bub *et al.* 1989). Since single letters can be analysed, this deficit may be closely related to simultanagnosia (Farah 1990; see the subsection on 'Balint's syndrome and simultanagnosia').

As mentioned earlier (in the subsection 'Associative agnosias: patient studies'), patients might be able to solve even the problem of matching representations of presently perceived objects with those encountered earlier in life but still be unable to tell the name of the object they are shown—while they can convey the identity of the object, e.g. by gesturing its use. But while, in the case of an associative agnosia, patients are unable to tell or gesture what the use of the object is, those patients able to solve the matching problem can tell us what the object is for—e.g. 'something used for locking doors' if they fail to find the word 'key'. They are just unable to connect the stored representation with its name—as sometimes occurs to all of us when searching for a word or for the name of a person we meet and whom we have not seen in a while: we may know where the person lives, works, etc., but the name escapes us nevertheless. (This fact by itself is an indication that the names of objects might be stored in a part of the brain differing from the one analysing visual input—not an implausible assumption given the inability to understand language after lesions of Wernicke's area in the superior temporal cortex, close to the auditory cortex.) To make sure that it is indeed the connection between the visual representation of an object and its name that is missing, for the above example, we can rattle a bunch of keys. If the patient then finds the correct noun, we can be sure that, indeed, only the connection between visual representations of objects and their names is missing—a syndrome called *optic aphasia*, or *anomia*, which is the inability to name objects.

Optic aphasia is not a real agnosia, since recognition of objects is possible and can be indicated, e.g. by gesturing (Assal and Regli 1980; Coslett and Saffran 1989; Gil *et al.* 1985; Larrabee *et al.* 1985; Poeck 1984; Riddoch and Humphreys 1987*b*; Sittig 1927; Spreen *et al.* 1966). Unlike for agnostic patients, perception is relatively unimpaired by the visual quality of the stimuli (and hence is similar for real objects, photographs, and line drawings) (Gil *et al.* 1985; Larrabee *et al.* 1985; Lhermitte and Beauvois 1973; Poeck 1984; Riddoch and Humphreys 1987*b*). Patients are not impaired regarding visual perception in everyday life, while associative agnostics are handicapped, e.g. by not recognizing other people. Usually, the deficit is caused by posterior left hemisphere stroke (Lhermitte and Beauvois 1973).

Associative agnosias and especially optic aphasias represent failures of visual analysis on the very last steps in the sequence of processing. But, as we will see in the next section, even if the processing of single object-representations can be finished, patients may still be impaired in using the results of this analysis.

Balint's syndrome and simultanagnosia

Defects of visual attention: Balint's syndrome

Balint's (1909) syndrome (see also Anton 1898, 1899; Holmes 1918*a*; Holmes and Horrax 1919; Michel *et al.* 1964; Friedman-Hill *et al.* 1995) is characterized by: (1) inability to perform directed voluntary saccades (eye movements) to targets in the periphery of the visual field ('psychic paralysis of gaze'); (2) inability to grasp or point to visual targets and to follow a moving target by means of smooth-pursuit eye movements ('optic ataxia'); and (3) inability to pay attention to more than one object at a time, while paying attention only to a central focus (and even the attended object may fade spontaneously over time). The patients behave as if blind—due to the bilateral narrowing of their field of attention and of the restriction of their exploratory space, similar to that in the simultanagnosias (see the next subsection). The underlying brain defect generally includes bilateral parieto-occipital cortex, possibly including destruction of underlying fibre tracts (Alexander and Albert 1983).

Failures to perceive more than one object at a time: simultanagnosia and spatial disorientation

Definition, symptoms, and tests

Patients suffering from simultanagnosia (Wolpert 1924) accurately perceive individual details or elements of a visual scene but are unable to combine these details to a meaningful entity. Hence, there are similarities to deficits in visual exploration, as stressed by some authors (Zihl and von Cramon 1986), and, in a way, to apperceptive agnosia, the failure to combine individual contours (rather than objects). Some authors use the term in a more literal sense, as the inability to perceive more than one object, or element, at any given time (Luria 1959). This symptom is usually part of Balint's syndrome (Balint 1909; see the preceding subsection). Single objects and faces are

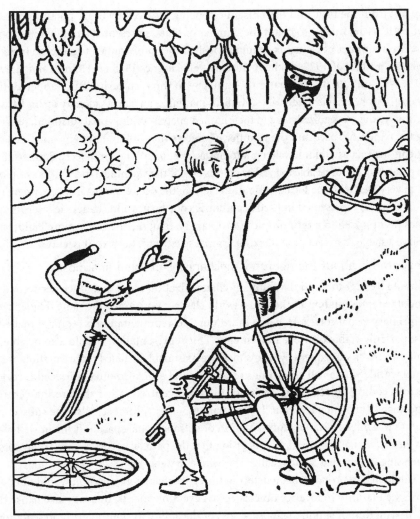

Fig. 7.17 The telegraph boy. Patients suffering from simultanagnosia or Balint's syndrome will only report the features they are presently looking at but will not be able to understand the contents of the scene.

readily identified and recognized but, in stimuli displaying several objects, only one object is recognized at a time (cf. Girotti *et al.* 1982; Rizzo and Hurtig 1987; Holmes 1918*a,b*; Holmes and Horrax 1919; Kase *et al.* 1977; Kosslyn *et al.* 1990; Luria 1959; Luria *et al.* 1963; Tyler 1968; Williams 1970; cf. also Godwin-Austen 1965).

A widely used test for simultanagnosia is the telegraph-boy picture (Fig. 7.17). Simultanagnosic patients only perceive parts of the picture without understanding the scene. For obvious reasons, these patients also suffer from severe reading problems (alexia; see the eponymous subsection) and report, for example, that words would pop out from the page and then disappear, being replaced by other portions of text. The patients are unable to count the number of objects presented simultaneously, but perceive a number of elements simultaneously if they are grouped together to form an object (Girotti *et al.* 1982; Godwin-Austen 1965; Holmes 1918*a,b*; Holmes and Horrax 1919; Williams 1970). The patients, similarly to those suffering from apperceptive agnosia, may be unable to identify stimuli, or may guess an object's identity on the basis of *one* feature they recognized. Due to their limited analysis of the visual surround, restricting the region of space and the number of objects they attend to at any one time, the patients may act as if blind, walking into obstacles and groping for objects. Furthermore, the patients may not be able to localize objects even if they identified them. This symptom fits in very well with the localization of the lesion: the occipitoparietal cortex where the visual world is represented in partly egocentric coordinates and changes less across saccades (as opposed to a retinotopic coordinate system; see the subsection 'Failures to achieve a stable representation of extrapersonal space' and the next subsection).

A hypothesis about the neuronal mechanisms in simultanagnosia

It should be kept in mind that humans change fixation more than once per second—hence the representation of the visual world changes position at the same frequency in the primary visual cortex. Hence, a more 'durable' representation is required that is at least partially stable over eye movements. This representation should also be able to synthesize, over subsequent eye movements, a reasonably detailed representation of the visual world. Single-cell recordings in the parietal lobe of monkeys indeed revealed neurons coding objects in partly head- or world-centred rather than retina-centred coordinates (cf. Andersen *et al.* 1997; Chapter 5, this volume; cf. also the subsection 'Failure to achieve a stable representation of extrapersonal space'). It fits in well with this view of visual information-processing that the parietal cortex is part of the dorsal processing stream that is often called the 'where' system.

I would like to propose that a defect in the egocentric representation would not only cause the inability to localize objects across eye movements, but may also cause the 'main' symptom of simultanagnosia—loss of the ability to *store* object representations across eye movements. As a consequence of the inability to store representation even for short periods the patient is unable to create a body-centred representation of the world (see the subsection 'Failures to achieve a stable representation of extrapersonal space' and Karnath *et al.* 2002; cf. Robertson *et al.* 1997). Intuitively, it also fits in very well that moving objects pose greater problems for these patients than stationary ones. If only a retinotopic representation is left, cortical object representations will undergo massive distortions if the object moves from the centre to the periphery. The finding that simultanagnosic patients are better able to perceive several objects if these are close together (hence do not require eye movements to be perceived in sufficient detail) would be compatible with this hypothesis. However, there are indications that not only eye movements, but also shifts of attention may lead to an extinction of the newly attended object and to an extinction of the previous concept (Luria 1959).

Many of the above arguments would also apply to the Balint syndrome (see eponymous section).

Visual disorientation in simultanagnosia

Another symptom of these patients is their visual disorientation, the inability to keep track of the position of a previous stimulus while analysing a new object and to code spatial relations between objects. The visual system codes spatial relations *within* objects differently from relations *between* objects. Therefore, simultanagnosic patients can preserve the ability to identify single objects, unlike those patients suffering from apperceptive agnosia.

The inability to code spatial relations is also apparent in the copies that simultanagnosic patients produce of drawings, which have an 'exploded' look even though the patient easily recognized the object (quite different from associative agnosiacs who produce exact copies without object recognition). As in the case of neglect patients, there has been some debate whether the deficit in simultanagnosia is primarily one of attention or of representation, but this seems more a semantic than a genuine discrepancy as we will see in the section on neglect (cf. Posner *et al.* 1984; Bisiach *et al.* 1979*a*; Shallice 1989; Farah 1990). The inability to keep track of previous positions will inevitably lead to problems of visual exploration and to a piecemeal type of perception (cf. Zihl and von Cramon 1986; Pötzl 1928; Newcombe *et al.* 1987).

Different subtypes of simultanagnosia

Some authors doubt the existence of an isolated deterioration in the detection of a whole (scene) with intact detection of its details, as postulated in simultanagnosia (Bay 1950; Weigl 1964; Rubens 1979), and some discriminate between two types of simultanagnosia: (1) dorsal simultanagnosia, a deficit in the spatial system that leads to the inability to *attend* to more than one item at a time (while single multipart objects, e.g. words, can still be perceived); (2) ventral simultanagnosia: inability to *recognize* more than one object at a time (however, since the attentional system is intact, patients have no problems in navigation; Farah 1990).

A subgroup of simultanagnosic patients, called 'ventral simultanagnosics' by Farah (1990), as opposed to the 'dorsal simultanagnosics' described above, suffer from lesions in the *left* inferior *temporo*-occipital region. By and large, symptoms of the two patient groups of ventral and dorsal simultanagnosias are very similar (Bauer 1993; de Renzi 1982; Frederiks 1969; Kertesz 1987; Williams 1970). But an important difference is that the patients suffering from ventral simultanagnosia due to unilateral lesions, fail to *recognize* multiple objects (as the bilateral parieto-occipital patients with the dorsal simultanagnosia do), but are able to *see* multiple objects and hence can count and manipulate objects and walk around without running into obstacles. This group of simultanagnosic patients seems still to possess an egocentric map of the outer world, but to have problems with *moving* 'attention' (or conscious analysis) from one object to the next. Reading is possible in a letter-by-letter way—synthesizing words by sequential analysis of letters.

Recognition of multiple objects is impaired even if these appear not strictly simultaneously, but in sequence: performance is determined by the total period available for processing (Kinsbourne and Warrington 1962; Levine and Calvanio 1978). Location pre-cues improve performance while postcues have no effect (Levine and Calvanio 1978).

Both types of simultanagnosiacs are often considered as suffering from a special type of apperceptive agnosia (see e.g. Farah 1990). Instead, I would argue that simultanagnosia should be considered as a class in-between associative agnosias and neglect (and Balint's syndrome), given the fact that recognition of single objects *is* possible in simultanagnosia (influenced by top–down influences), while not in apperceptive agnosia. In particular, the unilateral ventral type of defect (ventral simultanagnosia) shares the quality of an apparent deficit in 'attentional' allocation with the neglect syndrome, and may be better called 'bradygnosia' rather than agnosia (from Greek: *brady*, slow), since the most prominent symptom seems to be a problem of disengaging attention from an object, thus slowing down the progress of visual search (e.g. Posner *et al.* 1984; Baynes *et al.* 1986).

Blindsight and neglect

Failure of failed analysis within scotomata: blindsight

Legally, blindness of a part of the visual field is defined as an absolute scotoma in this part of the visual field. This means that patients are not able to consciously perceive a stimulus presented in this part of the visual world. However, as demonstrated in Chapter 9, this volume, at least some patients may still be able to react in a goal-directed way to stimuli presented within this blind part of the visual field. In this sense, the visual analysis fails, but in another sense, it succeeds (fails to fail) since the patient is still able to detect, localize, and analyse the stimulus, even if this analysis is not available to conscious insight. Patients usually are not pleased at all if asked to respond to stimuli that they do not subjectively see. As a new method of alleviating this problem when testing patients, we presented either two or three dots sequentially in the visual field and asked patients to discriminate between the directions of motion (Stoerig and Fahle 1995). In this task, the patient always saw two dots that were presented within the intact visual field and hence had no exceptional problem answering the question regarding motion direction between these two dots, even if the direction was not obvious. As to be expected, normal observers achieved significantly better results in this task when three dots were displayed rather than just two dots. The same was true for a patient suffering from a large scotoma caused by a brain trauma even though the additional third point was presented in the middle of his scotoma and hence was never consciously perceived (Fig. 7.18; Stoerig and Fahle 1995). However, in two other patients, suffering from large absolute scotomata due to cerebral infarctions, we did not find any sign of blindsight with this task (Spang and Fahle, unpublished). Hence, the gift of blindsight is not evident in all patients suffering from (absolute) visual field defects.

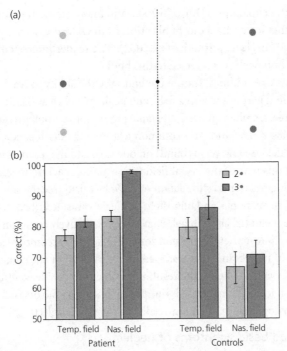

Fig. 7.18 Blindsight for motion direction. (a) The patient was asked to discriminate between upwards versus downwards motion. A least two stimulus dots were presented, one above and the other below the patient's scotoma (that had been caused by traumatic brain injury). The two dots were presented in sequence, with either the upper or the lower dot presented first. Presenting the upper dot first produced apparent motion downwards, starting with the lower dot resulted in the impression of upwards motion. In half of the presentations, a third dot was displayed midway between the outer dots, and at the appropriate time. Adding the third dot significantly improved direction discrimination in normal observers, and the same held true for the patient, in spite of him never consciously perceiving the middle dot that appeared in the middle of his scotoma. (b) So while the patient was unable to discriminate consciously between presentations containing two dots versus three dots, he nevertheless yielded better motion discrimination in the latter case even in the temporal field, with the third dot presented in his absolute scotoma. (From Stoerig and Fahle, unpublished.)

Neglect

Seeing but not perceiving: visual neglect

Visual neglect is a fascinating and still only partially understood phenomenon that has received renewed interest in recent years. Neglect, it must be said, probably is not just one homogeneous syndrome but a class of deficits with similar but distinct symptoms caused by defects in different parts of the brain but this view is by no means undisputed. It is impossible to give a full review of all the facets of this clinical syndrome here (such as discussions on compression of 'contralesional' subjective space (Bisiach *et al.* 1994), interactions with hemianopia (Doricchi 2002, and many more), but, fortunately, this is not necessary since a simultaneous publication from Oxford University Press covers in detail the topic of neglect (Karnath *et al.* 2002). The reader interested in a (far) more detailed account on neglect is referred to this book.

There is at least one common feature in blindsight, the ability to react to visual stimuli presented in a blind part of the visual field, and neglect (as well as Balint's syndrome and, to a certain degree, simultanagnosia), the *failure* to react to stimuli presented in a part of the visual field that is *not* blind. This common feature is the discrepancy between the status of the visual field (seeing versus blind) on one side, and the reaction to stimulus presentation within this part of the visual field (appropriate reaction to stimulation of the blind field, missing reaction to stimulation of the intact field (see the subsection 'Relation between neglect, hemianopia, and blindsight')). Neglect was described in patients as early as 1885 by Oppenheim (cf. also Poppelreuter 1917), is relatively common in patients with defects of the occipito-parietal-temporal zone, and is often accompanied by scotomata. The assessment of neglect in patients is greatly complicated by the coincidence of visual field defects and neglect—hence the resulting problem to decide whether the failure of visual stimulation to elicit a response is due to purely sensory factors such as blindness or else due to partly cognitive or attention-related factors as in neglect.

A definition and basic symptoms of neglect

Neglect is a failure of perception on the highest, supramodal level, namely, conscious perception, that is relatively common after strokes involving the (right) parietal and/or temporal brain hemisphere. As we will see in the following, most of the processes of visual pattern analysis discussed so far seem to be intact in these patients, and yet they behave as if they were blind in part of the visual field. Even worse: these patients behave as if the contralesional part of the world no longer existed; they seem not to be aware of it and not to explore it at all. Not surprisingly, this defect is quite disabling for the patient, much more so than an hemianopia. Neglect patients are unable to explore the neglected (sic!) part of the world while patients suffering from visual field defects can still explore the blind regions by using eye movements. Problems are greatest for those (not so rare) cases with large lesions leading to both sensory deficit (hemianopia or large scotomata) and neglect.

Unilateral neglect is thus characterized by a reduced ability of a patient—usually suffering from a lesion in the right hemisphere, thalamus, and/or basal ganglia—to detect and subsequently report stimuli presented to the contralesional, i.e. usually left half of the world. Neglect occurs for all sense modalities—hearing, touch, seeing, even pain—and, as mentioned above, involves an inability to explore the neglected space, corresponding well to the finding that patients very often are not aware of their deficit. In the present context, we will only deal with visual neglect.

Neglect has a unique role among the disorders on higher levels of processing. Like a scotoma, it prevents perception of all stimulus attributes—not just, e.g. their colour, or form. The object as a whole is not available to conscious perception, unlike in patients suffering from indiscriminations, or apperceptive or associative agnosias. Hence neglect, in a way, includes the symptoms of these other disorders. Neglect, therefore, is the most surprising of all failures of visual perception—a failure of conscious perception in spite of largely preserved visual pattern analysis. The neglect syndrome involves one of the basic categories of perception, one of the *a priori* of all perception and thinking in Kant's sense, namely, a partial loss of the concept of space—for the patient, a part of space no longer exists. In a way, the concept of the left part of the world for a neglect patient seems to be what the fourth dimension may be for a physicist: He or she knows that it must be there, but lacks a concept of what it looks like.

Relation between neglect, hemianopia, and blindsight

Contrasting neglect with blindsight and hemianopia leads to a better understanding of all three syndromes. As outlined above, neglect in a way is the reverse of blindsight. In blindsight, the primary visual cortex is defective (leading to hemianopia, see 'Complete failure to see: blindness and scotomata'), but patients can nevertheless detect and analyse stimuli presented in their scotoma (usually without a corresponding subjective awareness of the stimuli; see Chapter 9, this volume). It should be noted that blindsight is possible only in hemianopic patients with intact retinae and optic nerves. In severe neglect, the primary visual cortex is intact, but patients are nevertheless unable to react to stimuli in the contralesional visual field. Another difference is that the border of the scotoma is rather clear-cut in hemianopia and blindsight, reflecting the usually sharp border of the visual field defect, while no such sharp border exists in neglect, but rather a gradient (see Fig. 7.19). A third difference is the dependence on eye, head, and body posture. The defect in hemianopia and blindsight is defined strictly in retinotopic coordinates, while it depends on head and body posture in neglect where the defect seems to be in egocentric or even allocentric coordinates (see e.g. Pouget *et al.* 1993). This difference is due to the fact that neglect involves a defect on a higher level of representation than the retinotopic lesion that leads to a scotoma and may leave blindsight within the scotoma intact. The fourth difference concerns the dependence on additional stimuli in the intact visual field. These seem to have only marginal influence on perception in all blindsight patients. Patients suffering from mild forms of neglect, on the other side, can usually detect a stimulus displayed in the neglected portion of the visual field if the ipsilesional visual field is empty, i.e. homogeneous. However, presentation of stimuli in the ipsilesional visual field usually 'extinguishes' perception of stimuli presented in the neglected, contralesional part of the visual field. A fifth difference, again underlining the higher level of underlying defect in neglect, is the occurrence of neglect for nearby objects only (Halligan and Marshall 1991*b*), or else for far objects only (Vuilleumier *et al.* 1998), indicating that there may be different cortical representations for the space immediately accessible to grasping movements versus space farther away. This finding is in line with differences in response qualities of single neurons in the parietal cortex of monkeys, some of which code for nearby objects only (Colby and Goldberg 1999; Berti and Frassinetti 2000). A sixth difference is that scotomata are strictly visual and patients will react to auditory stimuli in the contralesional side of the outer world, while neglect often involves several sense modalities. A seventh difference is that neglect may also concern the contralesional side of objects and places recalled from memory from a specific vantage point (Bisiach and Luzzatti 1978; see the subsection 'Spatial neglect in allocentric, object-centred coordinates and for remembered landscapes').

Given all these differences, the reader may wonder what blindsight, cortical scotoma and neglect have in common at all. The answer is quite straightforward: all three types of patients are not normally reacting to stimuli presented to their contralesional side. They behave in a standard ophthalmological test as if they were blind or had defective vision, in the contralesional visual field. Moreover, blindsight and neglect share the property that considerable visual processing and analysis of the visual input occurs without reaching awareness (unlike in patients suffering from a retinal scotoma). In several ways, hemianopias caused by defects of the visual afferents and neglect are similar, since patients do not consciously perceive objects in the defective part of the world. But while hemianopia in patients without blindsight does not lead to any detectable effects of the stimuli on the cortex, this is not true in neglect nor in hemianopia caused by cortical defects for the patients showing blindsight.

Symptoms typical of visual neglect

We have already given an overview of the typical symptoms present in neglect patients. In the following, a more detailed account follows, while the reader is again referred to an even more detailed account in the book by Karnath *et al.* (2002; see also Heilman *et al.* 1993).

Neglect, as we know, is characterized by a lack of responsiveness to visual stimulation in the contralesional visual field in the absence of scotomata or at least with scotomata not covering the whole contralesional hemifield. Typically, the patients ignore all stimuli on the contralesional side, both visual stimuli and those from other sense modalities. Symptoms are usually far more severe after lesions of the right cortical hemisphere and hence in the left half-field. (As we will see in the subsection 'Neuronal and neuropsychological mechanisms of spatial neglect: deficit of attention versus representation?', the right hemisphere may contain a representation not only of the left side of the outer world, but also at least a rudimentary representation of the right side.) The cortical lesions underlying neglect seem to bias perception towards fine local details of visual scenes, leading to a loss of overview over more global properties and to a centripetal bias in addition to a horizontal (left/right) bias (Robertson *et al.* 1988; Lamb *et al.* 1990; Halligan and Marshall 1991*a,b*, 1993). Patients suffering from neglect caused by right hemispheric lesions may only eat the food on the right side of their plate and complain of having not enough food, while the left part of the plate is still not emptied. Just rotating the plate, thus exchanging its right and left sides, can satisfy them. Patients may read only the right side of a newspaper, or of isolated words, or describe and copy only the right half of a figure. When searching through a page of paper and marking all lines, or all shapes of a specific form, they may mark only those lines or shapes on the ipsilesional side of the paper. Anecdotal reports include a woman who after suffering a stroke and coming back from the hospital put formidable make-up on her face, but only on one side. Patients sometimes develop surprising strategies to search for objects, e.g. by turning to the right until the required object might turn up in their right visual field, i.e. shortly before they finish a complete circle.

Generally, neglect patients are not aware of and have little or no insight into their deficits, especially shortly after the injury and for large insults, a symptom sometimes called anosognosia (cf. already Redlich and Bonvicini 1909; Babinski 1914).

Graduation of spatial neglect and extinction of stimuli

Defects of the primary visual cortex, or in the pathways leading there, usually cause reasonably sharply delineated scotomata, reproducibly testable by perimetry. This is not the case for the failure of analysis observed in neglected parts of the outer world. There is no sharp spatial divide between positions where stimuli are consciously perceived and those where they are neglected, but rather a gradient in probability of detection and perception. In the most severe cases, stimuli in the neglected half are completely invisible for the patient, even if there are no simultaneous stimuli in the ipsilesional visual field, as is the case during perimetric testing. The probability of detecting a stimulus increases for stimuli presented more towards the ipsilesional side. For less severe neglect, the overall probability of stimulus detection in the contralesional visual half-field increases, but a gradient between the contra- and ipsilesional sides persists. As detailed in the next section, the gradient may also shift in horizontal direction depending on the position of eyes, head, and body.

Probability of stimulus detection also depends on whether other stimuli are simultaneously displayed, and where. The defect of spatial vision as evidenced in neglect is most obvious during competition between stimuli. Generally, the stimulus presented more to the contralesional side will not be perceived. It is suppressed or extinguished by the stimulus further towards or further within the ipsilesional field. Natural scenes usually contain a multitude of objects, so suppression will occur permanently, leading to extinction of objects on the neglected side, possibly due to attraction of attention by the objects on the ipsilesional, usually right side. As we will discuss in detail (in the subsection 'Evidence for preserved processing of visual input'), suppression of some stimuli occurs even in healthy observers if their attention is focused on other objects—we cannot consciously perceive all objects that are processed at least up to primary visual cortex. The extinction observed in neglect may be a special case of the suppression also experienced in healthy observers due to a limited conscious visual capacity, just with a strong spatial bias. However, healthy observers still have the concept that there are objects outside their focus of attention, while at least some neglect patients seem to lack the very concept of space on their contralesional side. A related phenomenon is simultanagnosia, a strong restriction in the number of objects that a patient simultaneously perceives (see the eponymous subsection; Holmes and Horrax 1919; Rafal 1997; cf. also Gorea and Sagi 2000).

Dependence on eye, head, and body posture

Failures of visual analysis caused by defects of the primary visual cortex cause retino-topically defined scotomata involving a fixed portion of the retinal image and hence, depending on eye position, covering quite different portions of a visual scene. In sharp contrast, the spatial disregard in neglect patients concerns predominantly a defined part of the surround, on the contralesional side. Therefore, the failure to respond to visual stimuli in neglect patients is less dependent on eye position than in hemianopia, even though a certain dependence exists (Fig. 7.19). As outlined in the preceding

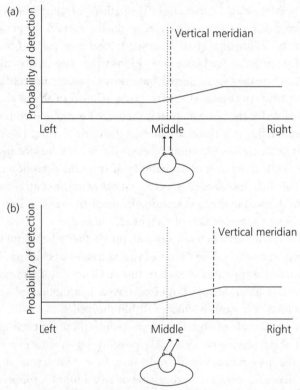

Fig. 7.19 Dependence of neglect on eye and head position. A patient suffering from a defect of the right hemisphere may suffer from neglect of the left side of the world. The border between the normal and the neglected part of the (visual) world is not sharp but follows a gradient and hence there is a gradient in the probability to detect a stimulus. The location of this gradient in the outer world is defined mostly by egocentric position, more specifically, by the position of the trunk. (a) For eyes straight ahead, the midline in egocentric coordinates and the vertical meridian, i.e. the midline of the retina, are superimposed. (b) Eye position is far less important than trunc position, so the position of the gradient does not strongly change after movements of the eyes while the visual vertical meridian is shifted to the right. Hence, unlike with a scotoma that is defined in retinotopic coordinates, neglect may or may not lead to extinction of a stimulus on a given retinal position, depending on eye position.

subsection, there is no sharp border in neglect between those spatial locations attended to and those where stimuli are neglected, but rather a gradient, with stimuli further towards the ipsilesional side detected more often than those shifted more towards the contralesional side (even if both stimuli lie in the same hemifield).

Surprisingly, the gradient is not defined in retinal coordinates, but more in egocentric ones. When the eyes are moved, the gradient may stay almost constant in the outer world. This is to say that it depends on the location of objects relative to the body, whether or not they are neglected, not on their location on the retina, as is the case in patients with scotomata (Fig. 7.19). So, rotating the body in a contralesional direction while simultaneously moving the eyes in the opposite direction, keeping the gaze on the same object, may switch a near-midline part of the visual field from the 'neglect' mode to a 'perception' mode. In the new body position, this visual field position belongs to the ipsilesional part of the outer world, and the stimuli it receives are far less neglected, though they fall of the same part of the retina.

Basically, the same holds true for movements of the head. Turning only the head rather than the body also shifts the gradient of neglect in retinal terms (either by shifting the entire reference system or predominantly the subjective straight ahead). This is even true for intended, rather than real head movements or if a head movement is simulated by stretch reflexes of the neck muscles (Karnath *et al.* 1991). Hence, it is, to a first approximation, body posture more than eye or head position that determines whether a stimulus at a given location succeeds or fails to reach awareness in a neglect patient: egocentric rather than retinotopic localization is the crucial parameter.

Spatial neglect in allocentric, object-centred coordinates and for remembered landscapes

Another symptom that strongly sets apart the failure of visual stimulation as measured by object identification in neglect from that in scotomata is the dependence of neglect on object-centred coordinates. The left side of a flower may be neglected, irrespective of whether it is presented in vertical orientation (left side is neglected, cf. Driver 1999) or rotated clockwise, to a horizontal orientation (upper side is neglected). This astonishing symptom can be understood in the framework of neglect as a disorder of object-centred spatial representations and/or of spatially selective attention. This is to say that some type of constancy-mechanism (see 'Failures to achieve object constancy') readjusts the object to the normal, upright position, and only thereafter may the neuronal mechanisms underlying conscious perception come into full play.

The ground-breaking experiments of Bisiach and colleagues (e.g. Bisiach and Luzzatti 1978) demonstrated convincingly that spatial neglect is not caused by sensory deficits or by deficits in memory consolidation or recall. Patients were asked to imagine standing on one side of a square they knew well in Milan, looking at the opposite side of the square. Their task was to name all the buildings they saw. Patients suffering from a neglect caused by a right-sided brain lesion would only name buildings located in the right half of the patient's imagined visual field. Then, patients were asked to imagine standing on the opposite side of the square, looking at the location they had just imagined to be. Again, they tried to name all the buildings they perceived with their mind's eye. This time, they would name only buildings on the opposite side of the square—again the ones in the right part of the visual field of their mind's eye. This experiment clearly shows that neglect is not primarily a defect of information-processing and storage, but of information retrieval by the aware subject.

Evidence for preserved processing of visual input

Three lines of evidence support the claim that neglected stimuli failing to reach conscious perception nevertheless are processed in some detail in the patient's visual system. This evidence relies on: (1) the clear effects of grouping and priming by neglected stimuli; (2) the presence of visually evoked sum potentials; as well as, (3) the evidence for stimulus-evoked changes of cortical blood oxygenation levels as evidenced by functional magnetic resonance imaging (fMRI).

Neglect (as well as simultanagnosia) can be considered as a severe form of the inability even of normal observers to process more than about five stimuli presented simultaneously, just with a spatial bias in the case of neglect. Grouping the stimuli presented in the neglected part of the visual field with others presented in the ipsilesional field into a *single* object should alleviate the suppression in the neglected hemifield. And suppression indeed decreased when two stimuli in the neglected half-field represented corners of a large illusory square whose other two corners were located in the normal half of the visual field. Hence, some type of *grouping* and categorization is still possible, including that of stimuli presented in the neglected part of the visual field. The grouping process has to be pre-attentive since, per definition, attentive vision is defective in the neglected half-field (Mattingley *et al.* 1997; Ward *et al.* 1994; cf. also Davis and Driver 1998; Gilchrist *et al.* 1996; cf. Luria 1959; Berti *et al.* 1992; Vuilleumier *et al.* 2001; Godwin-Austen 1965, for similar effects in simultanagnosic patients).

This finding strongly argues for a model of neglect as a competition between *object representations* rather than between retinotopic locations (see 'Neuronal and neuropsychological mechanisms of spatial neglect: deficit of attention versus representation?'). The same holds true for the fact that some patients asked to *enumerate* multiple objects presented simultaneously in both hemifields were able to take into account the stimuli in the neglected hemifield, while they suppressed and hence ignored these stimuli when asked to indicate their position in bilateral displays (Vuilleumier and Rafal 1999). Presented with the picture of a house with smoke coming from the contralesional side of the roof, the patients would not appreciate anything unusual with this house. Yet, when presented with two houses, one normal and one burning on the contralesional side, they would nevertheless choose the normal one if asked where they would prefer to live (Marshall and Halligan 1988). However, this result is not undisputed.

Priming effects of neglected (or suppressed) stimuli are evident in a number of experimental situations. One such effect is the decrease of reaction times after bilateral stimulus presentations as compared to unilateral presentations. This is to say that patients responded faster to stimuli presented to both hemifields than to stimuli presented to the ipsilesional hemifield alone—even if they were not aware of the stimulus in their contralesional field, this stimulus increased their speed of responding (Marzi *et al.* 1996). Not only can the presence of a stimulus in the contralesional visual field (unconsciously) influence reaction times but also rather complex features of this neglected stimulus such as its shape and colour may have an influence, as well as its identity and even its semantic contents do (Audet *et al.* 1991; Cohen *et al.* 1995; di Pellegrino and de Renzi 1995; Berti and Rizzolatti 1992; cf. also Baylis *et al.* 1993; McGlinchey-Berroth *et al.* 1993; Ladavas *et al.* 1993; 1997).

Processing of neglected stimuli does not only lead to improvement of reaction times. Patients suffering from neglect and extinction of contralesional stimuli were also able to discriminate between same and different stimulus presentations in both hemifields and hence could identify the stimulus in the neglected hemifield (Volpe *et al.* 1979; Berti *et al.* 1992; cf. Farah *et al.* 1991). Stroop effects, i.e. an interference of a coloured stimulus with reading a colour name, are exerted by stimuli in the neglected hemifield, similar to the effects in healthy observers—though the stimuli themselves are neglected (cf. Logan 1980; MacLeod 1991; Berti *et al.* 1994; Sharon *et al.* 1999). Presentation of stimuli in the neglected halffield, moreover, may lead to perceptual learning, i.e. improvement of perceptual capabilities for the stimuli displayed. To sum up, stimuli presented in the neglected hemifield can influence the response of the patient even though they are not consciously perceived and their effect may differ from that exerted by stimuli presented in the ipsilesional hemifield.

Objects and faces that were presented in the contralesional hemifield and were not subjectively perceived nevertheless evoked ERPs in sum potential recordings on the scalps of patients suffering from neglect. First, unspecific potentials arise about 100 ms after stimulus onset, followed at 170 to 200 ms latency by potentials specific for, e.g. presentation of faces. The potentials evoked by presentation in the contralesional visual field, however, sometimes differ considerably from those evoked by stimulus display in the ipsilesional field (Spinelli *et al.* 1994; Angelelli *et al.* 1996; Vallar *et al.* 1991; Sagiv *et al.* 2000; Bentin *et al.* 1996; Eimer 1998; cf. however Marzi *et al.* 2000; Hämäläinen *et al.* 1999; Deouell *et al.* 2000; Doricchi *et al.* 1996; Viggiano *et al.* 1995). This difference between the potentials evoked in the ipsi- versus contralateral hemifields is not surprising given the fact stressed in the subsection 'Visual information- processing in the cortex: parallel processing and feedback' that visual information- processing involves strong feedback connections. Thus, defects of 'higher' stages of processing will also have detrimental influences on the performance of 'lower' areas—unlike in a strictly hierarchical feedforward system.

Presentation of objects and faces in the contralesional hemifield also significantly increased fMRI signal strength in the primary visual cortex of neglect patients as well as in early extrastriate areas and the fusiform region of the lesioned cortical hemisphere (Rees *et al.* 2000; Vuilleumier *et al.* 2000, cf. also de Haan *et al.* 1987*a, b* for a behavioural correlate in prosopagnosia).

The evidence presented in this section clearly proves that stimuli presented in the neglected part of the outer world nevertheless activate not only the primary visual cortex, but also extrastriate and ventral temporal areas. These neglected stimuli are at least partly analysed and categorized, but do not reach awareness, even if patients take them into account, e.g. in enumeration tasks. This is a fundamental difference to agnosias. Preserved analysis in the ventral stream (see Chapter 5, this volume) without awareness supports *in principle* the notion of two parallel streams of cortical processing only one of which is linked to awareness (cf. Milner and Goodale 1995; Goodale *et al.* 1991; Goodale and Milner 1992; Ettlinger 1990; Newcombe *et al.* 1987; Ratcliff 1982). Some of the details of this dichotomy are still under debate, since the simplistic dichotomy between conscious ventral processing and unconscious dorsal processing would only apply if neglect were, indeed, a defect caused by damage primarily of the parietal lobe.

Tests for detecting spatial neglect in patients

A number of clinical tests have been developed to diagnose neglect and to discriminate it from purely sensory disorders such as scotomata. A very widely used test consists of asking the patients to search for short lines on a sheet of paper and to cross them all with pencil strokes (cf. Lezak 1995). Neglect patients tend to cross only those targets displayed on their ipsilesional side. A somewhat more difficult task is to search for a specific shape, say, a star or circle, among squares, stars, and rhombi, and to cross only the circles, or to search for a specific letter. In the first task, patients have 'just' to detect that there are stimuli on their neglected side, while in the second type they must discriminate between different shapes. Patients may not be able to perform this discrimination even though they may be partly aware of the presence of these objects.

Another class of tests requires the patients to bisect, by a pencil mark, a line presented on a sheet of paper. When bisecting a horizontal line, patients suffering from neglect often deviate towards the ipsilesional side, sometimes dramatically (e.g. Ferber and Karnath 2001). Hence, they do not take into account most of the line length presented on their contralesional, neglected side. In a third type of test the patients are asked to describe and/or copy a picture. Usually, they will exclusively or predominantly describe the ipsilesional part of the picture, and likewise omit parts of the contralesional part when copying it. The same holds true when the patient draws the object from memory, another indication that neglect is *not* exclusively or predominantly a defect in processing of *sensory* information (see Bisiach and Luzzatti 1978; see also 'Spatial neglect in allocentric, object-centred coordinates and for remembered landscapes').

Localization of lesions

Typically, the lesions in patients suffering from neglect involve the parietal cortex, with much more severe symptoms in patients suffering from right-sided cortical lesions than in those suffering from lesions of the left hemisphere. Typically, the lesions are located in the inferior parietal lobe, particularly in the angular and supramarginal gyri, i.e. Brodmann's areas 39 and 40, as well as the frontal lobe and/or the basal ganglia (Heilman and Valenstein 1972; Heilman *et al.* 1993; Leibovitch *et al.* 1998; Husain and Kennard 1996; Perenin 1997; Vallar 1993, 1998; Vallar and Perani 1986; cf. also Colombo *et al.* 1976). However, this view has been disputed recently with the claim that it is the temporal, not the parietal cortex that is responsible for spatial awareness (Karnath *et al.* 2001; cf. Driver 1996; Samuelsson *et al.* 1997). In the following, I will continue to ascribe neglect to injury of the parietal lobe, but this may have to be changed or extended to the temporal lobe in a later edition of this book. As with other neuropsychological syndromes, fibre-of passage damage may contribute to the symptoms, here through damage to fibre bundles running in the white matter beneath the parieto-temporo-occipital junction causing a disconnection syndrome (Leibovitch *et al.* 1998; Gaffan and Hornak 1997; Samuelsson *et al.* 1997).

It is difficult to more precisely specify the brain defect causing neglect by analogy to lesion studies in monkeys (cf. Chapter 5, this volume) since neglect deficits in monkeys are less persistent and less severe than in humans (for a recent review on this somewhat controversial problem, see Wardak *et al.* 2002). The parietal cortex of monkeys contains neurons not only with the usual contralateral but also with ipsilateral receptive fields (contrary to striate and extrastriate occipital cortex). The representation is strongest for regions close to the midline, i.e. close to the part of the outer world mainly represented by this side of cortex, and diminishes with distance from the midline, i.e. towards the periphery (Andersen *et al.* 1990; cf. also Pouget and Sejnovski 1997; Rizzolatti and Berti 1990). This graded representation is reminiscent of the spatially graded nature of neglect (see 'Graduation of spatial neglect and extinction of stimuli') and leads to less severe symptoms after unilateral (one-sided) cortical lesions.

Patients sometimes suffer from neglect-like symptoms without parietal damage, especially after lesions of frontal (Damasio *et al.* 1980*b*; Heilman and Valenstein 1972; Husain and Kennard 1996) or subcortical areas (Bogousslavsky *et al.* 1988; cf. also Rafal and Posner 1987; Vallar 1993; Vallar and Perani 1987; Watson and Heilman 1979; Hildebrandt *et al.* 2002). Hence, whatever the neuronal structures may be whose defects underlie neglect of the contralesional part of the world, they are part of an extended network involving both subcortical structures and different parts of cortex, such as frontal, cingulate, and—most notably—inferior parietal and/or superior temporal cortex.

Neuronal and neuropsychological mechanisms of spatial neglect: deficit of attention versus representation?

It seems fair to say that the neuronal and neuropsychological mechanisms causing spatial neglect are not completely understood. Broadly speaking, there are two views regarding the underlying cause that are not necessarily mutually exclusive: lack of attentional resources on the one side, and lack of (spatial) representation on the other. Let's first deal with the hypothesis that neglect is caused by a failure to attend to stimuli that are processed and relatively precisely analysed in the visual system but fail to reach consciousness, since *attention* is engaged in the ipsilesional part of the world. This phenomenon is not restricted to neglect patients, but applies to (neurologically) healthy observers as well in situations of sensory overload (e.g. Gorea and Sagi 2000). Human observers are unable to consciously process all of the information collected by the sense organs and transmitted to the brain. Hence, a selection has to take place, and one of the processes underlying this selection process is related to attention. We do have a certain control over where to direct our attention, but no total control—salient stimuli will automatically attract attention. Thresholds for detecting an object depend, to a certain degree, on whether or not they are attended to. In the extreme case, when our attention is engaged completely in analysing a specific aspect of a scene, or of an object (hence we are highly concentrated on this object or task), we may fail to perceive another aspect or object in spite of its being signalled to our primary visual cortex (e.g. change-blindness: Rensink *et al.* 1997).

The effect of attention on the processing of a stimulus can be measured not just by behavioural and, more specifically, psychophysical methods, but also by more objective ones. On the single-cell level, the responses of neurons in macaque monkey cortex to a specific stimulus increase when the animal attends the stimulus. The increase is more pronounced in higher, parietal and frontal areas than in the primary visual cortex (Wurtz *et al.* 1982; McAdams and Maunsell 1999; Desimone and Duncan 1995; Moran and Desimone 1985; see Giesbrecht and Mangun 2002 for a recent review on top–down attentional control), and neurons in the lateral interparietal (LIP) area of monkey cortex only respond to the attended stimulus or behaviourally relevant ones while ignoring all others (Gottlieb *et al.* 1998; Snyder *et al.* 1997). A similar increase of responses appears both in evoked sum-responses to visual stimuli (Chapter 3, this volume), and in the level of cortical blood oxygenation as measured by fMRI (e.g. Kastner and Ungerleider 2000; Corbetta 1998; Corbetta and Shulman 1998; for PET and event-related potentials, cf. Nobre *et al.* 1997, 2000; Neville and Lawson 1987). These examples of 'neglected' stimuli in normal observers with their psychophysical, electrophysiological, and imaging correlates are similar to the symptoms of neglect in patients. Hence, the problems that patients experience in directing their attention to the contralesional side of the outer world might be related to difficulties in steering attention in the visual field. This difficulty comes in graded specifications, from less severe forms that allow patients to attend to the contralesional side if no competitive stimuli are presented to the ipsilateral side, to more severe forms where, even under these artificial conditions with only one stimulus present, patients are not aware of a stimulus presented to their neglected side. So it seems fair to say that whatever causes neglect does have a *spatial* component.

A few details may not fit smoothly into this otherwise tempting and elegant model. One is the difference between defects of the two hemispheres. Injuries of the right parietal brain cause far more severe symptoms than those of the left hemisphere. So should only the right brain be able to steer attention? In that case, we would also expect severe attentional problems in patients' ipsilesional hemifield after right parietal injury. So we must conclude that right parietal lesions impair the ability to shift the 'spotlight of attention' into the left half of extrapersonal space, while it can be moved within the right half of this space. This, however, is a notion less intuitively convincing than the more general notion of a defect in directing attention.

There is a tradition of contrasting the hypothesis that neglect is due to a disturbance of attention with the view that (quite to the contrary) neglect is due to a disturbance of spatial *representation* of contralesional space (Battersby *et al.* 1956; Bisiach and Berti 1987; Bisiach *et al.* 1979a; Denny-Brown and Banker 1954; Hecaen 1972; Paterson and Zangwill 1944; Scheller and Seidemann 1931). It should be clear by now that neglect is not a defect of representation by neurons that are retinotopically organized. Neuronal defects on the retinotopic level lead to scotomata, the relative position of which moves with the eyes. On the other hand, the defect does not decrease a general ability such as that needed to direct attention but restricts this ability to a part of the outer world. Based on these facts, and on the results of electrophysiological and imaging techniques that find the strongest effects of attention in the parietal lobes rather than in the primary or secondary visual cortices, we can assume that neglect is caused by damage to those representations of the outer world that are organized in egocentric (and possibly partly in allocentric) coordinates and whose neurons show strong influences of attention. This hypothesis is supported by the fact that the neurons in the cortical regions involved in neglect do have these ego- or allo-centric receptive fields and are, by nature, to a large extent, polysensory, i.e. they integrate information from several sense modalities. Hence, these neurons would account also for multimodal forms of neglect (Andersen *et al.* 1997; Vallar 1998).

The symptoms encountered in neglect patients suggest that the internal representations of extrapersonal space in the parietal lobe are the neuronal basis for the subjective perceptual experience of this space—or that, at least, they are an essential prerequisite for this experience (cf. Bisiach and Berti 1987; Robertson *et al.* 1997; Driver and Vuilleumier 2001 for similar views). This is to say that neglect is caused by loss of the neuronal representation of the contralesional part of the outer world on an abstraction level characterized, to a first approximation, by an egocentric rather than retinotopic representation. A strong reciprocal inhibition between *object* representations exists at this representational level which is partly under volitional control (top–down attention) and which has access to awareness (or underlies the subjective experience of awareness; cf. Driver & Vuilleumier 2001).

One may go on and speculate that one of the reasons for this winner-take-all mechanism of attentional control that allows only one object representation at a time to reach awareness is related to the fact that, at any time, most of us are only capable of generating conscious motor output related to a single object. But the principle of one single representation and the exclusion of alternative interpretations seems to be a more general principle of cortical information-processing, as evidenced, for example, in binocular rivalry (see e.g. Blake and Logothetis 2002; Fahle 1982) and bistable figures (such as the Necker-cube).

Hence, the two seemingly contradictory views regarding the cause underlying neglect just stress two different aspects of the defect. One might well reconcile the two models presented above by postulating that neglect is a defect on a level of information-processing at which there is a strong competition between different object representations (influenced both by volition and stimulus attributes) in an egocentrically organized map that is linked to conscious perception.

Failure of visual analysis on very different levels of processing

In the course of this chapter, we have encountered quite different reasons as to why visual analysis may fail. The most straightforward causes of failed analysis are defects of the retina, the optic nerve, optic tract, LGN, and optic radiation as well as primary visual cortex, which all lead to complete blindness, with the possibility of blindsight in some patients suffering from defects of the LGN or 'higher up'. But analysis may fail in the sense that the patient is unable to analyse a visual stimulus and to react adequately even though the visual information reaches an intact primary visual cortex. Patients may be unable to analyse specific categories (or submodalities) of the visual input such as colour, motion, or depth and to extract borders between different areas of the visual field defined by the corresponding submodalities of vision. These defects such as cerebral achromatopsia, motion blindness, or stereoblindness may be referred to collectively as indiscriminations (see 'Visual indiscriminations').

On the next level of analysis, all elementary submodalities may still be intact, all contours in a scene are detected, and the neighbouring areas are perceived in the correct colour, speed, and depth, but the binding together of contours to surfaces and objects fails. This syndrome is usually called apperceptive agnosia.

Patients suffering from defects on the next level of analysis are able to bind together objects from contours located at different positions in the visual field, but these object representations cannot be related to stored representations. Hence, visual objects can be copied, but categorization fails. The patient could be considered to suffer from a complete visual amnesia, i.e. as having lost all memories for visual objects encountered previously—or having lost access to these memories due to fibre damage, and hence cannot make sense of the objects he or she perceives. This inability can be restricted to certain classes of visual objects, such as faces (prosopagnosia), letters (alexia), or tools, while sparing other object classes. But even if categorization of an object has been achieved—at least partly—analysis may nevertheless fail in the sense that patients suffering from neglect, Balint's syndrome or simultanagnosia may still not consciously perceive a stimulus in the neglected part of the visual field and may be unable to react to it.

'Positive' symptoms: illusions and hallucinations

In strong contrast to all the 'defective' symptoms presented in this chapter so far, injuries of cortical substance can also yield 'productive' or 'positive' symptoms—in addition to the 'negative' scotomata and failures of visual analysis described—and even real hallucinations. The most common example is the 'migraine ophthalmique', consisting of vivid phosphenes that start at an arbitrary position in the visual field and proceed, over several minutes, to neighbouring locations until they stop, most often at the visual field border (for a review, see Lauber 1944, and for visual imaginery, Kosslyn 1980; Sergeant 1990). They are thought to be triggered by vascular processes and may have caused some of the reports of 'burning bushes' and 'unidentified flying objects' (UFOs).

Other examples of positive visual symptoms are the hallucinations experienced by some during high fever, alcohol withdrawal delirium, and productive schizophrenic episodes as well as the ones produced by transcranial magnetic stimulation (see Chapter 6, this volume). But, even after strokes involving the visual areas and leading to visual field defects, a certain percentage of patients start to experience visual hallucinations, as indicated by sporadic evidence in the literature and the shy reports of some of our own patients. Many patients probably are too reluctant to even mention these symptoms for fear of being considered 'crazy'. The same is true for patients suffering from (age-related) macular degeneration who often experience rather vivid hallucinations for up to a year after loss of central acuity (Charles-Bonnet syndrome). Systematic investigation of these symptoms is sparse due to the difficulties involved in quantifying such subjective experiences (but compare Santhouse *et al.* 2000). I would like to discriminate between positive symptoms on the one hand and hallucinations on the other.

Positive symptoms or *hallucinations* can have quite different underlying causes—cerebral bleedings, trauma, tumours, vascular disorders, or possibly afferent (sensory) deprivation or epileptic foci. They are quite common although most often only reported subsequent to explicit questioning (Lenz 1909; Gloning *et al.* 1968; Becke 1904; Kölmel 1985; Vorster 1893; Lamy 1895; Laehr 1896). Wilbrand and Sänger (1904) discriminated between simple and complex positive symptoms. *Simple* positive symptoms consist, for example, of small or extended light flashes, simple features, or colour tinges, usually caused by disturbances of occipital cortex (Meadows 1974*b*; Pötzl 1928; Bodamer 1947; Gloning *et al.* 1962, 1968; Lenz 1905; Horrax and Putnam 1932; Kölmel 1984; Hughlings-Jackson 1889; Jackson 1932; Jaspers 1973; cf. also Critchley 1966; Kandinsky 1881). *Complex* positive symptoms consist in the perception of objects, complex patterns, humans, animals, or scenes and are the symptoms one normally associates with the noun 'hallucination'. They are quite common after injuries of the occipital cortex, and always occur *after* the injury, while simple positive symptoms may precede the injury, as a warning sign of e.g. insufficient blood supply. Patients are always aware of the unreal nature of these perceptions, which they usually experience in defective (or blind) parts of their visual field, unlike psychotic patients, and hence the term pseudo-hallucinations might be better suited.

Five types of *visual illusion* are generally discriminated (e.g. Zihl and von Cramon 1986). The first is palinopsia or *visual perseveration* (Robinson and Watt 1947; Critchley 1951; Pötzl 1954; Bender *et al.* 1968). Patients perceive an object for several seconds or even minutes after the object has disappeared, or after they have performed a saccade to a new visual field position. Hence, this illusion is a kind of cortical afterimage (but without contrast reversal!). The underlying cause is always a bilateral defect, caused by infarctions or tumours (Critchley 1951; Bender *et al.* 1968) or else cortical hypoxia (Adler 1944). This type of illusion is always associated with other visual illusions or positive symptoms (Kinsbourne and Warrington 1963; Brust and Behrens 1977; Kömpf *et al.* 1983).

The second type of illusion is visual *allesthesia*, the illusory transportation of stimuli to (a mirror-symmetric part of) the contralateral visual half field—or, more rarely, in vertical direction into the corresponding quadrant of the visual field (Beyer 1895; Herrman and Pötzl 1928; Jacobs 1980; Gloning *et al.* 1968). The third type of illusion is *metamorphopsia*, i.e. short-lived but repeatedly occurring qualitative changes of perception, usually experienced as deformations in the form of objects, and often associated with changes in perceived orientation (Klopp 1951, 1955; Pichler 1957; Critchley 1966). Metamorphopsias are often associated with other illusions (Kömpf *et al.* 1983; Gloning *et al.* 1968; Hecaen and Angelergues 1963; Hoff and Pötzl 1935*a*).

The fourth type of illusion is visual *dysmetropsia*, i.e. a change in the perceived distance of objects, usually combined with a change of perceived size. Macropsia means that objects appear as larger; micropsia that they appear as smaller. Both are usually experienced in the contralesional hemifield (if at all) after defects in the temporo-occipital cortex, and sometimes in migraine attacks (Gloning *et al.* 1968). The last illusion to be mentioned is *polyopsia*, or *polyopia*. It differs from diplopia caused, for example, by eye muscle disorders in that it persists even monocularly, after closure of one eye (Mingazzini 1908; Pötzl 1928; Hoff and Pötzl 1935*b*; Gloning *et al.* 1968; Kömpf *et al.* 1983; Bender 1945; Meadows 1973). Typically, several representations of an object are arranged around the real position of this object. The symptoms are usually caused by bilateral lesions of occipital cortex (Gloning *et al.* 1968).

Some types of epilepsy, especially of the temporal lobes, can lead to short visual hallucinations, as can electrical stimulation of the cortex during brain operations (Penfield 1947, 1965, 1972). Surprisingly, some patients undergoing electrical stimulation reported seeing objects and even scenes without any feelings of strangeness. These reports are consistent with the generally accepted belief that our feelings and thoughts rely on the electrical activity in neuronal ensembles of the central nervous system. Still, it is surprising that such a coarse manipulation as injecting a current into a circumscribed brain region leads to well-structured hallucinations.

These observations in humans are supported by better-controlled experiments in monkeys. As a first step, Salzman *et al.* (1990) identified cells in monkey area MT or V5 in the middle temporal lobe (see Fig. 7.5) sensitive for detecting one direction of stimulus motion. The monkey was trained to discriminate between different directions of stimulus motion and to indicate the corresponding direction after each stimulus presentation. Injection of small electrical currents during the presentation of these moving stimuli significantly changed the response behaviour of the monkey in favour of the direction signalled by the neurons stimulated electrically. Control experiments ruled out any direct influence of these cells and of this electrical stimulation on motor centres of the brain. This is to say that, obviously, injection of current, leading to rather unspecific stimulation probably of both excitatory and inhibitory neurons in a small part of cortex, cannot be distinguished by the cortex—and by its owner—from excitation through the correct channels, namely, the optic nerves, but changes perception of the outer world (not just the motor response). This result was corroborated by additional experiments in which the monkeys were required to make exactly this discrimination between purely visual stimuli and those accompanied by electrical cortical stimulation, and failed to distinguish between the two situations.

To conclude, analysis of visual signals can fail on very different levels of processing, from the retina to higher levels of cortical processing, producing a variety of different symptoms from blindness to disorders of contour or form perception, and from neglect of part of the world to production of perceptions without correlates in the outer world. Knowledge of the normal functioning of the (visual) brain helps us to understand these symptoms and syndromes, and the study of patients suffering from visual disturbances sheds some light on the processes underlying normal perception in healthy observers.

References

Adler, A. (1944). Disintegration and restoration of optic recognition in visual agnosia: analysis of a case. *Arch. Neurol. Psychiatry* 51, 243–59.

Albert, M.L., Reches, A., and Silverberg, R. (1975). Associative visual agnosia without alexia. *Neurology* 25, 322–6.

Alexander, M.P. and Albert, M.L. (1983). The anatomic basis of visual agnosia. In *Localization in neuropsychology* (ed. A. Kertesz). Academic Press, New York.

Andersen, R.A. (1995). Coordinate transformations and motor planning in posterior parietal cortex. In *The cognitive neurosciences* M.S. Gazzaniga (Ed), pp. 519–32. MIT Press, Cambridge, Massachusetts.

Andersen, R.A., Asanuma, C., Essick, G., and Siegel, R.M. (1990). Corticocortical connections of anatomically and physiologically defined subdivisions within the inferior parietal lobule. *J. Comp. Neurol.* 296, 65–113.

Andersen, R.A., Snyder, L.H., Bradley, D.C., and Xing, J. (1997). Multimodal representation of space in the posterior parietal cortex and its use in planning movements. *Ann. Rev. Neurosci.* 20, 303–30.

Angelelli, P., De Luca, M., and Spinelli, D. (1996). Early visual processing in neglect patients: a study with steady-state VEPs. *Neuropsychologia* 34, 1151–7.

Anton, D.G. (1898). Über Herderkrankungen des Gehirns, welche vom Patienten nicht wahrgenommen werden. *Wiener Klin. Wochenschr.* 11, 227–9.

Anton, D.G. (1899). Beiderseitige Erkrankung der Scheitelgegend des Grosshirnes. *Wiener Klin. Wochenschr.* 12, 1193–9.

Assal, G. and Regli, F. (1980). Syndrome de disconnexion visuo-verbale et visuo-gesturelle. *Rev. Neurologique* 136, 365–76.

Assal, G., Eisert, H.G., and Hécaen, H. (1969). Analyse des résultats du test de Farnsworth D15 chez 155 malades atteints de lésions hémisphériques droites ou gauches. *Acta Neurol. Belg.* 69, 705–17.

Assal, G., Favre, C., and Anderes, J.P. (1984). Non-reconnaissance d' animaux familiers chez un paysan. *Rev. Neurologique* **140**, 580–4.

Aubert, H. (1857). Beiträge zur kenntniss des indirecten Sehens. II Über die Gränzen der Farbenwahrnehmung auf den seitlichen Theilen der Retina. *Graefes Arch. Opthalmol.* **3**, II, 38–67.

Aubert, H. and Foerster, R. (1857). Beiträge zur Kenntniss des indirecten Sehens. Untersachungen über den Raumsinn der Retina. *Graefes Arch. Ophthalmol.* **3**, II, 1–37.

Audet, T., Bub, D., and Lecours, A.R. (1991). Visual neglect and left-sided context effects. *Brain and Cogn.* **16**, 11–28.

Aulhorn, E. and Harms, H. (1972). Visual perimetry. In *Handbook of sensory physiology* (ed. D. Jameson and L.M. Hurvich), Vol. 7/4, pp. 102–45. Springer-Verlag, Berlin.

Aulhorn, E. and Köst, G. (1988). RauschfeldKampimetrie. *Klin. Monatsblätt. Augenheilk.* **192**, 284–8.

Axenfeld, D. (1894). Eine einfache Methode Hemianopsie zu constatiren. *Neurolog. Centralbl.* **13**, 437–8.

Babinski, M.J. (1914). Contribution à l'étude des troubles mentaux dans l'hémiplégie organique cérébrale (anosognosie). *Rev. Neurologique* **27**, 845–8.

Bach, F.A., Hebb, D.O., Morgan, C.T., and Nissen, W. (eds.) (1960). *The neuropsychology of Lashley.* McGraw-Hill, New York.

Bachmann, G. and Fahle, M. (1998). Component perimetry: a fast visual field test for different visual functions. In *Beiträge zur 1. Tübinger Wahrnehmungskonferenz* (ed. H.H. Bülthoff, M. Fahle, K.R. Gegenfurtner, and H.A Mallot), p. 158. Knirsch Verlag.

Bachmann, G. and Fahle. M. (2000). Component perimetry: a fast method to detect visual field defects caused by brain lesions. *Invest Ophthalmol. Vis. Sci.* **41**, 2870–86.

Bálint, R. (1909). Seelenlähmung des "Schauens", optische Ataxie, räumliche Störung der Aufmerksamkeit. *Monatsschr Psychiatrie Neurol.* **25**, 51–81.

Barbur, J.L. (1995). A study of pupil response components in human vision. In *Basic and clinical perspectives in vision research* (ed. J.G. Robbins, M.B.A Djamgoz, and A. Taylor), pp. 3–18. Plenum Publishing Company, New York.

Battersby, W.S., Bender, M.B., Pollack, M., and Kahn, R.L. (1956). Unilateral 'spatial agnosia' ('inattention') in patients with cerebral lesions. *Brain* **79**, 68–93.

Bauer, R.M. (1982). Visual hypoemotionality as a symptom of visual-limbic disconnection in man. *Arch. Neurol.* **39**, 702–8.

Bauer, R.M. (1984). Autonomic recognition of names and faces in prosopagnosia: a neuropsychological application of the guilty knowledge test. *Neuropsychologia* **22**, 457–69.

Bauer, R.M. (1993). Agnosia. In *Clinical neuropsychology* (ed. K.M. Heilman and E. Valenstein), 3rd edn, pp. 215–78. Oxford University Press, New York.

Bauer, R.M. and Verfaellie, M. (1988). Electrodermal discrimination of familiar but not unfamiliar faces in prosopagnosia. *Brain Cogn.* **8**, 240–52.

Bay, E. (1950). *Agnosie und Funktionswandel,* Monographien aus dem Gesamtgebiet der Neurologie und Psychiatrie, no. 73. Springer-Verlag, Berlin.

Baylis, G.C., Driver, J., and Rafal, R.D. (1993). Visual extinction and stimulus repetition. *J. Cogn. Neurosci.* **5**, 453–66.

Baynes, K., Holtzman, J.D., and Volpe, B.T. (1986). Components of visual attention. Alterations in response pattern to visual stimuli following parietal lobe infarction. *Brain* **109**, 99–114.

Becke. (1904, 1917). *Inauguraldissertation,* Marburg. Cited after Wilbrand and Saenger.

Bender, M.B. (1945). Polyopia and monocular diplopia of cerebral origin. *Arch. Neurol. Psychiatry* **54**, 323–38.

Bender, M.B. and Bodis-Wollner, I. (1978). Visual dysfunctions in optic tract lesions. *Ann. Neurol.* **3**, 187–93.

Bender, M.B., Feldman, M. and Sobin, A.J. (1968). Palinopsia. *Brain* **91**, 321–38.

Bender, M.B. and Feldman, M. (1972). The so-called 'visual agnosias'. *Brain* **9**, 173–86.

Bender, M.B. and Jung, R. (1948). Abweichungen der subjektiven optischen Vertikalen und Horizontalen bei Gesunden und Hirnverletzten. *Arch. Psychiatrie Nervenkrankh.* **181**,193–212.

Bender, M.B. and Teuber, H.L. (1946). Phenomena of fluctuation, extinction and completion in visual perception. *Arch. Neurol. Psychiatry* **55**, 627–58.

Benson, D.F. and Greenberg, J.P. (1969). Visual form agnosia. *Arch. Neurol.* **20**, 82–9.

Benson, D.F., Segarra, J., and Albert, M.L. (1974). Visual agnosia-prosopagnosia. *Arch. Neurol.* **30**, 307–10.

Bentin, S., Allison, T., Puce, A., Perez, E., and McCarthy, G. (1996). Electrophysiological studies of face perception in humans. *J. Cogn. Neurosci.* **8**, 551–65.

Benton, A.L. (1980). The neuropsychology of facial recognition. *Am. Psychol.* **35**, 176–86.

Benton, A.L. and Hécaen, H. (1970). Stereoscopic vision in patients with unilateral cerebral disease. *Neurology* **20**, 1084–8.

Benton, A.L. and van Allen, M.W. (1968). Impairment in facial recognition in patients with cerebral disease. *Cortex* **4**, 344–58.

Benton, A.L. and van Allen, M.W. (1972). Prosopagnosia and facial discrimination. *J. Neurol. Sci.* **15**, 167–72.

Benton, A.L., Hannay, H.J., and Varney, N.R. (1975). Visual perception of line direction in patients with unilateral brain disease. *Neurology* **25**, 907–10.

Benton, A.L. and Tranel, D. (1993). Visuoperceptual, visuospatial, and visuoconstructive disorders. In *Clinical Neuropsychology* (eds. K.M. Heilman and E. Valenstein), 3rd edn, pp. 165–213. Oxford University Press, New York.

Berti, A. and Rizzolatti, G. (1992). Visual processing without awareness: evidence from unilateral neglect. *J. Cogn. Neurosci.* **4**, 345–51.

Berti, A., Allport, A., Driver, J., Dienes, Z., Oxbury, J., and Oxbury, S. (1992). Levels of processing for stimuli in an 'extinguished' field. *Neuropsychologia* **30**, 403–15.

Berti, A., Frassinetti, F., and Umiltà, C. (1994). Nonconscious reading? Evidence from neglect dyslexia. *Cortex* **30**, 181–97.

Berti, A. and Frassinetti, F. (2000). When far becomes near: remapping of space by tool use. *J. Cogn. Neurosci.* **12**, 415–20.

Beyer, E. (1895). Ueber Verlagerungen im Gesichtsfeld bei Flimmerskotom. *Neurol. Centralblatt* **14**, 10–15.

Beyn, E.S. and Knyazeva, G.R. (1962). The problem of prosopagnosia. *J. Neurol. Neurosurg. Psychiatry* **25**, 154–8.

Birkmayer, W. (1951). *Hirnverletzungen.* Springer-Verlag, Vienna.

Bisiach, E. and Berti, A. (1987). Dyschiria: an attempt at its systematic explanation. In *Neurophysiological and neuropsychological aspects of spatial neglect* (ed. M. Jeannerod), Vol. 45, pp. 183–202. North-Holland, Amsterdam.

Bisiach, E. and Luzzatti, C. (1978). Unilateral neglect of representional space. *Cortex* **14**, 129–33.

Bisiach, E., Luzzatti, C., and Perani, D. (1979a). Unilateral neglect, representational schema and consciousness. *Brain* **102**, 609–18.

Bisiach, E., Nichelli, P., and Sala, C. (1979b) Recognition of random shapes in unilateral brain damaged patients; a reappraisal. *Cortex* **15**, 491–9.

Bisiach, E., Rusconi, M.L., Peretti, V.A., and Vallar, G. (1994). Challenging current accounts of unilateral neglect. *Neuropsychologia* **32**, 1431–4.

Blake, R. and Logothetis, N.K. (2002). Visual competition. *Nat. Rev. Neurosci.* **3**, 13–23.

Bodamer, J. (1947). Die Prosop-Agnosie. *Archi. Psychiatrie Nervenkrankhe.* **179**, 6–54.

Bogousslavsky, J., Miklossy, J., Regli, F., Deruaz, J.P., Assal, G., and Delaloye, B. (1988). Subcortical neglect: neuropsychological, SPECT, and neuropathological correlations with anterior choroidal artery territory infarction. *Ann. Neurol.* 23, 448–52.

Bornstein, B. (1963). Prosopagnosia. In *Problems of dynamic neurology* (ed. L. Halpern), pp. 283–318. Hadassah Medical Organization, Jerusalem.

Bornstein, B. and Kidron, D.P. (1959). Prosopagnosia, *J. Neurol. Neurosurg. Psychiatry* 22, 124–31.

Bornstein, B., Stroka, H., and Munitz, H. (1969). Prosopagnosia with animal face agnosia. *Cortex* 5, 164–9.

Boudouresques, J., Poncet, M., Sebahoun, M., and Alicherif, A. (1972). Deux cas d' alexie sans agraphie avec troubles de la denomination des couleurs et des images. *Oto-Neuro-Ophthalmol.* 44, 297–303.

Boudouresques, J., Poncet, M., Cherif, A., and Balzamo, M. (1979). L'agnosie des visages: un témoin de la désorganisation fonctionelle d' un certain type de connaissance des éléments du monde extérieur. *Bull. Acad. Nat. Méd.* 163, 695–702.

Brand, A., Groeger, T., Kopmann, S., Knak, S., and Herzog, M.H. (2001). Deficits of early visual processing in schizophrenia. In *Proceedings of the Conference on Negative Symptoms in Schizophrenia and Organic Brain Disease.* Bremen.

Braun, D., Petersen, D., Schönle, P., and Fahle, M. (1998). Deficits and recovery of first- and second-order motion perception in patients with unilateral cortical lesions. *Eur. J. Neurosci.* 10, 2117–28.

Brodmann, K. (1909). *Vergleichende Lokalisationslehre der Grosshirnrinde in ihren Prinzipien dargestellt auf Grund des Zellenbaues.* Barth, Leipzig.

Brown, J.W. (1975). *Aphasie. Apraxie und Agnosie.* Gustav Fischer Verlag, Stuttgart.

Brust, J.C.M. and Behrens, M.M. (1977). "Release hallucinations" as the major symptom of posterior cerebral artery occlusion: A report of 2 cases. *Ann. Neurol.* 2, 432–6.

Bruyer, R., Laterre, C., Seron, X., Feiereisen, P., Strypstein, E., Pierrard, E., and Rectem, D. (1983). A case of prosopagnosia with some preserved covert remembrance of familiar faces. *Brain Cogn.* 2, 257–84.

Bub, D.N., Black, S., and Howell, J. (1989). Word recognition and orthographic context effects in a letter-by-letter reader. *Brain Lang.* 36, 357–76.

Bülthoff, H.H., Edelman, S.Y., and Tarr, M. (1995). How are three-dimensional objects represented in the brain? *Cereb. Cortex* 5, 247–60.

Campion, J. (1987). Apperceptive agnosia: the specification and description of constructs. In *Visual object processing: a cognitive neuropsychological approach.* (ed. G.W. Humphreys and M.J. Riddoch), Lawrence Erlbaum Associates, London.

Campion, J. and Latto, R. (1985). Apperceptive agnosia due to carbon monoxide poisoning. An interpretation based on critical band masking from disseminated lesions. *Behav. Brain Res.* 15, 227–40.

Clifford, C.W.G. and Vaina, L.M. (1999). Anomalous perception of coherence and transparency in moving plaid patterns. *Cogn. Brain Res.* 8, 345–53.

Cohen, A., Ivry, R.B., Rafal, R.D., and Kohn, C. (1995). Activating response codes by stimuli in the neglected visual field. *Neuropsychology* 9, 165–73.

Cohn, R., Neumann, M.S., and Wood, D.H. (1977). Prosopagnosia: a clinicopathological study. *Ann. Neurol.* 1, 177–82.

Colby, C.L. and Goldberg, M.E. (1999). Space and attention in parietal cortex. *Ann. Rev. Neurosci.* 22, 319–49.

Cole, M. and Perez-Cruet, J. (1964). Prosopagnosia. *Neuropsychologia* 2, 237–46.

Colombo, A., de Renzi, E., and Faglioni, P. (1976). The occurrence of visual neglect in patients with unilateral cerebral disease. *Cortex* 12, 221–31.

Corbetta, M. (1998). Frontoparietal cortical networks for directing attention and the eye to visual locations: Identical, independent, or overlapping neural systems? *Proc. Natl. Acad. Sci.* 95, 831–8.

Corbetta, M. and Shulman, G.L. (1998). Human cortical mechanisms of visual attention during orienting and search. *Phil. Trans. R. Soc. Lond. B.* 353, 1353–62.

Corkin, S. (1979). Hidden-figures-test performance: lasting effects of unilateral penetrating head injury and transient effects of bilateral cingulotomy. *Neuropsychologia* 17, 585–605.

Coslett, H.B. and Saffran, E.M. (1989). Preserved object recognition and reading comprehension in optic aphasia. *Brain* 112, 1091–110.

Cowey, A. and Vaina, L.M. (2000). Blindness to form from motion despite intact static form perception and motion detection. *Neuropsychologia* 38, 566–78.

Critchley, M. (1951). Types of visual perseveration: "Palinopsia" and "illusory visual spread." *Brain* 74, 267–99.

Critchley, M. (1964). The problem of visual agnosia. *J. Neurol. Sci.* 1, 274–90.

Critchley, M. (1966). The parietal lobes. Hafner Publishing Company: New York, London.

Cronin-Golomb, A., Sugiura, R., Corkin, S. and Growdon, J.H. (1993). Incomplete achromatopsia in Alzheimer's disease. *Neurobiology of Aging* 14, 471–7.

Damasio, A.R. (1985). Disorders of complex visual processing: agnosias, achromatopsia, Balint's syndrome, and related difficulties of orientation and construction. In *Principles of behavioral neurology* (ed. M.M. Mesulam), pp. 259–88. F.A. Davis Co, Philadelphia.

Damasio, A.R. and Damasio, H. (1983). The anatomic basis of pure alexia. *Neurology* 33, 1573–83.

Damasio, A.R., Damasio, H., and Chui, H.C. (1980b). Neglect following damage to frontal lobe or basal ganglia. *Neuropsychologia* 18, 123–32.

Damasio, A.R., Damasio, H., and van Hoesen, G.W. (1982). Prosopagnosia: anatomic basis and behavioral mechanisms. *Neurology* 32, 331–41.

Damasio, A.R., Damasio, H., and Tranel, D. (1990a). Impairments of visual recognition as clues to the processes of categorization and memory. In *Signal and sense: local and global order in perceptual maps* (ed. G.M. Edelman, W.E. Gall, and W.M. Cowan), pp. 451–73. Wiley-Liss, New York.

Damasio, A.R., Tranel, D., and Damasio, H. (1990b). Face agnosia and the neural substrates of memory. *Ann. Rev. Neurosci.* 13, 89–109.

Damasio, A.R., Yamada, T., Damasio, H., Corbett, J., and McKee, J. (1980a). Central achromatopsia: Behavioral, anatomic, and physiologic aspects. *Neurology* 30, 1064–71.

Danta, G., Hilton, R.C., and O'Boyle, D.J. (1978). Hemisphere function and binocular depth perception. *Brain* 101, 569–89.

Davidoff, J. and Wilson, B. (1985). A case of visual agnosia showing a disorder of presemantic visual classification. *Cortex* 21, 121–34.

Davidoff, J. and Warrington, E.K. (1993). A dissociation of shape discrimination and figure-ground perception in a patient with normal acuity. *Neuropsychologia* 31, 83–93.

Davis, G. and Driver, J. (1998). Kanizsa subjective figures can act as occluding surfaces at parallel stages of visual search. *J. Exp. Psychol. Hum. Perception Perform.* 24, 169–84.

Denny-Brown, D. and Banker, B.Q. (1954). Amorphosynthesis from left parietal lesion. *Arch. Neurol. Psychiatry* 72, 643–4.

de Haan, E.H.F., Young, A., and Newcombe, F. (1987a). Faces interfere with name classification in a prosopagnosic patient. *Cortex* 23, 309–16.

de Haan, E.H.F., Young, A., and Newcombe, F. (1987b). Face recognition without awareness. *Cogn. Neuropsychol.* 4, 385–415.

Deouell, L.Y., Bentin, S., and Soroker, N. (2000). Electrophysiological evidence for an early (pre-attentive) information processing deficit in patients with right hemisphere damage and unilateral neglect. *Brain* 123, 353–65.

de Renzi, E. (1982). *Disorders of space exploration and cognition.* John Wiley and Sons, New York.

de Renzi, E. (1986*a*). Prosopagnosia in two patients with CT scan evidence of damage confined to the right hemisphere. *Neuropsychologia* 24, 385–9.

de Renzi, E. (1986*b*). Slowly progressive visual agnosia or apraxia without dementia. *Cortex* 22, 171–80.

de Renzi, E. (1986*c*). Current issues in prosopagnosia. In *Aspects of face processing* (ed. H.D. Ellis, M.A. Jeeves, F. Newcombe, and A. Young). Martinus Nijhoff, Dordrecht.

de Renzi, E. and Spinnler, H. (1967). Impaired performance on color tasks in patients with hemispheric damage. *Cortex* 3, 194–216.

de Renzi, E., Scotti, G., and Spinnler, H. (1969). Perceptual and associative disorders of visual recognition: Relationship to the side of the cerebral lesion. *Neurology* 19, 634–42.

de Renzi, E., Faglioni, P., and Scotti, G. (1971). Judgment of spatial orientation in patients with focal brain damage. *J. Neurol. Neurosurg. Psychiatry* 34, 489–95.

de Renzi, E., Faglioni, P., Scotti, G., and Spinnler, H. (1972). Impairment of color sorting behavior after hemispheric damage: An experimental study with the Holmgren skein test. *Cortex* 8, 147–63.

de Renzi, E., Faglioni, P., and Spinnler, H. (1986). The performance of patients with unilateral brain damage on face recognition tasks. *Cortex* 4, 17–34.

Desimone, R. and Duncan, J. (1995). Neural mechanisms of selective visual attention. *Ann. Rev. Neurosci.* 18, 193–222.

di Pellegrino, G. and de Renzi, E. (1995). An experimental investigation on the nature of extinction. *Neuropsychologia* 33, 153–70.

Dill, M. and Fahle, M. (1999). Display symmetry affects positional specificity in *same-different* judgment of pairs of novel visual patterns. *Vision Research* 39, 3752–60.

Doricchi, F. (2002). The contribution of retinotopic and mulitmodal coding of space to horizontal space misrepresentation in neglect and hemianopia. *The cognitive and neural bases of spatial neglect* (H.O. Karnath, D. Milner, and G. Vallar, eds.). Oxford University Press, Oxford.

Doricchi, F., Angelelli, P., De Luca, M., Spinelli, D. (1996). Neglect for low luminance contrast stimuli but not for high colour contrast stimuli: a behavioural and electrophysiological study. *Neuroreport* 7, 1360–4.

Driver, J. (1996). What can visual neglect and extinction reveal about the extent of 'preattentive' processing? In *Convergent operations in the study of visual selective attention* (ed. A.F. Kramer, M.G.H. Cole, and G.D. Logan), pp. 193–224. APA Press, Washington, DC.

Driver, J. (1999). Egocentric and object-based visual neglect. In *The hippocampal and parietal foundations of spatial cognition* (ed. N.K. Burgess and J.O'Keefe). Oxford University Press, Oxford.

Driver, J. and Vuilleumier (2001). Perceptual awareness and its loss in unilateral neglect and extinction. *Cognition* 79, 39–88.

Duensing, F. (1952). Beitrag zur Frage der optischen Agnosie. *Arch. Psychiatrie und Zeitschrift Neurologie.* 188, 131–61.

Duensing, F. (1953). Raumgnostische und ideatorisch-apraktische Störung des gestaltenden Handelns. *Dtsch. Z. Nervenheilk.* 170, 72–94.

Efron, R. (1968). What is perception? *Boston Studies Phil. Sci.* 4, 137–73.

Eimer, M. (1998). Does the face-specific N170 component reflect the activity of a specialized eye processor? *NeuroReport* 9, 2945–8.

Etcoff, N.L. (1984). Selective attention to facial identity and facial emotion. *Neuropsychologia* 22, 281–95.

Ettlinger, G. (1990). 'Object vision' and 'spatial vision': the neuropsychological evidence for the distinction. *Cortex* 26, 319–41.

Eysel, U.T. (2002). Plasticity of receptive fields in early stages of the adult visual system. In *Perceptual learning* (M. Fahle and T. Poggio, eds.), MIT Press, Cambridge, Massachusetts.

Fahle, M. (1982). Binocular rivalry: suppression depends on orientation and spatial frequency. *Vis. Res.* 22, 787–800.

Fahle, M. (1993). Figure–ground discrimination from temporal information. *Proc. R. Soc. Lond. B* 254, 199–203.

Fahle, M. (2003a). Visuelle Täuschungen. In *Neuropsychologie* (eds. H.O. Karnath and P. Thier), pp. 47–66. Springer, Heidelberg.

Fahle, M. (2003b). Gesichtssinn und Okulomotorik. In *Lehrbuch Vorklirik* (R.F. Schmidt and K. Unsicker (eds.)). Deutscher Arzte – Verlag, Köln.

Fahle, M. and Poggio, T. (eds.) (2002). *Perceptual learning*. MIT Press, Cambridge, Massachusetts.

Fahle, M. and Troscianko, T. (1991). Limiting factors of texture and stereoscopic depth perception in humans. In *Limits of vision. (Vision and visual dysfunction, Vol. 5)*. (J. Kulikowski, V. Walsh and I. Murray, Eds.) London: Macmillan, pp. 120–32.

Fahle, M. and Westheimer, G. (1995). On the time-course of inhibition in the stereoscopic perception of rows of dots. *Vis. Res.* 35, 1393–9.

Farah, M.J. (1990). *Visual agnosia*. MIT Press, Cambridge, Massachusetts.

Farah, M.J., Monheit, M.A., and Wallace, M.A. (1991). Unconscious perception of 'extinguished' visual stimuli: reassessing the evidence. *Neuropsychologia* 29, 949–58.

Faust, C. (1947). Über Gestaltzerfall als Symptom des parieto-occipitalen Übergangsgebietes bei doppelseitiger Verletzung nach Hirnschuss. *Nervenarzt* 18, 103–15.

Feinberg, T.E., Gonzalez-Rothi, L.J., and Heilman, K.M. (1986). Multimodal agnosia after unilateral left hemisphere lesion. *Neurology* 36, 864–7.

Ferber, S. and Karnath, H.-O. (2001). How to assess spatial neglect—line bisection or cancellation tasks? *Journal of Clinical and Experimental Neuropsychology* 23, 599–607.

Ferree, C.E. and Rand, G. (1920). The extent and shape of the zones of color sensitivity in relation to the intensity of the stimulus light. *Am. J. Physiol. Optics* 1, 185–213.

Ferrier, D. (1881). Cerebral amblyopia and hemiopia. *Brain* 3, 456–77.

Fine, I., Smallman, H.S., Doyle, P., and MacLeod, D.I.A. (2002). Visual function before and after the removal of bilateral congenital cataracts in adulthood. *Vision Res.* 42, 191–210.

Foerster, R. (1890). Ueber Rindenblindheit. *Graefes Arch. Ophthalmol.* 36, 94–108.

Frederiks, J.A.M. (1969). The agnosias. In *Handbook of clinical neurology* (ed. P.J. Vinken and G.W. Bruyn). North Holland, Amsterdam.

Freud, S. (1891). *Zur Auffassung der Aphasien*. F. Deuticke, Leipzig.

Friedman-Hill, S.R., Robertson, L.C. and Treisman, A. (1995). Parietal contributions to visual feature binding: evidence from a patient with bilateral lesions. *Science* 269, 853–5.

Gaffan, D. and Hornak, J. (1997). Visual neglect in the monkey. Representation and disconnection. *Brain* 120, 1647–57.

Gelb, A. (1926). Die psychologische Bedeutung pathologischer Störungen der Raumwahrnehmung. *Bericht über den IX. Kongress für Experimentelle Psychologie*, pp. 23–80. Fischer Verlag, Jena.

Gelb, A. and Goldstein, K. (1922). Psychologische Analysen hirnpathologischer Fälle auf Grand ven Untersuchinger Himverletzter VII. Über Gesichtsfeldbefunde bei abnormer 'Ermüdbarkeit' des Auges (sog. 'Ringskotome'). *Arch. Ophthalmol.* 109, 387–403.

Gelpke, T. (1899). Zur Casuistik der einseitigen homonymen Hemianopsie corticalen Ursprungs, mit eigenartigen Störungen in den sehenden Gesichtsfeldhälften. *Arch. Augenheilk.* 39, 116–26.

Giesbrecht, B. and Mangun, G.R. (2002). The neural mechanisms of attentional control. In *The cognitive and neural bases of spatial neglect.* (H.O. Karnath, D. Milner, and G. Vallar Eds). Oxford University Press, Oxford.

Gil, R., Pluchon, C., Toullat, G., Michenau, D., Rogez, R., and Lefevre, J.P. (1985). Disconnexion visuo-verbale (aphasie optique) pour les objets, les images, les couleurs et les visages avec alexie 'abstractive'. *Neuropsychologia* 23, 333–49.

Gilbert, C.D. and Wiesel, T.N. (1992). Receptive field dynamics in adult primary visual cortex. *Nature* 356, 150–2.

Gilchrist, I.D., Humphreys, G.W., and Riddoch, M.J. (1996). Grouping and extinction: evidence for low-level modulation of visual selection. *Cogn. Neuropsychol.* 13, 1223–49.

Girotti, F., Milanese, C., Casazza, M., Allegranza, A., Corridori, F., and Avanzini, G. (1982). Oculomotor disturbances in Balint's syndrome: anatomoclinical findings and electrooculographic analysis in a case. *Cortex* 18, 603–14.

Glickstein, M. and Fahle, M. (2000). Visual disturbances following gunshot wounds of the cortical visual area. *Brain* 123 (special suppl.), 1–101.

Gloning, I., Gloning, K., and Tschabitscher, H. (1962). Die occipitale Blindheit auf vasculärer Basis. *Von Graefes Arch. Ophthalmol.* 165, 138–77.

Gloning, I., Gloning, K., Hoff, H., and Tschabitscher, H. (1966). Zur Prosopagnosie. *Neuropsychologia* 4, 113–32.

Gloning, I., Gloning, K., and Hoff, H. (1968). *Neuropsychological symptoms and syndromes in lesions of the occipital lobe and the adjacent areas.* Gauthier-Villars, Paris.

Gloning, K. (1965). Die cerebral bedingten Störungen des räumlichen Sehens und des Raumerlebens. W. Maudrich Verlag, Vienna.

Godwin-Austen, R.B. (1965). A case of visual disorientation. *J. Neurol. Neurosurg. Psychiatry* 28, 453–8.

Goldstein, K. and Gelb, A. (1918). Psychologische Analysen hirnpathologischer Fälle auf Grand von Untersuchungen Hirnverletzter Zur Psychologie des optischen Wahrnehmungs- und Erkennungsvorganges. *Z. Gesamte Neurol. Psychiatrie* 41, 1–142.

Gollin, E.S. (1960). Developmental studies of visual recognition of incomplete objects. *Percep. Motor Skills* 11, 289–98.

Gomori, A.J. and Hawryluk, G.A. (1984). Visual agnosia without alexia. *Neurology* 34, 947–50.

Goodale, M.A., Milner, A.D., Jakobson, L.S. and Carey, D.P. (1991). A neurological dissociation between perceiving objects and grasping them. *Nature* 349, 154–6.

Goodale, M.A. and Milner, A.D. (1992). Separate visual pathways for perception and action. *Trends Neurosci.* 15, 20–5.

Gorea, A. and Sagi, D. (2000). Failure to handle more than one internal representation in visual detection tasks. *Proc. Natl. Acad. Sci., USA* 97, 12380–4.

Gottlieb, J.P., Kusunoki, M., and Goldberg, M.E. (1998). The representation of visual salience in monkey parietal cortex. *Nature* 391, 481–4.

Green, G.J. and Lessell, S. (1977). Acquired cerebral dyschromatopsia. *Arch. Ophthalmol.* 95, 121–8.

Greenlee, M.W. and Smith, A.T. (1997). Detection and discimination of first- and second-order motion in patients with unilateral brain damage. *Journal of Neuroscience* 17, 804–18.

Gregory, R.L. and Wallace, J.G. (1963). *Recovery from early blindness: a case study,* Experimental Psychology Society monograph 2. Heffer and Sons, Cambridge.

Grossberg, S. (1991). Why do parallel cortical systems exist for the perception of static form and moving form? *Percept. Psychophys.* 49, 117–41.

Grüsser, V.O.J. and Landis, T. (1991). Visual agnosias and other disturbances of visual perception and cognition. In *Vision and visual dysfunction, Vol. 12.* (J. Cronly-Dillon Ed.), Macmillan, London.

Haarmeier, T., Thier, P., Repnow, M., and Petersen, D. (1997). False perception of motion in a patient who cannot compensate for eye movements. *Nature* **389**, 849–52.

Halligan, P.W. and Marshall, J.C. (1991*a*). Figural modulation of visuo-spatial neglect: a case study. *Neuropsychologia* **29**, 619–28.

Halligan, P.W. and Marshall, J.C. (1991*b*). Left neglect for near but not far space in man. *Nature* **350**, 498–500.

Halligan, P.W. and Marshall, J.C. (1993). Homing in on neglect: a case study of visual search. *Cortex* **29**, 167–74.

Hämäläinen, H., Pirilä, J., Lahtinen, E., Lindroos, J., and Salmelin, R. (1999). Cognitive ERP components in neglect. *J. Cogn. Neurosci.* **11** (Suppl., Abstracts of the Annual Meeting of the Society of Cognitive Neuroscience), 58.

Hamsher, K de S. (1978). Stereopsis and unilateral brain disease. *Invest. Ophthalmol. Vis. Sci.* **17**, 336–43.

Hamsher, K de S., Levin, H.S., and Benton, A.L. (1979). Facial recognition in patients with focal brain lesions. *Arch. Neurol.* **36**, 837–9.

Hamsher, K de S., Capruso, D.X., and Benton, A.L. (1992). Visuospatial judgment and right hemisphere disease. *Cortex* **28**, 493–95.

Hannay, H.J., Varney, N.R., and Benton, A.L. (1976). Visual localization in patients with unilateral brain disease. *J. Neurol., Neurosurg., Psychiatry* **39**, 307–13.

Hart, C.T. (1969). Disturbances of fusion following head injury. *Proc. R. Soc. Med.* **62**, 704–6.

Hécaen, H. (1972). *Introduction à la neuropsychologie*. Larousse, Paris.

Hécaen, H. and Angelergues, R. (1962). Agnosia for faces (prosopagnosia). *Arch. Neurol.* **7**, 92–100.

Hécaen, H. and Angelergues, R. (1963). *La cécité psychique*. Masson et Cie, Paris.

Hécaen, H. and de Ajuriaguerra, J. (1956). Agnosie visuelle pour les objects inanimés par lésion unilatérale gauche. *Rev. Neurologique* **94**, 222–33.

Hécaen, H., Goldblum, M.C., Masure, M.C., and Ramier, A.M. (1974). Une nouvelle observation d'agnosie d'objet. Deficit de l'association ou de la categorisation, specifique de la modalite visuelle? *Neuropsychologia* **12**, 447–64.

Heidenhain, A. (1927). Beitrag zur Kenntnis der Seelenblindheit. *Monatsschr. Psychiatrie Neurol.* **66**, 61–116.

Heilman, K.M. and Valenstein, E. (1972). Frontal lobe neglect in man. *Neurology* **22**, 660–4.

Heilman, K.M., Watson, R.T., and Valenstein, E. (1993). Neglect and related disorders. In *Clinical neuropsychology* (ed. K.M. Heilman and E. Valenstein), pp. 279–336. Oxford University Press, New York.

Henschen, S.E. (1896). *Klinische und anatomische Beiträge zur Anatomie des Gehirns*, Teile 1–3. Almquist and Wikesell, Upsala.

Herrman, G. and Pötzl, O. (1928). Die optische Allaesthesie. Abhandlungen aus der Neurologie, Psychiatrie, Psychologie and ihren Grenzgebieten, Helft 47. Berlin: S. Karger.

Herzog, M.H., Fahle, M., and Koch, C. (2001). Spatial aspects of object formation revealed by a new illusion, shine-through. *Vision Res.* **41**, 2325–35.

Herzog, M.H. and Fahle, M. (2002). Effects of grouping in contextual modulation. *Nature* **415**, 433–6.

Hildebrandt, H., Spang, K., and Ebke, M. (2002). Visuospatial hemi-inattention following cerebellar/brain stem bleeding, *Neurocase* **8**, 323–9.

Hinton, G.E. (1981). A parallel computation that assigns canonical object-based frames of reference. *Proceedings of the International Joint Conference on Artificial Intelligence*, 683–5. Vancouver, Canada.

Hoff, H. and Pötzl, O. (1935*a*). Über Störungen des Tiefensehens bei zerebraler Metamorphopsie. *Monatsschr. Psychiatrie Neurol.* 90, 305–26.

Hoff, H. and Pötzl, O. (1935*b*). Zur diagnostischen Bedeutung der Polyopie bei Tumoren des Occipitalhirnes. *Z. gesamte Neurol. Psychiatries* 152, 433–50.

Holmes, G. (1918*a*). Disturbances of vision by cerebral lesions. *Br. J. Ophthalmol.* 2, 353–84

Holmes, G. (1918*b*). Disturbances of visual orientation. *Br. J. Ophthalmol.* 2, 449–68, 506–16

Holmes, G. and Horrax, G. (1919). Disturbances of spatial orientation and visual attention, with loss of stereoscopic vision. *Arch. Neurol. Psychiatry* 1, 385–407.

Horrax, G. and Putnam, T.J. (1932). Distortions of the visual fields in cases of brain tumour. *Brain* 55, 499–523.

Hughlings-Jackson, J. (1889). On a particular variety of epilepsy ("intellectual aura"), one case with symptoms of organic brain disease. *Brain* 11, 179–207.

Humphrey, G.K., Goodale, M.A., Corbetta, M., Aglioti, S. (1995). The McCollough effect reveals orientation discrimination in a case of cortical blindness. *Curr Biol.* 5, 545–51.

Humphrey, G.K., Symons, L.A., Herbert, A.M., Goodale, M.A. (1996). A neurological dissociation between shape from shading and shape from edges. *Behav Brain Res.* 76, 117–25.

Humphreys, G.W. and Riddoch, M.J. (1984). Routes to object constancy: implications from neurological impairments of object constancy. *Quart. J. Exp. Psychol.* 36A, 385–415.

Humphreys, G.W. and Riddoch, M.J. (1985). Author's correction to 'Routes to object constancy'. *Quart. J. Exp. Psychol.* 37A, 493–5

Humphreys, G.W. and Riddoch, M.J. (1987*a*) *To see but not to see: a case study of visual agnosia.* Lawrence Erlbaum Associates, Hillsdale, New Jersey.

Humphreys, G.W. and Riddoch, M.J. (1987*b*) The fractionation of visual agnosia. In *Visual object processing: a cognitive neuropsychological approach* (ed. G.W. Humphreys and M.J. Riddoch). Lawrence Erlbaum Associates, London.

Husain, M. and Kennard, C. (1996). Visual neglect associated with frontal lobe infarction. *J. Neurol.* 243, 652–7.

Jackson, J.H. (1932). *Selected writings of John Hughlings Jackson. Vol. 2: Evolution and dissolution of the nervous system.* London: Hodder and Stoughton.

Jacobs, L. (1980). Visual allesthesia. *Neurology* 30, 1059–63.

Jaspers, K. (1973). *Allgemeine Psychopathologie.* 9th Edition. Berlin, Heidelberg, New York: Springer.

Julesz, B. (1971). *Foundations of cylopean perception.* Universityof Chicago Press, Chicago.

Kandinsky, V. (1881). Zur Lehre von den Hallucinationen. *Archiv für Psych. und Nervenkrankheiten* 11/26, 453–64.

Karnath, H.O., Schenkel, P., and Fischer, B. (1991). Trunk orientation as the determining factor of the 'contralateral' deficit in the neglect syndrome and as the physical anchor of the internal representation of body orientation in space. *Brain* 114, 1997–2014.

Karnath, H.O., Ferber, S., and Himmelbach, M. (2001). Spatial awareness is a function of the temporal not the posterior parietal lobe. *Nature* 411, 950–3.

Karnath, H.O., Milner, D.A., and Vallar, G. (2002). *The cognitive and neural bases of spatial neglect.* Oxford University Press, Oxford.

Kartsounis, L.D. and Warrington, E.K. (1991). Failure of object recognition due to a breakdown of figure-ground discrimination in a patient with normal acuity. *Neuropsychologia* 29, 969–80.

Kase, C.S., Troncoso, J.F., Court, J.E., Tapia, F.J., and Mohr, J.P. (1977). Global spatial disorientation. *J. Neurol. Sci.* 34, 267–78.

Kastner, S. and Ungerleider L.G. (2000). Mechanisms of visual attention in the human cortex. *Ann. Rev. Neurosci.* 23, 315–41.

Kay, M.C. and Levin, H.S. (1982). Prosopagnosia. *Am. J. Ophthalmol.* 94, 75–80.

Kertesz, A. (1979). Visual agnosia: the dual deficit of perception and recognition. *Cortex* 15, 403–19.

Kertesz, A. (1987). The clinical spectrum and localization of visual agnosia. In *Visual object processing: a cognitive neuropsychological approach* (ed. G.W. Humphreys and M.J. Riddoch). Lawrence Erlbaum Associates, London.

Kinsbourne, M. and Warrington, E.K. (1962). A disorder of simultaneous form perception. *Brain* 85, 461–86.

Kinsbourne, M. and Warrington, E.K. (1963). A study of visual perseveration. *J. Neurol. Neurosurg. Psychiatr.* 26, 468–75.

Kleist, K. (1923). Kriegsverletzungen des Gehirns in ihrer Bedeutung für die Hirnlokalisation und Hirnpathologie. In *Handbuch der Ärztlichen Erfahrung im Weltkriege, 1914/1918* (ed. O. von Schjerning), Vol. 4. Barth, Leipzig.

Klopp, H.W. (1951). Über Umgekehrt- und Verkehrtsehen. *Deutsche Zeitschrift für Nervenheilkunde* 165, 231–60.

Klopp, H.W. (1955). Verkehrtsehen nach kurzdauernder Erblindung. *Nervenarzt* 26, 438–41.

Kölmel, H.W. (1984). Visuelle Halluzinationen im hemianopen Feld. *Schriftenreihe Neurologie, Bd.* 26, Berlin, Heidelberg, New York, Toyko: Springer-Verlag.

Kölmel, H.W. (1985). Complex visual hallucinations in the hemianopic field. *J Neurology, Neurosurgery, and Psychiatry* 48, 29–38.

Kömpf, D., Piper, H.F., Neundörfer, B. and Dietrich, H. (1983). Palinopsie (visuelle Perseveration) und zerebrale Polyopie-klinische Analyse und computertomographische Befunde. *Fortschritte der Neurologie Psychiatrie* 51, 270–81.

Konorski, J. (1967). *Integrative activity of the brain.* University of Chicago Press, Chicago.

Kosslyn, S.M. (1980). *Image and mind.* Harvard University Press, Cambridge, Massachusetts.

Kosslyn, S.M., Flynn, R.A., Amsterdam, J.B., and Wang, G. (1990). Components of high-level vision: a cognitive neuroscience analysis and accounts of neurological syndromes. *Cognition* 34, 203–77.

Kramer, F. (1907). Über eine partielle Störung der optischen Tiefenwahrnehmung. *Monatsschr. Psychiatrie. Neurol.* 22, 189–202.

Kurucz, J. and Feldmar, G. (1979). Prosopo-affective agnosia as a symptom of cerebral organic disease. *J. Am. Geriatr. Soci.* 27, 225–30.

Ladavas, E., Paladini, R., and Cubelli, R. (1993). Implicit associative priming in a patient with left visual neglect. *Neuropsychologia* 31, 1307–20.

Ladavas, E., Shallice, T. and Zanella, M.T. (1997). Preserved semantic access in neglect dyslexia. *Neurospsychologia* 35, 257–70.

Laehr, M. (1896). Zur Symptomatologie occipitaler Herderkrankungen. *Charite-Annalen* 21, 790–814.

Lamb, M.R., Robertson, L.C., and Knight, R.T. (1990). Component mechanisms underlying the processing of hierarchically organized patterns: inference from patients with unilateral cortical lesions. *J. Exp. Psychol.: Learning, Mem. Cogn.* 16, 471–83.

Lamy, H. (1895). Hemianopsie avec hallucinations dans la partie abolie du champ de la vision. *Revue Neurologique* 3, 129–35.

Landis, T., Graves, R., Benson, D.F., and Hebben, N. (1982). Visual recognition through kinaesthetic mediation. *Psychol. Med.* 12, 515–31.

Landis, T., Cummings, J.L., Christen, L., Bogen, J.E., and Imhof, H.G. (1986). Are unilateral posterior cerebral lesions sufficient to cause prosopagnosia? *Cortex* 22, 243–52.

Landis, T., Regard, M., Bliestle, A., and Kleihues, P. (1988). Prosopagnosia and agnosia for non-canonical views. An autopsied case. *Brain* 111, 1287–97.

Larrabee, G.J., Levin, H.S., Huff, F.J., Kay, M.C., and Guinto, F.C. (1985). Visual agnosia contrasted with visual-verbal disconnection. *Neuropsychologia* 23, 1–12.

Lauber, H. (1944). *Das Gesichtsfeld*. München: J.F. Bergmann.

Leber, T. (1869). Ueber das Vorkommen von Anomalien des Farbensinnes bei Krankheiten des Auges, nebst Bemerkungen über einige Formen von Amblyopie. *Grafe's Arch. Ophthalmol.* 15 (Abtheilung I), 26–107.

Lehmann, D. and Wälchi, P. (1975). Depth perception and location of brain lesions. *J. Neurol.* 209, 157–64.

Leibovitch, F.S., Black, S.E., Caldwell, C.B., Ebert, P.L., Ehrlich, L.E., and Szalai, J.P. (1998). Brain-behavior correlations in hemispatial neglect using CT and SPECT. The Sunnybrook Stroke Study. *Neurology*, 50, 901–8.

Lenz, G. (1905). Beiträge zur Hemianopsie. *Klinische Monatsblätter für Augenheilkunde* 43, 263–326 (Beilageheft).

Lenz, G. (1909). *Zur Pathologie der cerebralen Sehbahn unter besonderer Berücksichtigung ihrer Ergebnisse für die Anatomie und Physiologie*. Verlag von Wilhelm Engelmann, Leipzig.

Lenz, H. (1944). Raumsinnstörungen bei Hirnverletzten. *Dtsch. Z. Nervenheilk.* 157, 22–64.

Levine, D.N. (1978). Prosopagnosia and visual object agnosia: a behavioral study. *Brain and Language* 5, 341–65.

Levine, D.N. and Calvanio, R. (1978). A study of the visual defect in verbal alexia-simultanagnosia. *Brain* 101, 65–81.

Levine, D.N. and Calvanio, R. (1989). Prosopagnosia: A defect in visual configural processing. *Brain Cogn.* 10, 149–70.

Lewandowsky, M. (1908). Ueber Abspaltung des Farbensinnes. *Monatsschr. Psychiatr. Neurol.* 23, 488–510.

Lezak, M.D. (1995). *Neuropsychological assessment*. Oxford University Press, New York.

Lhermitte, F. and Beauvois, M.F. (1973). A visual-speech disconnexion syndrome. Report of a case with optic aphasia, agnosic alexia and colour agnosia. *Brain* 96, 695–714.

Lhermitte, F. and Pillon, B. (1975). La prosopagnosie. Role de l'hemisphere droit dans la perception visuelle. *Rev. Neurol., Paris* 131, 791–812.

Lhermitte, F., Chain, F., Aron, D., Leblanc, M., and Souty, O. (1969). Les troubles de la vision des couleurs dans les lésions postérieures du cerveau. *Rev. Neurol., Paris* 121, 5–29.

Lhermitte, F., Chain, F., Escourolle, R., Ducarne, B., and Pillon, B. (1972). Etude anatomo-clinique d'un cas de prosopagnosie. *Rev. Neurol., Paris* 126, 329–46.

Liepmann, H. and Kalmus, E. (1900). Ueber eine Augenmaassstörung bei Hemianopikern. *Berliner Klin. Wochenschr.* 37(38), 838–42.

Lissauer, H. (1890). Ein Fall von Seelenblindheit nebst einem Beitrage zur Theorie derselben. *Arch. Psychiatrie Nervenkrankh.* 21, 222–70.

Logan, G.D. (1980). Attention and automaticity in Stroop and priming tasks: theory and data. *Cogn. Psychol.* 12, 523–53.

Luria, A.R. (1959). Disorders of 'simultaneous perception' in a case of bilateral occipito-parietal brain injury. *Brain* 83, 437–49.

Luria, A.R., Pravdina-Vinarskaya, E.N., and Yarbuss, A.L. (1963). Disorders of ocular movement in a case of simultanagnosia. *Brain* 86, 219–28.

Mack, J.L. and Boller, F. (1977). Associative visual agnosia and its related deficits: the role of the minor hemisphere in assigning meaning to visual perceptions. *Neuropsychologia* 15, 345–49.

MacLeod, C.M. (1991). Half a century of research on the Stroop effect: an integrative review. *Psychol. Bull.* 109, 163–203.

Macrae, D. and Trolle, E. (1956). The defect of function in visual agnosia. *Brain* 79, 94–110.

Marr, D. (1982). *Vision.* Freeman, San Francisco.

Marshall, J.C. and Halligan, P.W. (1988). Blindsight and insight in visuo-spatial neglect. *Nature* 336, 766–7.

Marzi, C.A., Smania, N., Martini, M.C., Gambina, G., Tomelleri, G., Palamara, A., Alessandrini, F., and Prior, M. (1996). Implicit redundant-targets effect in visual extinction. *Neuropsychologia* 34, 9–22.

Marzi, C.A., Girelli, M., Miniussi, C., Smania, N., and Maravita, A. (2000). Electrophysiological correlates of conscious vision: evidence from unilateral extinction. *J. Cogn. Neurosci.* 12, 869–77.

Massironi, M., Guariglia, C., Pizzamiglio, L., Zoccolotti, P., Spinelli, D. (1990). Shape, size and relative space position perception in neglect patients. *Int J Neurosci.* 54, 13–20.

Mattingley, J.B., Davis, G., and Driver, J. (1997). Preattentive filling-in of visual surfaces in parietal extinction. *Science* 275, 671–4.

Mauthner, L. (1881). *Gehirn und Auge.* J.F. Bergmann, Wiesbaden.

Mazzucchi, A. and Biber, C. (1983). Is prosopagnosia more frequent in males than in females? *Cortex* 19, 509–16.

McAdams, C.J. and Maunsell, J.H.R. (1999). Effects of attention on the reliability of individual neurons in monkey visual cortex. *Neuron* 23, 765–73.

McCarthy, R.A. and Warrington, E.K. (1986). Visual associative agnosia: a clinico-anatomical study of a single case. *J. Neurol., Neurosurg., Psychiatry* 49, 1233–40.

McGlinchey-Berroth, R., Milberg, W.P., Verfaellie, M., Alexander, M., and Kilduff, P.T. (1993). Semantic processing in the neglected visual field: evidence from a lexical decision task. *Cogn. Neuropsychol.* 10, 79–108.

Meadows, J.C. (1973). Observations on a case of monocular diplopia of cerebral origin. *Journal of the Neurological Sciences* 18, 249–53.

Meadows, J.C. (1974*a*). The anatomical basis of prosopagnosia. *J. Neurol., Neurosurg., Psychiatry* 37, 489–501.

Meadows, J.C. (1974*b*). Disturbed perception of colors associated with localized cerebral lesions. *Brain* 97, 615–32.

Mendez, M.F. (1988). Visuoperceptual function in visual agnosia. *Neurology* 38, 1754–9.

Mendola, J.D., Rizzo, J.F., Cosgrove, G.R., Cole, A.J., Black, P., and Corkin, S. (1999). Visual discrimination after anterior temporal lobectomy in humans. *Neurology* 52, 1028–37.

Mendola, J.D. and Corkin, S. (1999). Visual discrimination and attention after bilateral temporal-lobe lesions: A case study. *Neuropsychologia* 37, 91–102.

Mesulam, M.M. (1985). Patterns in behavioral neuroanatomy. In *Principles of behavioral neurology* (ed. M.M. Mesulam), pp. 1–70. F.A. Davis Co, Philadelphia.

Michel, F., Jeannerod, M., and Devic, M. (1965). Trouble de l'orientation visuelle dans les trois dimensions de l'espace. *Cortex* 1, 441–66.

Michel, F., Perenin, M.T., and Sieroff, E. (1986). Prosopagnosie sans hémianopsie après lésion unilatérale occipito-temporale droite. *Rev. Neurol., Paris* 142, 545–9.

Milner, A.D. and Goodale, M.A. (1995). *The visual brain in action.* Oxford University Press, Oxford.

Mingazzini, G. (1908). Über Symptome infolge von Verletzungen des Occipitallappens durch Geschosse. *Neurologisches Zentralblatt* 27, 1112–23.

Mooney, C.M. (1957). Closure as affected by configural clarity and contextual consistency. *Can. J. Psychol.* 11, 80–8.

Moran, J. and Desimone, R. (1985). Selective attention gates visual processing in the extrastriate cortex. *Science* 229, 782–4.

Munk, H. (1878). Weitere Mittheilungen zur Physiologie der Grosshirnrinde. *Arch. Anat. Physiol.* 2, 162–78.

Nardelli, E., Buonamo, F., Coccia, G., Fiaschi, H., Terzian, H., and Rizzuto, N. (1982). Prosopagnosia: report of four cases. *Eur. Neurol.* 21, 289–97.

Neville, H.J. and Lawson, D. (1987). Attention to central and peripheral visual space in a movement detection task: an event-related potential and behavioral study. I. Normal hearing adults. *Brain Res.* 405, 253–67.

Newcombe, F. (1979). The processing of visual information in prosopagnosia and acquired dyslexia: functional versus physiological interpretation. In *Research in Psychology and Medicine* (ed. D.J. Oborne, M.M. Gruneberg, and J.R. Eiser), pp. 315–22. Academic Press, London.

Newcombe, F., Ratcliff, G., and Damasio, H. (1987). Dissociable visual and spatial impairments following right posterior cerebral lesions: clinical, neuropsychological and anatomical evidence. *Neuropsychologia* 25, 149–61.

Newcombe, F., Young, A.W., and de Haan, E.H.F. (1989). Prosopagnosia and object agnosia without covert recognition. *Neuropsychologia* 27, 179–91.

Nobre, A.C., Sebestyen, G.N., Gitelman, D.R., Mesulam, M.M., Frackowiak, R.S.J. and Frith, C.D. (1997). Functional localization of the system for visuospatial attention using positron emission tomography. *Brain* 120, 515–33.

Nobre, A.C., Sebestyen, G.N. and Miniussi, C. (2000). The dynamics of shifting visuospatial attention revealed by event-related potentials. *Neuropsychologia* 38, 964–74.

Oppenheim, H. (1885). Ueber eine durch eine klinisch bisher nicht verwerthete Untersuchungsmethode ermittelte Form der Sensibilitätsstörung bei einseitigen Erkrankungen des Grosshirns. *Neurol. Centralbl.* 4, 529–33.

Palm, G. (1982). *Neural assemblies. An alternative approach to artificial intelligence.* Berlin: Heidelberg, Springer.

Pallis, C.A. (1955). Impaired identification of faces and places with agnosia for colors. *J. Neurol. Neurosurg. Psychiatry* 18, 218–24.

Paradiso, M.A. and Nakayama, K. (1991). Brightness perception and filling-in. *Vis. Res.* 31, 1221–36.

Paterson, A. and Zangwill, O.L. (1944). Disorders of visual space perception associated with lesions of the right cerebral hemisphere. *Brain* 67, 331–58.

Patla, A.E., Goodale, M.A. (1996). Obstacle avoidance during locomotion is unaffected in a patient with visual form agnosia. *Neuroreport* 8, 165–8.

Pearlman, A.L., Birch J., and Meadows, J.C. (1975). Cerebral color blindness: An acquired defect in hue discrimination. *Ann. Neurol.* 5, 253–61.

Penfield, W. (1947). Some observations on the cerebral cortex of man. *Proc. R. Soc. Lond. B* 134, 329–49.

Penfield, W. (1965). Conditioning the uncommitted cortex for language learning. *Brain* 88, 787–98.

Penfield, W. (1972). The electrode, the brain and the mind. *Z. Neurol.* 201, 297–309.

Perenin, M.-T. (1997). Optic ataxia and unilateral neglect: clinical evidence for dissociable spatial functions in posterior parietal cortex. In *Parietal lobe contributions to orientation in 3D space* (ed. H.-O. Karnath and P. Thier), pp. 289–308. Springer, Berlin.

Peterhans, E. and von der Heydt, R. (1991). Subjective contours—bridging the gap between psychophysics and physiology. *Trends Neurosci.* 14, 112–19.

Pevzner, S., Bornstein, B., and Loewenthal, M. (1962). Prosopagnosia. *J. Neurol., Neurosurg., Psychiatry* 25, 336–8.

Pichler, E. (1957). Ueber Verkehrtsehen als Großhirnsymptom. *Wiener Klinische Wochenschrift* **69**, 625–30.

Pick, A. (1901). Neue Mittheilungen über Störungen der Tiefenlocalisation. *Neurologisches Zentralblatt* **20**, 338–43.

Pillon, B., Signoret, J.L., and Lhermitte, F. (1981). Agnosie visuelle associative. Role de l'hemisphere gauche dans la perception visuelle. *Rev. Neurol., Paris* **137**, 831–42.

Poeck, K. (1984). Neuropsychological demonstration of splenial interhemispheric disconnection in a case of 'optic anomia'. *Neuropsychologia* **22**, 707–13.

Poppelreuter, W. (1917). *Die psychischen Schädigungen durch Kopfschuss im Kriege 1914–1916. Bd. I. Die Störungen der niederen und höheren Sehleistungen durch Verletzungen des Okzipitalhirns* L. Voss, Leipzig.

Posner, M.I., Walker, J.A., Friedrich, F.J., and Rafal, R.D. (1984). Effects of parietal lobe injury on covert orienting of attention. *J. Neurosci.* **4**, 1863–74.

Pötzl, O. (1928). Die Aphasielehre vom Standpunkte der klinischen Psychiatrie. Erster Band: die optisch-agnostischen Störungen. F. Deuticke, Leipzig.

Pötzl, O. (1954). Über Palinopsie (und deren Beziehung zu Eigenleistungen Occipitaler Rindenfelder). *Wien. Z. Nerv. Heilk.* **8**, 161–86.

Pötzl, O. and Redlich, E. (1911). Demonstration eines Falles von bilateraler Affektion beider Occipitallappen. *Wiener Klin. Wochenschr.* **24**, 517–18.

Pouget, A. and Sejnowski, T.J. (1997). Spatial transformations in the parietal cortex using basis functions. *J. Cogn. Neurosci.* **9**, 222–37.

Pouget, A., Fisher, S.A., and Sejnowski, T.J. (1993). Egocentric spatial representation in early vision. *J. Cogn. Neurosci.* **5**, 150–61.

Rafal, R.D. (1997). Balint syndrome. In *Behavioral neurology and neuropsychology* (ed. T.E. Feinberg and M.J. Farah), pp. 337–56.

Rafal, R.D. and Posner, M.I. (1987). Deficits in human visual spatial attention following thalamic lesions. *Proc. Natl. Acad. Sci., USA* **84**, 7349–53.

Ratcliff, G. (1982). Disturbances of spatial orientation associated with cerebral lesions. In *Spatial abilities: development and physiological foundations* (ed. M. Potegal). Academic Press, New York.(1982)

Ratcliff, G. and Davies-Jones, G.A.B. (1972). Defective visual localization in focal brain wounds. *Brain* **95**, 49–60.

Ratcliff, G. and Newcombe, F. (1982). Object recognition: some deductions from the clinical evidence. In *Normality and pathology in cognitive functions* (ed. A.W. Ellis). Academic Press, New York.

Redlich, E. and Bonvicini, G. (1909). Über das Fehlen der Wahrnehmung der eigenen Blindheit bei Hirnkrankheiten. *Jahrbüch. Psychiatrie* **29**, 1–133.

Rees, G., Wojciulik, E., Clarke, K., Husain, M., Frith, C., and Driver, J. (2000). Unconscious activation of visual cortex in the damaged right hemisphere of a parietal patient with extinction. *Brain* **123**, 1624–33.

Renault, B., Signoret, J.L., Debruille, B., Breton, F., and Bolgert, F. (1989). Brain potentials reveal covert facial recognition in prosopagnosia. *Neuropsychologia* **27**, 905–12.

Rensink, R.A., O'Regan, J.K., and Clark, J.J. (1997). To see or not to see: the need for attention to perceive changes in scenes. *Psychol. Sci.* **8**, 368–73.

Repnow, M., Fahle, M., and Köst, G. (1995). Gaze perimetry—a new method based on monitoring eye position. *Perception* **24**, Supplement, 92.

Riddoch, G. (1917). Dissociation of visual perceptions due to occipital injuries, with especial reference to appreciation of movement. *Brain* **40**, 15–57.

Riddoch, G. (1935). Visual disorientation in homonymous half-fields. *Brain* **58**, 376–82.

Riddoch, M.J. and Humphreys, G.W. (1986). Disturbances of figure-ground discrimination.

Riddoch, M.J. and Humphreys, G.W. (1987a). A case of integrative visual agnosia. *Brain* 110, 1431–62.

Riddoch, M.J. and Humphreys, G.W. (1987b). Visual object processing in optic aphasia: a case of semantic access agnosia. *Cogn. Neuropsychol.* 4, 131–85.

Rizzo M. (1989). Asteropsis. In *Handbook of neuropsychology* (ed. F. Boller and J. Grafman), Vol. 2. Elsevier, Amsterdam.

Rizzo, M. and Damasio, H. (1985). Impairment of stereopsis with focal brain lesions. *Ann. Neurol.* 18, 147.

Rizzo, M. and Hurtig, R. (1987). Looking but not seeing: attention, perception, and eye movements in simultanagnosia. *Neurology* 37, 1642–8.

Rizzolatti, G. and Berti, A. (1990). Neglect as a neural representation deficit. *Rev. Neurol., Paris* 146, 626–34.

Robertson, L.C., Lamb, M.R., and Knight, R.T. (1988). Effects of lesions of the temporal-parietal junction on perceptual and attentional processing in humans. *J. Neurosci.* 8, 3757–69.

Robertson, L., Treisman, A., Friedman-Hill, S., and Grabowecky, M. (1997). The interaction of spatial and object pathways: evidence from Balint's syndrome. *J. Cogn. Neurosci.* 9, 295–317.

Robinson, P.K. and Watt, A.C. (1947). Hallucinations of remembered scenes as an epileptic aura. *Brain* 70, 440–8.

Rondot, P., Tzavaras, A. and Garcin, R. (1967). Sur un cas de prosopagnosie persistant depuis quinze ans. *Revue Neurologique* 117, 424–8.

Rothstein, T.B. and Sacks, J.G. (1972). Defective stereopsis in lesions of the parietal lobe. *Am. J. Ophthalmol.* 73, 281–4.

Rubens, A.B. (1979). Agnosia. In *Clinical neuropsychology* (ed. K.M. Heilman and E. Valenstein), pp. 233–67. Oxford University Press, Oxford.

Rubens, A.B. and Benson, D.F. (1971). Associative visual agnosia. *Arch. Neurol.* 24, 305–16.

Russo, M. and Vignolo, L.A. (1967). Visual figure–ground discrimination in patients with unilateral cerebral disease. *Cortex* 3, 113–27.

Rüttiger, L., Braun, D.I., Gegenfurtner, K.R., Petersen, D., Schönle P., and Sharpe, L.T. (1999). Selective color constancy deficits after circumscribed unilateral brain lesions. *J. Neurosci.* 19, 3094–106.

Sagiv, N., Vuilleumier, P., and Swick, D. (2000). Extinguished faces: Electrophysiological correlates of conscious and unconscious perception in unilateral spatial neglect. Cognitive Neuroscience Society Meeting, San Francisco. *J. Cogn. Neurosci.* 12 (suppl.), 95.

Salzman, C.D., Britten, K.H., and Newsome, W.T. (1990). Cortical microstimulation influences perceptual judgements of motion direction. *Nature* 346, 174–7.

Samelsohn, J. (1881). Zur Frage des Farbensinncentrums. *Centralblatt für die medicinischen Wissenschaften* 19, 850–3.

Samuelsson, H., Jensen, C., Ekholm, S., Naver, H., and Blomstrand, C. (1997). Anatomical and neurological correlates of acute and chronic visuospatial neglect following right hemisphere stroke. *Cortex* 33, 271–85.

Santhouse, A.M., Howard, R.J., and Fytche, D.H. (2000). Visual hallucinatory syndromes and the anatomy of the visual brain. *Brain* 123, 2055–64.

Scheller, H. and Seidemann, H. (1931). Zur Frage der optisch-räumlichen Agnosie (Zugleich ein Beitrag zur Dyslexie). *Monatsschr. Psychiatrie Neurol.* 81, 97–188.

Scotti, G. and Spinnler, H. (1970). Colour imperception in unilateral hemisphere-damaged patients. *J. Neurol., Neurosurg., Psychiatry* 33, 22–8.

Sergent, J. (1990). The neuropsychology of visual image generation: data, method, and theory. *Brain Cogn.* 13, 98–129.

Sergent, J. and Villemure, J.G. (1989). Prosopagnosia in a right hemispherectomized patient. *Brain* 112, 975–95.

Servos, P. and Goodale, M.A. (1995). Preserved visual imagery in visual form agnosia. *Neuropsychologia* 33, 1383–94.

Servos, P., Matin, L., and Goodale, M.A. (1995). Dissociation between two modes of spatial processing by a visual form agnosic. *Neuroreport* 6, 1893–6.

Shallice, T. (1989). *From neuropsychology to mental structure.* Cambridge University Press, New York.

Sharon, Z., Avishai, H., and Nachum, S. (1999). Dissociation between word and color processing in patients with unilateral neglect. *J. Cogn. Neurosci.* 11 (Suppl., Abstracts of the Annual Meeting of the Society of Cognitive Neuroscience), 58.

Shuttleworth, E.C., Syring, V., and Allen, N. (1982). Further observations on the nature of prosopagnosia. *Brain Cogn.* 1, 307–22.

Singer, W. (1999). Neuronal synchrony: a versatile code for the definition of relations? *Neuron* 24, 49–65, 111–125.

Sittig, O. (1921). Störungen im Verhalten gegenüber Farben bei Aphasischen. *Monatsschr. Psychiatr. Neurol.* 49, 63–8, 169–87.

Slotnick, S.D., Klein, S.A., Carney, T., and Sutter, E.E. (2001). Electrophysiological estimate of human cortical magnification. *Clin. Neurophysiol.* 112, 1349–56.

Smith, A.T., Greenlee, M.W., Singh, K.D., Kraemer, F.M., and Hennig, J. (1998). The processing of first- and second- order motion in human visual cortex assessed by functional magnetic resonance imaging (fMRI). *J. Neurosci.* 18, 3816–30.

Snyder, L.H., Batista, A.P., and Andersen, R.A. (1997). Coding of intention in the posterior parietal cortex. *Nature,* 386, 167–70.

Spang, K.M., Timm, C., Schwendemann, G., and Fahle, M. (2001). Subjective experience of visual field defects caused by cerebral infarctions. *IOVS* 42, S847.

Spinelli, D., Burr, D.C., and Morrone, M.C. (1994). Spatial neglect is associated with increased latencies of visual evoked potentials. *Vis. Neurosci.* 11, 909–18.

Spreen, O., Benton, A.L., and van Allen, M.W. (1966). Dissociation of visual and tactile naming in amnesic aphasia. *Neurology* 16, 807–14.

Stoerig, P. and Fahle, M. (1995). Apparent motion across a scotoma: an implicit test of blindsight. *Eur. J. Neurosci.* 8 (suppl.) 76.

Taylor, A. and Warrington, E.K. (1971). Visual agnosia: a single case report. *Cortex* 7, 152–61.

Taylor, A. and Warrington, E.K. (1973). Visual discrimination in patients with localized cerebral lesions. *Cortex* 9, 82–93.

Teuber, H.L. (1968). Alteration of perception and memory in man. In *Analysis of behavioral change* (ed. L. Weiskrantz). Harper and Row, New York.

Teuber, H.L. and Mishkin, M. (1954). Judgment of visual and postural vertical after brain injury. *J. Psychol.* 38, 161–75.

Teuber, H.L., Battersby, W., and Bender, M.B. (1960). *Visual field defects after penetrating missile wounds of the brain.* MIT Press, Cambridge, Massachusetts.

Thorpe, S., Fize, D., and Marlot, C. (1996). Speed of processing in the human visual system. *Nature* 381, 520–2.

Tootell, R.B.H., Silverman, M.S., Switkes, E., and de Valois, R.L. (1982). Deoxyglucose analysis of retinotopic organization in primate striate cortex. *Science* 218, 902–4.

Torii, H. and Tamai, A. (1985). The problem of prosopagnosia: report of three cases with occlusion of the right posterior cerebral artery. *J. Neurol.* **232** (suppl.) 140.

Tranel, D. and Damasio, A.R. (1985). Knowledge without awareness: an autonomic index of facial recognition by prosopagnosics. *Science* **228**, 1453–4.

Tranel, D. and Damasio, A.R. (1988). Non-conscious face recognition in patients with face agnosia. *Behav. Brain Res.* **30**, 235–49.

Tranel, D., Damasio, A.R., and Damasio, H. (1988). Intact recognition of facial expression, gender, and age in patients with impaired recognition of face identity. *Neurology* **38**, 690–6.

Treisman, A. and Schmidt, H. (1982). Illusory conjunctions in the perception of objects. *Cogn. Psychol.* **14**, 107–41.

Troscianko, T., Davidoff, J., Humphreys, G., Landis, T., Fahle, M., Greenlee, M., Brugger, P., and Phillips, W. (1996). Human color discrimination based on a non-parvocellular pathway. *Curr. Biol.* **6**, 200–10.

Tyler, H.R. (1968). Abnormalities of perception with defective eye movements (Balint's syndrome). *Cortex* **4**, 154–71.

Tzavaras, A., Hécaen, H., and LeBras, H. (1971). Troubles de la vision des couleurs après lésions corticales unilatérales. *Rev. Neurol. Paris* **124**, 396–402.

Ullman, S. (1995). Sequence seeking and counter streams: a computational model for bidirectional information flow in the visual cortex. *Cereb. Cortex* **5**, 1–11.

Ungerleider, L.G. and Mishkin, M. (1982). Two cortical visual systems. In *Analysis of visual behavior* (D.J. Ingle, M.A. Goodale and R.J.W. Mansfield Eds.), pp. 549–86. Cambridge, MA: MIT Press.

Vaina, L.M. (1989). Selective impairment of visual motion interpretation following lesions of the right occipito-parietal area in humans. *Biol. Cybern.* **61**, 347–59.

Vaina, L.M. (1994). Functional segregation of color and motion processing in the human visual cortex: clinical evidence. *Cereb Cortex* **4**, 555–72.

Vaina, L.M. (1998). Complex motion perception and its deficits. *Curr. Opin. Neurobiol* **8**, 494–502.

Vaina, L.M. and Cowey, A. (1996). Impairment of the perception of second order motion but not first order motion in a patient with unilateral focal brain damage. *Proc. R. Soc. Lond B Biol Sci* **263**, 1225–32.

Vaina, L.M., Cowey, A. and Kennedy, D. (1999). Perception of first- and second-order motion: separable neurological mechanisms? *Hum. Brain Mapp.* **7**, 67–77.

Vaina, L.M., Cowey, A., Eskew, R.T., LeMay, M., and Kemper, T. (2001a). Regional cerebral correlates of global motion perception: Evidence from unilateral cerebral brain damage. *Brain* **124**, 310–21.

Vaina, L.M., LeMay, M., Bienfang, D.C., Choi, A.Y. and Nakayama, K. (1990). Intact "biological motion" and "structure from motion" perception in a patient with impaired motion mechanisms: A case study. *Vis. Neurosci.* **5**, 353–69.

Vaina, L.M. and Rushton, S.K. (2000). What neurological patients tell us about the use of optic flow. *Int. Rev. Neurobiol.* **44**, 293–313.

Vaina, L.M., Solomon, J., Chowdhury, S., Sinha, P., and Belliveau, J.W. (2001b). Functional neuroanatomy of biological motion perception in humans. *Proc. Natl. Acad. Sci.* **25**, 11656–61.

Vaina, L.M., Soloviev, S., Bienfang, D.C. and Cowey, A. (2000). A lesion of cortical area V2 selectively impairs the perception of the direction of first-order visual motion. *Neuroreport* **11**, 1039–44.

Vallar, G. (1993). The anatomical basis of spatial neglect in humans. In *Unilateral neglect: clinical and experimental studies* (ed. I.H. Robertson and J.C. Marshall) pp. 27–62. Lawrence Erlbaum Associates, Hillsdale, New Jersey.

Vallar, G. (1998). Spatial hemineglect in humans. *Trends Cogn. Sci.* **2**, 87–97.

Vallar, G. and Perani, D. (1986). The anatomy of unilateral neglect after right-hemisphere stroke lesions: a clinical/CT-scan correlation study in man. *Neuropsychologia* 24, 609–22.

Vallar, G. and Perani, D. (1987). The anatomy of spatial neglect in humans. In *Neurophysiological and neuropsychological aspects of spatial neglect* (ed. M. Jeannerod), pp. 235–58. North-Holland, Amsterdam.

Vallar, G., Sandroni, P., Rusconi, M.L., and Barbieri, S. (1991). Hemianopia, hemianesthesia, and spatial neglect: a study with evoked potentials. *Neurology*, 41, 1918–22.

van Essen, D.C., Anderson, C.H., and Felleman, D.J. (1992). Information processing in the primate visual system: an integrated systems perspective. *Science* 255, 419–23.

Viggiano, M.P., Spinelli, D., and Mecacci, L. (1995). Pattern reversal visual evoked potentials in patients with hemineglect syndrome. *Brain Cogn.* 27, 17–35.

Volpe, B.T., Ledoux, J.E., and Gazzaniga, M.S. (1979). Information processing of visual stimuli in an 'extinguished' field. *Nature* 282, 722–4.

von Graefe, A. (1856). Ueber die Untersuchung des Gesichtsfeldes bei amblyopischen Affektionen. *Von Graefes Arch. Ophthalmol.* 2, 258–98.

von Holst, E. and Mittelstaedt, H. (1950). Das Reafferenzprinzip. *Naturwissenschaften* 37, 464–76.

Vorster, O. (1893). Ueber einen Fall von doppelseitiger Hemianopsie mit Seelenblindheit, Photopsien und Gesichtstäuschungen. *Allgemeine Zeitschrift für Psychiatrie und psychisch-gerichtliche Medizin* 49, 227–49.

Vuilleumier, P. and Rafal, R. (1999). 'Both' means more than 'two': localizing and counting in patients with visuospatial neglect. *Nat. Neurosci.* 2, 783–4.

Vuilleumier, P., Hazeltine, E., Poldrack, R.A., Sagiv, N., Rafal, R.D. and Gabrieli, J. (2000). The neural fate of neglected faces: An event-related fMRI study of visual extinction. Cognitive Neuroscience Society Meeting, San Francisco. *Journal of Cognitive Neuroscience* 12 (Suppl.), 97–8.

Vuilleumier, P., Valenza, N., Mayer, E., Reverdin, A., and Landis, T. (1998). Near and far visual space in unilateral neglect. *Ann. Neurol.* 43, 406–10.

Vuilleumier, P., Valenza, N., and Landis, T. (2001). Explicit and implicit perception of illusory contours in unilateral spatial neglect: behavioural and anatomical correlates of preattentive grouping mechanisms. *Neuropsychologia* 39, 597–610.

Walsh, F.B. and Hoyt, W.F. (1969). *Clinical neuro-ophthalmology*, 3rd edn, Williams and Wilkins, Baltimore.

Wapner, W., Judd, T., and Gardner, H. (1978). Visual agnosia in an artist. *Cortex* 14, 343–64.

Ward, R., Goodrich, S., and Driver, J. (1994). Grouping reduces visual extinction: neuropsychological evidence for weight-linkage in visual selection. *Vis. Cogn.* 1, 101–29.

Wardak, C., Olivier, E., and Duhamel, J.-R. (2002). Neglect in monkeys: effect of permanent and reversible lesions. In *Neglect* (ed. H.O. Karnath, D.A. Milner and G. Vallar). Oxford University Press, Oxford.

Warrington, E.K. (1982). Neuropsychological studies of object recognition. *Phil. Trans. R. Soc. Lond.* B. 298, 15–33.

Warrington, E.K. (1985). Agnosia: the impairment of object recognition. In *Handbook of clinical neurology* (ed. P.J. Vinken, G.W. Bruyn, and H.L. Klawans). Elsevier, Amsterdam.

Warrington, E.K. and James, M. (1967). An experimental investigation of facial recognition in patients with unilateral cerebral lesions. *Cortex* 3, 317–26.

Warrington, E.K. and Rabin, P. (1970). Perceptual matching in patients with cerebral lesions. *Neuropsychologia* 8, 475–87.

Warrington, E.K. and Taylor, A.M. (1973). The contribution of the right parietal lobe to object recognition. *Cortex* 9, 152–64.

Warrington, E.K. and Taylor, A.M. (1978). Two categorical stages of object recognition. *Perception* 7, 695–705.

Warrington, E.K. and Shallice, T. (1979). Semantic access dyslexia. *Brain* 102, 43–63.

Warrington, E.K. and Shallice, T. (1980). Word-form dyslexia. *Brain* 103, 99–112.

Watson, R.T. and Heilman, K.M. (1979). Thalamic neglect. *Neurology* 29, 690–4.

Weigl, E. (1964). Some critical remarks concerning the problem of so-called simultanagnosia. *Neuropsychologia* 2, 189–207.

Welpe, E., von Seelen, W., and Fahle, M. (1980). A dichoptic edge effect resulting from binocular contour dominance. *Perception* 9, 683–93.

Wertheim, T. (1894) Über die indirekte Sehschärfe. *Z. Psychol.* 7, 172–87.

Westwood, D.A., Danckert, J., Servos, P., Goodale, M.A. (2002). Grasping two-dimensional images and three-dimensional objects in visual-form agnosia. *Exp. Brain Res.* 144, 262–7.

Whiteley, A.M. and Warrington, E.K. (1977). Prosopagnosia: a clinical, psychological, and anatomical study of three patients. *J. Neurol. Neurosurg. Psychiatry* 40, 395–403.

Wilbrand, H. (1887). *Die Seelenblindheit als Herderscheinung und ihre Beziehungen zur homonymen Hemianopsie*. J.F. Bergmann, Wiesbaden.

Wilbrand, H. (1890). *Die hemianopischen Gesichtsfeld-Formen und das optische Wahrnehmungszentrum*. J.F. Bergmann, Wiesbaden.

Wilbrand, H. and Sänger, A. (1892). *Über Sehstörungen bei functionellen Nervenleiden*. Verlag von F.C.W. Vogel, Leipzig.

Wilbrand, H. and Sänger, A. (1904, 1917). *Die Neurologie des Auges*, Bd. 3, Bd. 7. J.F. Bergmann, Wiesbaden.

Williams, M. (1970) *Brain damage and the mind*. Penguin Books, Baltimore.

Wolpert, I. (1924) Die Simultanagnosie—Störung der Gesamtauffassung. *Z. Gesamte Neurol. Psychiatrie* 93, 397–415.

Wurtz, R.H., Goldberg, M.E., and Robinson, D.L. (1982). Brain mechanisms of visual attention. *Sci. Am.* 246, 100–7.

Young, A.W. (1988). Functional organization of visual recognition. In *Thought without language* (ed. L. Weiskrantz). Oxford University Press, Oxford.

Zanker, J.M., Patzwahl, D.P., Braun, D., and Fahle, M. (1998). Complex motion stimuli localize higher-order visual processing in normal observers and in patients with parietal lesions. *Aust. N. Z. J. Ophthalmol.* 26, 149–55.

Zihl, J. (1995). Eye movement patterns in hemianopic dyslexia. *Brain* 118, 891–912.

Zihl, J. and von Cramon, D. (1986). *Zerebrale Sehstörungen*. Kohlhammer, Mainz.

Zihl, J., von Cramon, D., and Mai, N. (1983). Selective disturbance of movement vision after bilateral brain damage. *Brain* 106, 313–40.

Zihl, J. and Schmid, C. (1989). Use of visually evoked responses in evaluation of visual blurring in brain-damaged patients. *Electroencephalography Clinical Neurophysiology* 74, 394–8.

Chapter 8

Colour vision and its disturbances after cortical lesions

C.A. Heywood and A. Cowey

Introduction

In 1671 the Bishop of Salisbury, Robert Hooke, and Robert Boyle were invited by the Royal Society to report on the contents of a letter from Isaac Newton to Henry Oldenberg. In the letter, Newton described the results of procuring a prism ' . . . to try therewith the celebrated Phaenomena of Colours', a presumed reference to an experiment described by Descartes in *Les météores* to account for the formation of the rainbow (Turnbull 1961). What Newton suggested was the existence of two sorts of colour, 'The one original and simple, the other compounded of these. The Original or primary colours are, Red, Yellow, Green, Blew, and a Violet-purple, together with Orange, Indigo, and an indefinite variety of Intermediate gradations.' He further suggested that sunlight 'Tis ever compounded, and to its composition are requisite all the aforesaid primary Colours, mixed in a due proportion.' Newton's proposal that the spectrum contains seven colours, analogous to the seven tones and semitones in an octave of the musical scale, was incorrect and almost certainly arose from his mystical temperament and the special significance of the number seven. Nevertheless, he was correct in concluding that sunlight contains various amounts of light energy from different regions of what we now know as the electromagnetic spectrum. But, as Newton pointed out, to determine ' . . . by what modes or actions it produceth in our minds the Phantasms of Colours, is not so easie.'

A plethora of physiological, psychological, and philosophical investigations have sought to establish the nature of our colour phenomenology. Along the way, this endeavour has addressed such questions as the following. What are the purposes of colour vision and how has it evolved? What are the dimensions of colour, commonly described as hue, saturation, and brightness? How are colours categorized? What are the mechanisms of colour vision? Since the subjective experience of colour is a product of our nervous system, it would seem profitable to turn to neuroscientific methods for answers to these questions. By probing the activity of single cells with a microelectrode, or using modern techniques of neuroimaging to gauge brain activity on a coarser scale, it has been possible to elucidate the neural basis of chromatic vision. Moreover, studies of patients who, as a result of brain damage, show impaired colour performance have revealed unexpected functional dissociations. Taken together, it is apparent that the neural machinery that supports our colour phenomenology shows an unexpected complexity that runs counter to our introspections about the ease with which we perceive a richly coloured world.

Human vision evolved in a sunlit environment. Unsurprisingly, the narrow band of wavelengths of electromagnetic radiation to which our visual system is sensitive, from 400 to 700 nm and barely one octave out of eighty, closely corresponds to the range of wavelengths of sunlight that best survives passage through the terrestrial atmosphere. Moreover, human spectral sensitivity parallels their distribution, peaking at a wavelength of 550 nm where the sunlight's intensity is greatest. However, the mixture of wavelengths that strikes the surface of an object in the visual scene varies considerably from moment to moment. Light passing through the atmosphere is scattered by particles, most notably the air molecules themselves or water droplets. On a cloudless day, in the absence of water vapour, short wavelengths are predominantly scattered and the sky appears blue. The spectral composition of light falling on an object in shadow will then be shifted to shorter wavelengths as direct sunlight is blocked and the object illuminated by reflected and scattered ambient light. A clouded sky provides diffuse illumination where longer wavelengths of sunlight are also scattered by water vapour, producing a white haze. A more gradual diurnal variation in the spectral power distribution of sunlight also occurs when the sun moves closer to the horizon and its rays penetrate the atmosphere tangentially rather than orthogonally. A longer suspension of particles must then be traversed, with increasing opportunity for differential wavelength absorption and scattering. Thus, the spectrum impinging on a surface has a shifting wavelength distribution. Moreover, the spectral reflectance function, describing the percentage of each wavelength that is reflected from that surface, is continuous across all wavelengths of the visible spectrum (Fig. 8.1).

The wavelength composition of the image on the retina is an apparently inextricable mixture of the spectral power distribution of the illuminant and the spectral reflectance function of a surface. To assign a constant colour to a surface requires that the visual system disentangle the two. If the perceived colour of an object were uniquely determined by the

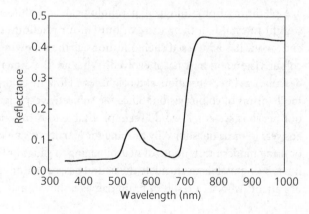

Fig. 8.1 A typical spectral reflectance function of foliage showing the relative reflectance of light of different wavelengths across the visible spectrum. The wavelength composition of reflected light will depend on the wavelength distribution of the illuminant. (Also see 'Plates' section.)

wavelength composition of light reflected from a surface, then we would live in a world of shifting colours. Our perceptual constancy, which enables us to view colour as an inherent property of a particular object, suggests that the visual system successfully 'discounts the illuminant' (Helmholtz 1911) in the assignment of surface colour.

The adaptive significance of colour constancy is self-evident, namely, it allows us to recognize and identify an object as the same when we repeatedly encounter it under varying conditions of illumination. Recognition of a permanent attribute of an object, namely, its spectral reflectance profile, can be used, e.g. in the identification of conspecifics, recognition of mood, sexual signalling, or assessing the ripeness of dietary fruits (Mollon 1989). Other putative advantages of chromatic vision include its contribution to segmenting, disambiguating, and searching the visual scene. An object can be distinguished from its background on the basis of differences in depth, texture, luminance, and chromaticity. Spatial and temporal luminance variation, as a result of shadow, can introduce spurious luminance contrast that masks the contours of an object in an achromatic image but chromatic contrast can reveal them. The addition of chromatic information can render a stationary object visible, or distinguish a moving object from a background of moving shadow. Moreover, chromatic vision improves visual recognition memory for natural scenes by facilitating the encoding and retrieval of images (Gegenfurtner and Rieger 2000). Finally, colour differences assist in the rapid detection of objects in the visual scene and are more effective than either shape or brightness differences in guiding visual search (Williams 1966).

In view of the advantages listed above, it is no surprise that the visual system is remarkably adept in the discrimination of colours. The eighteenth century astronomer Sir Frederick William Herschel noted that the mosaicists of the Vatican must have distinguished some 30 000 colours. While the number of discriminable steps in the visible spectrum is of the order of 150, when dimensions of hue, brightness, and saturation are systematically varied more recent estimates place the figure closer to one million (Boynton 1990).

In addition to telling colours apart, the human visual system classifies colours into basic colour categories that are a prerequisite for proficient colour naming. Such categories may include the four elemental opponent-colour sensations of Edward Hering and the 11 basic colour terms that are common to many languages (Berlin and Kay 1969). Moreover, we have the capacity to memorize colours, recall the colours of familiar objects, and engage in visual imagery. Each of these perceptual, mnemonic, and linguistic colour abilities can be disrupted as a result of brain damage, and the pattern of associations and dissociations among impairments has been informative with respect to their neural organization. For example, early reports drew attention to impairments in retrieving the colours of familiar objects from pictorial or verbal cues (Lewandowsky 1908a,b; Davidoff and Fodor 1989), or distinguished between a loss of colour names and an inability to sort colours into their categories, neither of which were necessarily accompanied by a loss of memory for object colour (Sittig 1921). It has since been confirmed many times that disorders, such as colour anomia (Oxbury *et al.* 1969) and colour agnosia (Beauvois and Saillant 1985), and deficits of colour imagery and memory (Kinsbourne and Warrington 1964; Luzzatti and Davidoff 1994), are quite distinct. Equally, the loss of colour vision as a result of brain damage can occur as a strikingly selective disorder. Whether colour constancy can be selectively impaired is less clear and will be discussed.

Visual pathways in the primate brain

It is now established that the primate brain contains multiple visual areas, although both their precise number and perceptual roles are far from clear. It is unnecessary to dwell at length on the organization of the primate visual system, which is described in Chapter 5, this volume and reviewed extensively elsewhere (see Livingstone and Hubel 1987*a,b*; Zeki and Shipp 1988; Schiller *et al.* 1990; Zeki 1990*a,b*). In brief, areas in the parietal and temporal lobes are associated with 'dorsal' and 'ventral' streams of visual processing. Dorsal stream areas play a crucial role in the visual control of action and are functionally distinct (which is not to say that they never interact) from those in the ventral stream, which convey information about colour and form to the temporal lobe (Milner and Goodale 1995). Moreover, electrophysiological studies have distinguished between P- and M-channels of visual processing, which cannot, however, be assigned to the two distinct groupings of visual cortical areas in a straightforward and exclusive manner.

The M- and P-channels originate in the Pα and Pβ ganglion cells of the primate retina, respectively. These different classes of cells send their axons to different laminae of the dorsal lateral geniculate nucleus (dLGN), the magnocellular and parvocellular layers, from which the channels derive their name. The M- and P-channels convey different properties of the visual image to primary visual cortex. Whereas the M-channel chiefly relays low-contrast, achromatic visual information at high temporal frequencies, the P-channel is principally concerned with the chromatic properties of the image and the processing of higher spatial, and lower temporal, frequencies.

More recently, a third pathway has been identified, arising from blue/yellow bistratified ganglion cells, and dubbed the koniocellular (K) pathway (Hendry and Yoshioka 1994; Dacey 1993: Dacey and Lee 1994). The interlaminar K-cells are much more numerous than previously thought and may be as common as the M-cells. It has been suggested that they play a major role in aspects of colour vision, but this remains to be established (for reviews see Dacey 1993, 2000; Hendry and Reid 2000).

The segregation between the retinocortical visual pathways of primates, so prominent in the dLGN, continues up to primary and secondary visual cortical areas. The parvocellular layers of the dLGN project to layer 4Cβ of V1 and then to the so-called 'blob' and 'interblob' regions in primary visual cortex, revealed by labelling with the metabolic marker, cytochrome oxidase. The blobs also receive a direct projection from interlaminar dLGN cells of the K-channel. The cells in the cytochrome oxidase blobs are selective for wavelength, but not orientation. In contradistinction, orientation, but not wavelength selectivity, is common in cells in the interblobs. The blobs and interblobs of V1 project to cytochrome oxidase-rich thin stripes and cytochrome oxidase-deficient interstripes in area V2, which, in turn, project to area V4.

In contrast, the magnocellular channel in dLGN projects primarily to layer 4Cα of area V1 and from there to layer 4B. Layer 4B projects both directly and, via the cytochrome oxidase-rich thick stripes in V2, to cortical area MT.

In summary, the blob and interblob regions provide two arms of the P-channel that project to visual areas assigned to the ventral stream. As the response properties of their constituent neurons suggest, the blob and interblob regions code wavelength and form, respectively. The orientation and direction selectivity of cells in the M-channel, along with their high luminance contrast gain, suggests that it plays a role in conveying motion and form information to visual areas in the parietal lobes.

Area V4 and colour

While the properties of single neurons cannot unambiguously provide a reliable indicator of the perceptual role of the visual area in which they reside (Cowey 1994), it has been argued that area V4 plays a pivotal role in colour processing, particularly in colour constancy (Zeki 1990b). This proposal is based on the early observation that V4 contains a relatively high proportion of cells that code colour (Zeki 1973). The later demonstration (Zeki 1983) that cells in V4, unlike those in V1, respond to the colour of a surface in a complex chromatic scene, regardless of the wavelength composition of the reflected light, i.e. that they appear to achieve colour constancy, has bolstered this view. There are, however, some detractors. For example, successive studies have, more recently, reported ever-declining estimates of the proportion of colour-coded cells in area V4 (see below). Furthermore, it has been suggested that cells exhibiting colour constancy are just as evident in V1 as long as the stimuli used to examine it are scaled to match the smaller receptive field in V1 (Wachtler et al. 1999). Notwithstanding, this conflicting evidence has not prevented V4 from being termed the 'colour area'. Certainly, the large receptive fields of cells in V4, and their widespread callosal connections, suggest this area engages in long-range processes of the sort required for mediating colour constancy. Such processes are thought to include the calculation of the relative ratios of the intensity of light of different wavebands from different surfaces. Ratios are independent of the absolute intensities, and therefore of the illuminant. Thus V4, the 'colour area', has been identified as an area where such ratios are computed and constant colours are assigned to surfaces.

If area V4 is critical for the ratio-taking processes outlined above, then its destruction should lead to a selective failing of colour constancy. The chromatic vision of the monkey should then rely on colour processes earlier in the visual pathway, namely, those in areas V1 and V2, where cells respond to the wavelength distribution of light falling in their receptive fields. The monkey should retain the ability to tell colours apart but the colour appearance of a surface will depend on the spectral power distribution of the illuminant. We shall return to this issue below but suffice it to say that the evidence that

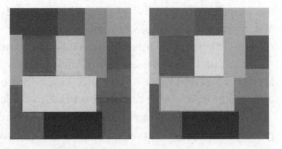

Fig. 8.2 To the left is a chromatic Mondrian pattern and, to the right, its achromatic counterpart. (See Plate 6, colour plate section.)

bilateral ablation of simian V4 results in colour impairment, especially of colour constancy, is slim. Meanwhile, it should be noted that there was a further reason that encouraged area V4 to be functionally dubbed the 'colour area'.

An early interpretation of the roles of multiple visual areas was that each is relatively specialized for the processing of a different perceptual attribute. However, attempts to assign perceptual functions to visual areas of the brain, either on the basis of the response properties of their cells, or from inferences made from the behavioural effects of selective ablation, have encountered considerable difficulties (see Cowey 1994 for review). In stark contrast to the absence of compelling evidence for selective visual disorders following the ablation of any single visual area in monkeys, naturally occurring brain lesions in man occasionally produce disorders that are strikingly selective. Most notable among these is the clinical condition of cerebral achromatopsia, where medial occipitotemporal damage can abolish colour vision (Brill 1882; Meadows 1974; Albert *et al.* 1975; Green and Lessell 1977; Heywood *et al.* 1987; Victor *et al.* 1989; Zeki 1993). The selectivity of the disorder is consistent with the notion of functional specialization within different regions of extrastriate visual cortex. The advent of neuroimaging allowed for a further supposition.

An early study demonstrated a hotspot of activation in the region of the lingual and fusiform gyri when normal observers passively viewed a display of coloured rectilinear patches (called a Mondrian; Fig. 8.2) compared with the viewing of an identical, but achromatic scene of equivalent lightnesses (Zeki *et al.* 1991).

The activation was located within the region invariably damaged in the brains of achromatopsic patients, albeit their lesions are a great deal more extensive. It was a short step to equate this 'colour centre' with the macaque colour area identified by other means, and designate it 'human V4'. The step may have been premature.

Cerebral achromatopsia

Cerebral achromatopsia refers to the loss of colour vision as a result of brain damage. Patients retain three functional cone mechanisms (Mollon *et al.* 1980) as shown by the increment threshold technique of Stiles (1978) and the deficit is clearly of central origin. Patients are unable to match, discriminate, sort, or name colours and perform poorly on the Farnsworth–Munsell 100-Hue test, which requires placing in chromatic

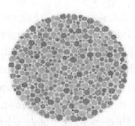

Fig. 8.3 An Ishihara plate is composed of small circles with random luminance variation. The numeral is defined by colour difference. (See Plate 7, colour plate section.)

order a number of equiluminant coloured chips (at least they are equiluminant for the average, young, male observer). The deficit exists in varying degrees of severity where in cases of incomplete achromatopsia there is frequently a greater loss of blues and greens and a relative sparing of reds (Pearlman *et al.* 1979). On another conventional test of colour vision, the Ishihara pseudoisochromatic plates (Fig. 8.3), results are variable. Some patients are able to read some or all of the plates (Meadows 1974; Victor *et al.* 1989), while others only succeed under particular testing conditions, notably viewing distance (Green and Lessell 1977; Albert *et al.* 1975; Heywood *et al.* 1987).

It is often stated that patients complain that their visual world is drained of colour and consists of 'dirty' shades of grey. However, it is unclear and, to our knowledge, never yet discussed whether such subjective reports of visual phenomenology are possible only in cases of incomplete loss, the so-called dyschromatopsias. Just as a severe visual field loss may go unreported, the complete absence of the processing system that underlies our visual phenomenology may render an achromatopsic patient incapable of reporting the absence of a perceptual attribute that is normally the product of the missing neural machinery. This may account for the strange reluctance on the part of patients to assign labels to their perceptions of chromatic or achromatic surfaces, unless their achromatopsia affects only one hemifield, in which case the normal hemifield preserves their conceptual knowledge about colour. There is little reason to suppose that their phenomenal experience is akin to a chromatic image stripped of colour variation, i.e. as a normal observer may experience a monochrome display. Indeed, the putative mechanisms that have been lost are presumed to undertake computations just as essential for determining the greyness of a surface as any other colour tone. Some patients retain visual imagery of colours (Shuren *et al.* 1996), and it is unknown whether such sparing relates to a greater readiness to describe the nature of their colourless world.

Achromatopsia is frequently, though not invariably (Duvelleroy *et al.* 1997), accompanied by impaired facial recognition (prosopagnosia) and altitudinal visual field defects (Meadows 1974). This is a straightforward consequence of the proximity of the 'colour centre' to face-processing regions in the fusiform gyrus and the lip and lower bank of area V1, which topographically represents the upper visual field. However, there are occasional reports where the impairment is restricted to the perception of colour (Mackay and Dunlop 1899; Kölmel 1988; Damasio *el al.* 1980; Sacks *et al.* 1988). Without doubting any of the observations made in these reports it should not be forgotten that the examination of non-chromatic vision was hardly extensive.

As noted by Verrey (1888), achromatopsia can be confined to one hemifield or a single quadrant (Wilbrand 1884; Kölmel 1988). In such cases patients may be unaware of their loss, again implying that the activity normally elicited in the damaged region perhaps mediates attention to colour, or is the neural correlate of conscious colour experience.

It is becoming increasingly clear that, while achromatopsia patients have depleted colour vision, they can nevertheless use wavelength variation to determine other aspects of the visual scene. In this respect, those with complete achromatopsia are particularly informative and one such patient, M.S., has been studied extensively. An early indication that, paradoxically, the loss of colour vision does not prevent the segmentation of the visual scene on the basis of colour differences was provided by Mollon *et al.* (1980). Patient M.S. was unable to read the Ishihara pseudoisochromatic plates at conventional reading distance but could do so when they were presented at 2 m. The test requires the identification of a numeral that is defined by coloured dots embedded in similar dots of varying lightness. At normal reading distance, the chromatic border that defines the numeral is masked by the luminance contour of individual dots. At a distance where the latter can no longer be resolved, or when the plate is optically blurred (Heywood *et al.* 1991), M.S. can detect the now dominant chromatic boundary and report the concealed figure. In a further test (Heywood *et al.* 1991), M.S. was presented with two rows of equi-luminant coloured patches. In each row the colours abutted each other, but in one row they were in chromatic order and in the other they were jumbled (Fig. 8.4(a)). M.S. could tell the difference between jumbled and ordered arrays, presumably by detecting, and distinguishing the salience of, chromatic boundaries. In the jumbled array, adjacent equi-luminant hues were inevitably more widely separated in colour space and the greater chromatic contrast presumably made them more salient. Chromatic borders between two equiluminant hues are therefore visible to M.S. even when the two hues cannot be told apart. And when the colours were all moved a few mm apart, creating a conspicuous white border between all adjacent colours, he became unable to discriminate the ordered from disordered series (Fig. 8.4(b)). It would be interesting to see whether the widely

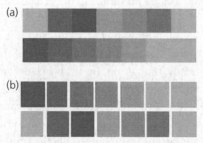

Fig. 8.4 (a) The upper figure is a row of abutting equiluminant patches ordered in chromaticity. Below, the identical patches are presented as a jumbled array. Although M.S. was unable to discriminate between any of the constituent patches, he was able to discriminate between the ordered and jumbled arrays. In (b) the patches no longer abut and M.S. can no longer tell the arrays apart. (See Plate 8, colour plate section.)

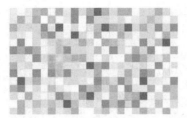

Fig. 8.5 The figure is composed of an achromatic checkerboard (draught board) in which a green cross is embedded. When the luminance of each square is rapidly varied from moment to moment, M.S. effortlessly detects the location of the green cross. The rapid fluctuation in luminance, to which the M-channel is sensitive, would render it ineffective in detecting the chromatic contour. Detection must presumably be mediated by a preserved P- or K-channel. (See Plate 9, colour plate section.)

used Farnsworth–Munsell 100-Hue test would become possible for achromatopsic patients if the prominent black border round every colour were removed!

These abilities are consistent with the properties of broad-band cells in the M-channel, i.e. those that sum the output of long- and middle-wavelength cones, rather than acting in an opponent fashion, which can signal chromatic contour without coding information about the constituent colours (Saito *et al.* 1989). One possible interpretation of achromatopsia is that it results from selective destruction of the P-channel. However, several lines of evidence argue against this attractively simple proposal. The introduction of rapid and spurious spatial and temporal luminance fluctuations (luminance noise) into chromatic visual displays prevents the broad-band system from distinguishing between chromatic and luminance contrast. Such random luminance masking did not prevent M.S. from segregating figure and ground on the basis of chromatic cues alone (Fig. 8.5), suggesting preservation of the colour-opponent P-channel and/or the K-channel (Heywood *et al.* 1994). Thus, M.S. can use wavelength to extract form despite lacking any phenomenal experience of colour itself. Moreover, M.S. has essentially normal chromatic contrast sensitivity for the detection of sinusoidally modulated equiluminant chromatic gratings, i.e. he can detect gratings composed of colour differences he cannot tell apart (Heywood *et al.* 1996). A similar dissociation has been reported in cases of incomplete achromatopsia (Barbur *et al.* 1994). Unlike in normal observers, thresholds for the detection of colour change differ from those for revealing chromatic form suggesting that different and independent processes contribute to perceived object colour and form derived from chromatic signals.

A second reason to suspect P-channel involvement stems from measurements of spectral sensitivity (Heywood *et al.* 1991). As illustrated in Fig. 8.6, M.S. does not show the single peak at ~550 nm characteristic of the sensitivity of the broadband channel, but shows sensitivity peaks at three different wavelengths, indicative of colour-opponent mechanisms of the P-channel (Sperling and Harwerth 1971). One consequence of colour-opponency is that mixtures of red and green light result in a yellow

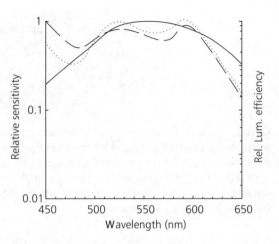

Fig. 8.6 The solid curve shows the luminous efficiency curve (Vλ) indicating the sensitivity of the broad-band, M-channel to lights of different wavelength. The dotted and dashed lines show the increment threshold relative spectral sensitivity of a normal observer and patient M.S., respectively (scaled to unity). The peaks and troughs are indicative of colour-opponent processes.

that appears conspicuously dimmer than would be expected on the basis of simple brightness additivity (Guth 1965). A colour-opponent (e.g. red$^+$/green$^-$) receptive field will be maximally excited by long-, and inhibited by middle-wavelength light. The reverse occurs for cells showing opposite opponency (green$^+$/red$^-$). The excitatory and inhibitory receptive field mechanisms will be placed in equilibrium for a red/green mixture. This is the basis for the 'troughs' in the spectral sensitivity profiles shown in Fig. 8.6.

While few would deny that chromatic contrast contributes to visual form, the issue of its role in motion-processing remains controversial. The common view is that colour and motion undergo independent processing, consistent with the allotted roles of the P- and M-channels, respectively. The observation that drifting chromatic gratings appear to move considerably more slowly than their luminance-modulated counterparts is consistent with this view. Furthermore, the threshold luminance contrast to determine the direction of motion of a grating is greater than that required to detect it. Recent evidence now suggests that the motion pathway is not colour-blind (Cropper and Derrington 1996; Gegenfurtner and Hawken 1996; Derrington 2000). Specifically, there is a colour-opponent mechanism, with high sensitivity to colour, that responds to slow speeds, is sensitive to direction of motion, but does not code velocity veridically. This is distinct from a mechanism that deals with faster speeds, has a high sensitivity to luminance contrast, treats colour signals like low-contrast luminance variation, and codes motion veridically.

Functional imaging has confirmed that area MT, the likely site of the latter mechanism, is activated by chromatic motion (ffytche *et al.* 1995). Cells in this region in the macaque monkey respond to equiluminant gratings presented in a manner whereby the phase of the grating is shifted by 90° from moment to moment (Dobkins and Albright 1994). Each change results in the replacement of a border (e.g. red/green) with one of opposite sign (e.g. green/red). The direction of motion should thus be ambiguous to a cell immune to the sign of the colour and to a colour-blind observer (Fig. 8.7). M.S. had no difficulty in reporting the 'correct' direction of apparent movement,

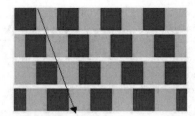

Fig. 8.7 The figure shows four successively presented frames of an equiluminant display where the phase of the pattern is shifted a quarter of a cycle. The direction of motion (left-to-right) can only be ascertained by matching successive green/red borders. If red/green and green/red borders cannot be distinguished, the direction of motion will be ambiguous. (See Plate 10, colour plate section.)

even though he was unable to tell apart the constituent colours of the grating (Heywood *et al.* 1994).

There are two further reports of spared motion processes in achromatopsia. In the first (Cavanagh *et al.* 1998), three achromatopsic patients were presented with moving, high-contrast, equiluminant chromatic gratings. It was possible to measure the strength of the preserved motion response based on colour by gauging the equivalent luminance contrast countermotion required to null it. Unlike M.S., these achromatopsic patients had grossly impaired sensitivity to chromatic contrast. Nevertheless, high-contrast equiluminant gratings produced a robust motion response equivalent to that of normal observers. The response was five to ten times stronger than that expected from the chromatic mechanism identified with area MT and was presumably mediated elsewhere. The second report (Heywood *et al.* 1998) provides indirect evidence for an intact P-channel contribution to motion in achromatopsia.

The 'slow' chromatic motion pathway is highly sensitive to chromatic contrast but does not code velocity veridically. This perhaps accounts for the phenomenon of 'motion slowing', where drifting, sinusoidal chromatic gratings are perceived as moving considerably more slowly than an achromatic grating drifting at the same speed. When sinusoidal gratings are constructed by the addition of middle- and long-wavelength light in spatial antiphase (as in Fig. 8.8(a)), the effects of brightness subadditivity will result in unintended brightness variation. This is most conspicuous midway between the red and green peaks, where red and green are mixed in equal proportion. The slow-motion channel receives a colour-opponent input and will therefore be susceptible to the sort of subadditive brightness responses described above, i.e. it is plausible that such brightness variation might influence perceived speed. When this brightness variation was corrected, by the addition of an appropriate amount of frequency-doubled luminance (Fig. 8.8(b)), there was a further reduction in the apparent speed of the grating in 10 observers with normal colour vision (Heywood *et al.* 1998). However, the same occurred for patient M.S., indicating processing of slow equiluminant chromatic motion even when, for M.S., the colours are indistinguishable.

Fig. 8.8 (c) shows an equiluminant chromatic grating constructed by sinusoidally modulating red and green in spatial antiphase, as shown in (a). Where red and green are mixed in equal proportion, creating yellow, the grating will appear dimmer because of brightness subadditivity. (d) and (e) show two examples of gratings where luminance had been added as shown in (a) to compensate for the effects of subadditivity. A drifting equiluminant grating will appear to move considerably more slowly than a luminance grating (f) drifting at the same speed. By adding an appropriate amount of luminance compensation, the grating is perceived as moving even *more* slowly by both M.S. and normal observers. Since subadditivity is the result of P-channel colour-opponency, this implies that M.S. retains intact colour input into the motion system. (See Plate 11, colour plate section.)

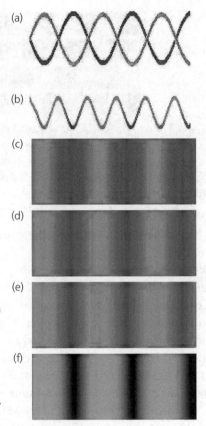

(a)

(b)

(c)

(d)

(e)

(f)

In summary, the loss of colour vision in achromatopsia can leave other wavelength-based processing intact. The syndrome is consistent with the loss of a 'colour centre', or mechanism, the purpose of which is to provide the phenomenal experience of hue. However, some authors have proposed that a 'colour centre' need not exist at all, at least in the conventional sense of a region that maps phenomenal colour space and assigns coordinates that determine our colour experience (Akins 2000; Akins and Hahn 2000). Instead, they suggest that colour vision evolved, not to provide the phenomenal features of our colour experience, but to encode chromatic contrast. Furthermore, the visual system is considered to be chiefly concerned with using chromatic contrast in a manner that is parallel and complementary to the use of luminance contrast. It has already been noted that chromatic contrast is an additional aid to image segmentation when, for example, shadows mask edges provided by local luminance contrast, or can resolve ambiguity, as when shadows move in a direction that conflicts with that of a moving object. On this account, the primary function of the visual system is to use spectral contrast in a variety of processes including those, for example, that signal motion, depth, form, and texture. The authors correctly point out (Akins 2000) that, if the *raison d'être* of spectral processing is to assign colour, and colours are assigned prior to subsequent processing to extract motion and form, then residual abilities based on spectral processing in cases of cortical colour blindness are unexpected. Instead, they propose that phenomenal colour is a secondary consequence of these several dissociable spectral processes, damage to which could delete some, but not all, aspects of conscious visual experience. These proposals are consistent with the nature of residual chromatic processing, described above, in a case of complete achromatopsia, patient M.S. (Heywood *et al.* 1994). They are also in agreement with accounts elsewhere (Cowey and Heywood 1997; Heywood *et al.* 1998), where we argued that residual abilities are mediated, not by what remains of a damaged 'colour centre', but by other independent spectral processes that use wavelength differences to derive other visual attributes. Each of these remaining processes has a conscious correlate.

The studies described above suggest that wavelength variation in the visual scene can be used, not only to produce colour experience, but also to determine further attributes such as form and motion. In achromatopsia, colour experience can be obliterated while the latter remain intact. Such cases provide important clues about the organization of the colour pathways, which, more recently, have been more closely examined by imaging the brains of normal observers viewing a variety of chromatic displays.

Functional neuroimaging of the colour pathways

The location of an extrastriate focus of activation concerned with chromatic processing has now been confirmed in a number of neuroimaging studies using markedly different paradigms. They can broadly be divided into those that entail passive viewing of chromatic displays, where residual cortical activation (as revealed by cerebral blood flow) after appropriate subtraction of an achromatic reference condition identifies regions responding to chromaticity, and those that involve a discrimination task in each of the two conditions. In the first category, the study mentioned earlier (Zeki *et al.* 1991) used positron emission tomography (PET) and required subjects to passively view 'Mondrian' patterns composed of chromatic patches of different hue and brightness. The reference condition was an identical arrangement of grey patches with the same corresponding luminance (Fig. 8.2). The activation of the fusiform gyrus revealed by PET has been demonstrated in several subsequent studies. Sakai *et al.* (1995) replicated this finding using functional magnetic resonance imaging (fMRI), where a focal signal increase in the posterior part of the fusiform gyrus correlated with the percept of colour, most notably with the perception of afterimages. Activation in response to the passive viewing of an array of coloured circles was compared with that in response to an identical array of achromatic circles, equiluminant with their coloured counterparts. Activation was bilateral in some subjects and unilateral in others. Similarly, Kleinschmidt *et al.* (1996) demonstrated bilateral activation, using fMRI, in the collateral sulci and extending into the lingual and fusiform gyri, when subjects viewed equiluminant chromatic modulation, but not isochromatic luminance modulation, and the reference condition was a uniform field of the same mean luminance and chromaticity. Such studies provide evidence for a 'colour centre'.

More recent studies have described a greater complexity of the organization of cortical areas engaged in colour-processing. Beauchamp *et al.* (1999) used a colour-ordering task akin to the clinical test commonly used to assess colour vision, the Farnsworth–Munsell 100-Hue test. In addition to the 'colour area' identified in earlier studies, these authors found robust activations in the more anterior and medial territory of the collateral sulcus and fusiform gyrus (see also Kastner *et al.* 1998). This was confirmed by Zeki and Bartels (1999a) who distinguished V4 from a smaller anterior region they termed V4α. Both areas contain a representation of the upper and lower quadrant of the contralateral visual field which, in the case of V4, is retinotopically mapped. Retinotopy was absent from V4α, or possibly too coarse to be revealed by the methods employed. Independent component analysis, on data derived from functional imaging, suggest that the areas act cooperatively in colour-processing and the latter authors therefore refer to them as the human 'V4 complex'.

Colour in the natural world is chiefly a property of objects that are endowed with meaning and associated with knowledge, learning, and memory. In contrast, the relatively simple abstract designs of Mondrian patterns were originally used in imaging studies of colour to minimize such cognitive factors. A recent study (Zeki and Marini 1998) sought to identify brain regions involved in object colour. The activity evoked by passive viewing of chromatic scenes, compared with their grey-level counterparts, extended anteriorly to include the posterior two-thirds of the fusiform gyrus. However, and remarkably, this was only the case if objects were invested with their natural colours. An identical procedure, using abnormally coloured scenes, revealed activation strikingly similar to that obtained using Mondrian patterns. The use of natural and unnatural colouring was further distinguished by activation in the dorsolateral and ventrolateral frontal cortex, respectively. A re-analysis of these data (Bartels and Zeki 2000) showed that V4 and V4α are co-active during the viewing of unnaturally coloured scenes, whereas naturally coloured scenes elicit activity in both V4α and anterior regions implicated in face and object recognition.

Functional imaging has charted a number of areas concerned with colour- or, more properly, wavelength-processing. Doubtless, as techniques are improved, a further fractionation and a finer parcellation of the fusiform gyrus will be achieved. Such a distributed arrangement of colour areas perhaps explains the varied nature of colour imperceptions, and different instances of their recovery, produced by cerebral lesions (Rizzo *et al.* 1993). However, the involvement of several areas in colour processing also begs the question as to why area V4, or its putative homologue in the human brain, should be reified as the 'colour area' or 'colour centre'? Perhaps it is meant to imply that it is more involved than other areas in the perception of colours. Alternatively, and less plausibly, it may suggest that it alone is necessary and sufficient for colour phenomenology. Yet, in the monkey, bilateral and total ablation of area V4 led to no impairment in ordering equiluminant colour patches, or in selecting the chromatically different patch concealed among an array of equiluminant distracters (Heywood *et al.* 1992). Nevertheless, a profoundly achromatopsic patient was severely impaired on these tasks, but performed well when the tasks entailed making judgements on the basis of luminance differences (Heywood *et al.* 1991). This suggests that in achromatopsia the damage cannot be restricted to area V4 but must encroach on other regions engaged in colour-processing, even indirectly by white matter damage beneath the collateral sulcus.

To designate area V4 as the 'colour area' may also serve to ignore its contribution to other visual processes. While colour discrimination remains intact following V4 removal in the monkey, form vision is grossly impaired (Heywood and Cowey 1987; Heywood *et al.* 1992; Schiller and Lee 1991). This is consistent with the prominent role in form vision indicated by neuronal sensitivity in V4 to this attribute (Desimone and Schein 1987). Moreover, Tootell and Hadjikhani (1998) have pointed out the decreasing estimates of the percentage of reported colour-selective cells over the succeeding years (87%, Zeki 1977; 68%, Zeki 1978; 32%, Van Essen and Zeki 1978; 20%, Fischer *et al.* 1981; 10%, Van Essen *et al.* 1981; and 18%, Schein *et al.* 1982).

As already alluded to, the notion of V4, or its presumed human homologue, as a 'colour centre' stems from the view that the V4 complex is the site of the ratio-taking operations that 'are at the heart of the colour-generating system' (Bartels and Zeki 2000). We now turn to this problem.

Achromatopsia and colour constancy

A significant contributor to the maintenance of constancy is the calculation of cone contrast, namely, the relative activity of each class of cones that is elicited by light reflected from two, or usually more, surfaces. These signals, which represent the ratio of cone excitation between two surfaces, for the three respective cone outputs, are invariant with respect to shifts in the illuminant. Normal observers interpret colour changes in the visual scene that preserve cone ratios as changes in the illuminant. Those that alter cone ratios are perceived as changes in the surface property. When two isolated patches, viewed dichoptically and eliciting different cone excitation, are presented against different backgrounds, they will appear identical as long as they produce identical cone ratios with their backgrounds. An important contributor (reflected in many accounts of colour constancy) to this constancy mechanism is retinal adaptation to the prevailing illumination, for example, during the course of the day. Adaptive colour constancy remained intact in a case of complete achromatopsia, albeit with raised thresholds (Hurlbert *et al.* 1998). The ability of an achromatopsic observer to compare *local* cone contrasts did not extend to judgements of complex scenes containing many surfaces, where the ability to make global comparisons of cone contrasts is abolished (Hurlbert *et al.* 1998).

Slow adaptation is unable to account for constancy under more rapid changes in the illuminant, e.g. when a cloud passes across the sun. The latter requires global comparisons among non-adjacent surfaces. Similarly, when two identical surfaces are viewed successively against different backgrounds, cone ratios can change markedly but the appearance of the surface changes very little. The background-independent, as opposed to illumination-independent, nature of the surface of an object, regardless of its position in a visual scene, is termed type II constancy. Such constancy also requires a mechanism that makes global comparisons among non-adjacent surfaces. A failure of type II constancy in an achromatopsic patient was reported by D'Zmura et al. (1998). A colour sample was assigned to different categories depending on whether it was presented against a lighter or darker background. Categorization was therefore largely determined by the sign and magnitude of luminance contrast.

Neurons in V4 show many of the properties expected in a mechanism computing colour constancy. For example, their extensive callosal connections (Van Essen and Zeki 1978; Desimone et al. 1993) allow for long-range interactions required to ascertain the ratio of reflectances of light of different wavebands from different surfaces in the visual scene that straddle the vertical midline of the visual field. The large inhibitory surrounds of the receptive fields of cells in V4, tuned to the same wavelengths as the excitatory centre, make them ideal candidates for 'discounting the illuminant'. This could result from a nulling of the response of the cell when diffuse illumination of light of the appropriate waveband falls simultaneously on centre and surround (Schein and Desimone 1990). Confirmatory evidence that V4 plays such a role would be provided if it were established that its removal results in a failure of constancy. But when this was attempted (Wild et al. 1985; Walsh et al. 1993), the results were inconclusive in that more than one interpretation was possible. Nevertheless, in the absence of firm evidence to the contrary, it is plausible that area V4 in the monkey undertakes computations that are essential for the constancy of colours. If this were the case, then, following the removal of V4, monkeys would lose colour constancy but nevertheless retain phenomenal experience of the colour of a surface, albeit the perceived colour would shift with changes in the prevailing illumination.

Achromatopsic patients lose the perceptual experience of hue and this has been interpreted by some as a consequence of a failure of constancy mechanisms essential for the 'synthesis' or 'construction' of colour (Zeki 1990a; Bartels and Zeki 2000). This suggests that the system that performs the ratio-taking operations may be the same as the one resulting in the phenomenal experience of colour (Zeki and Bartels 1999b). This would cast doubt on the functional equivalence between area V4 and its putative homologue, the 'colour centre'. If V4 is crucial for the ratio-taking mechanism that underlies both colour constancy and phenomenal colour vision, then its removal in the monkey should result in an inability to discriminate among equiluminant hues. Clearly, it does not. Instead, large anterior inferotemporal, rather than area V4, ablations in the monkey result in substantial and enduring colour impairment (Heywood et al. 1995). Alternatively, it is possible that the ratio-taking operation is distinct from the one generating object colour. Disruption of the former could result in a selective failure of colour constancy with preserved colour discrimination, whereas damage to the latter process could result in achromatopsia. There are reports of a dissociation between achromatopsia and loss of colour constancy. For example, defective colour constancy without any accompanying impairment in colour-matching has been reported in three patients with large ventral occipitotemporal lesions (Clarke *et al.* 1998). A further study by Rüttiger *et al.* (1999) of 27 patients with unilateral parietotemporal cortical lesions reported five with colour constancy deficits in the absence of impairments of hue discrimination. The region of brain damage common to all was in the vicinity of the superior and medial temporal gyri, distal and anterior to the 'colour centre'.

In a remarkable case (Zeki *et al.* 1999), patient P.B., rendered virtually blind as a result of vascular insufficiency, was unable to perceive form but could discriminate wavelengths. Colour constancy was lost in that responses varied with changes in the distribution of reflected wavelengths. Neuroimaging revealed activity chiefly in V1 and V2, suggesting that early visual areas contributed to, and were sufficient for, this residual capacity. In a case of incomplete achromatopsia, a single study (Kennard *et al.* 1995) described a patient who reported predictable changes in perceived colour with systematic changes in the illuminant. In both cases wavelength discrimination was accompanied by a conscious experience of colour. If activity in areas V1 and V2 can give rise to conscious, albeit nonconstant, colour experiences then it argues against the proposal that constancy and conscious hue perception are subserved by a single mechanism. It also raises the question as to why signals in intact V1 and V2 of achromatopsic patients do not have conscious correlates.

Functional neuroimaging and colour constancy

The human 'colour centre' was identified by imaging brain regions preferentially activated by passive viewing of coloured Mondrians compared with their achromatic counterparts. Natural scenes characteristically vary in both chrominance and luminance. If the colour centre plays a role in the construction of colour via a ratio-taking process, then it is the output of the process that assigns a neutral grey or a particular hue to a surface. It is therefore likely that brain regions responsible for colour constancy are *the same* as those for lightness constancy. It may then be supposed that these regions would be activated both by luminance and chrominance and not readily revealed in imaging studies that compare activation as a result of passive viewing of chromatic and achromatic stimuli, where the activation is similar in each condition. A more direct test of the role in perceptual constancy of colour regions in the fusiform gyrus has recently been reported (Bartels and Zeki 2000). Functional imaging was carried out while observers viewed chromatic or achromatic Mondrian patterns, presented under three conditions. In the first, static mode, the wavelength composition and intensity of each component patch remained unaltered during viewing. In the second and third, dynamic modes, either the intensity of the illumination, or its wavelength composition, were continuously changed. On the assumption that the dynamic modes would make more demands on constancy mechanisms, brain activation was compared with that elicited by viewing in the static mode. Given the sensitivity of their constituent neurons to changes in wavelength composition, surprisingly little activation was seen in areas V1 and V2. However, both V4 and V4α were strongly activated in the dynamic, compared with the static condition and this was true for coloured and for achromatic displays. There was only weak fusiform activity when a comparison was made between viewing dynamic changes in wavelength composition and intensity within either the chromatic or achromatic condition. In short, activity in the 'V4 complex' did not distinguish between changes in either the intensity or wavelength composition of light illuminating a chromatic or achromatic visual scene. Yet the authors conclude that it is the 'V4 complex' that undertakes the required ratio-taking operations that yield the perceptually unchanging nature of colour in the face of such changes. Another way of expressing the result is that the V4 complex is as much involved in lightness as in colour constancy.

It is not known whether the visual system computes the spectral reflectance profile of surfaces from moment to moment, or when confronted with a change in wavelength composition. Certainly, the former possibility would be computationally costly. Selective attention to colour modulates activity in the colour centre (Corbetta et al. 1991a,b), in both its posterior and anterior divisions (Bartels and Zeki 2000). It is possible that hues are only made explicit when attention demands it.

Conclusion

Complete cerebral achromatopsia, where colour vision is entirely abolished, has been described as the loss of colour constancy mechanisms responsible for the construction of colour. The human 'colour centre' is invariably damaged in achromatopsic observers. Based on the fact that neuronal properties in area V4 of the macaque monkey are consistent with mechanisms of constancy, it has been proposed that the human 'colour centre' is the homologue of simian V4. Yet ablation of area V4 does not delete spectral vision in the monkey, which is a persuasive reason to doubt that the 'colour centre' is 'human V4'. It is uncertain whether colour constancy is disrupted following V4 removal. If it is, then, in the monkey at least, the constancy mechanism cannot be synonymous with the perceptual system since monkeys can still discriminate hue. It would further require an explanation as to why the deficit in achromatopsia extends to a complete loss of the phenomenal experience of colour where equiluminant hues appear indistinguishable. If constancy remains unaffected by V4 damage then it is difficult to sustain the notion that V4 is the 'colour centre'. It is plausible that V4 indeed plays a role in the ratio-taking operations thought to underlie constancy. However, frank achromatopsia may require either direct additional damage to more anterior colour areas, as in the monkey, or destruction of the white matter which connects them. In short, colour constancy and phenomenal colour experience are likely to be dissociable. Varieties of achromatopsia are then the result of different patterns of involvement of a number of areas engaged in spectral processing.

Notwithstanding the loss of colour experience, achromatopsic observers can continue to process wavelength variation in the visual scene to derive information about form and motion. Thus, chromatic information plays a manifold role in vision. It remains to be seen whether other chromatic processes, such as the processing of depth or texture segmentation or attentional capture, can be preserved in cases of cerebral achromatopsia.

References

Akins, K. (2001). More than mere coloring: a dialog between philosophy and neuroscience on the nature of spectral vision. In *Carving our destiny: scientific research faces a new millenium*, (ed. S.M. Fitzpatrick and J.T. Bryer), pp. 77–116. Joseph Henry Press, Washington, DC.

Akins, K. and Hahn, M. (2000). The peculiarity of color. In *Color* (ed. S. Davis), Vancouver Studies in Cognitive Science, Vol. 9, pp. 215–47. New York/Oxford: OUP.

Albert, M.L., Reches, A., and Silverberg, R. (1975). Hemianopic color blindness. *J. Neurol., Neurosurg., Psychiatry* 38, 546–9.

Barbur, J.L., Harlow, A.J., and Plant, G. (1994). Insights into the different exploits of colour in the visual cortex. *Proc. R. Soc. Lond. B* 258 (1353), 327–34.

Bartels, A. and Zeki, S. (2000). The architecture of the colour center in the human visual brain: new results and a review. *Eur. J. Neurosci.* 12, 172–93.

Beauchamp, M.S., Haxby, J.V., Jennings, J.E., and DeYoe, E.A. (1999). An fMRI version of the Farnsworth–Munsell 100-Hue test reveals multiple color-selective areas in human ventral occipitotemporal cortex. *Cereb. Cortex* 9 (3), 257–63.

Beauvois, M.F. and Saillant, B. (1985). Optic aphasia for colors and color agnosia—a distinction between visual and visuo-verbal impairments in the processing of colors. *Cognitive Neuropsychology* 2, 1–48.

Berlin, B. and Kay, P. (1969). *Basic color terms: their universality and evolution*. University of California Press, Berkeley.

Boynton, R.M. (1990). Human color perception. In *Science of color vision* (ed. K.N. Leibovic), pp. 211–53. Springer Verlag, New York.

Brill, N.E. (1882). A case of destructive lesion in the cuncus, accompanied by color blindness. *Am. J. Neurol. Psychiatry* 1, 356–68.

Cavanagh, P., Hénaff, M-A., Michel, F., Landis, T., Troscianko, T., and Intriligator, J. (1998). Complete sparing of high-contrast color input to motion perception in cortical color blindness. *Nat. Neurosci.* 1 (3), 242–7.

Clarke, S., Walsh, V., Schoppig, A., Assal, G., and Cowey, A. (1998). Colour constancy impairments in patients with lesions of the prestriate cortex. *Exp. Brain Res.* 123, 154–8.

Corbetta, M., Miezin, F.M., Shulman, G.L., and Petersen, S.E. (1991a). Selective attention modulates extrastriate visual regions in humans during visual feature discrimination and recognition. In *Exploring brain functional anatomy with positron tomography*, Ciba Foundation Symposium, Vol. 163 (ed. D.J. Chadwick and J. Whelan), pp. 165–80. John Wiley, Chichester.

Corbetta, M., Miezin, F.M., Dobmeyer, S., Shulman, G.L., and Petersen, S.E. (1991b). Selective and divided attention during visual discriminations of shape, color and speed: functional anatomy by positron emission tomography. *J. Neurosci.* 11, 2383–402.

Cowey, A. (1994). Cortical visual areas and the neurobiology of higher visual processes. In *The neuropsychology of high-level vision* (ed. M.J. Farah and G. Ratcliff), pp. 3–31. Lawrence Erlbaum, Hillsdale, New Jersey.

Cowey, A. and Heywood, C.A. (1997). Cerebral achromatopsia: colour blindness despite wavelength processing. *Trends Cogn. Sci.* 1 (4), 133–9.

Cropper, S.J. and Derrington, A.M. (1996). Rapid colour-specific detection of motion in human vision. *Nature* 379, 72–4.

Dacey, D.M. (1993). The mosaic of midget ganglion cells in the human retina. *J. Neurosci.* 13, 5334–55.

Dacey, D.M. (2000). Parallel pathways for spectral coding in primate retina. *Ann. Rev. Neurosci.* 23, 743–75.

Dacey, D.M. and Lee, B.B. (1994). The blue-ON opponent pathway in primate retina originates from a distinct bistratified ganglion cell type. *Nature* 367, 731–5.

Damasio, A., Yamada, T., Damasio, H., Corbett, J., and McKee, J. (1980). Central achromatopsia: behavioral, anatomic, and physiologic aspects. *Neurology* 30, 1064–71.

Davidoff, J.B. and Fodor, G. (1989). An annotated translation of Lewandowsky (1908). *Cogn. Neuropsychol.* 6, 165–77.

Derrington, A.M. (2000). Can colour contribute to motion? *Curr. Biol.* 10, 268–70.

Desimone, R. and Schein, S.J. (1987). Visual properties of neurons in area V4 of macaque: sensitivity to stimulus form. *J. Neurophysiol.* 57, 835–68.

Desimone R., Moran, J., Schein, S.J., and Mishkin, M. (1993). A role for the corpus collosum in visual area V4 of the macaque. *Vis. Neurosci.* 10, 159–71.

Dobkins, K.R. and Albright, T.D. (1994). What happens if it changes color when it moves?: the nature of chromatic input to macaque visual area MT. *J. Neurosci.* 14 (8), 4854–70.

Duvelleroy Hommet, C., Gillet, P., Cottier, J.P., de Toffol, B., Sandeau, D., Corcia, P., and Autret, A. (1997). Achromatopsie cérébrale sans prosopagnosie ni alexie ni agnosie des objets. *Rev. Neurol. Paris* 153, 554–60.

D'Zmura, M., Knoblauch, K., Henaff, M.-A., and Michel, F. (1998). Dependence of color on context in a case of cortical color deficiency. *Vision Res.* 38, 3455–9.

ffytche, D.H., Skidmore, B.D., and Zeki, S. (1995). Motion-from-hue activates area V5 of human visual cortex. *Proc. R. Soc. Lond. B Biol. Sci.* 260 (1359), 353–8.

Fischer, B., Boch, R., and Bach, M. (1981). Stimulus versus eye-movements—comparison of neural activity in the striate and prelunate visual-cortex (a17 and a19) of trained rhesus-monkey. *Exp. Brain Res.* 43, 69–77.

Gegenfurtner, K.R. and Hawken, M.J. (1996). Interaction of motion and color in the visual pathways. *Trends Neurosci.* 19 (9), 394–401.

Gegenfurtner, K.R. and Rieger, J. (2000). Sensory and cognitive contributions to the recognition of natural scenes. *Curr. Biol.* 10, 805–8.

Green, G.J. and Lessell, S. (1977). Acquired cerebral dyschromatopsia. *Arch. Ophthalmol.* 95, 121–8.

Guth, S.L. (1965). Luminance addition: general considerations and some results at foveal threshold. *J. Opt. Soc. Am.* 55, 718–22.

Helmholtz, H.V. (1911). *Handbuch der physiologischen Optik.* Leopold Voss, Hamburg.

Hendry, S.H.C. and Reid, R.C. (2000). The koniocellular pathway in primate vision. *Ann. Rev. Neurosci.* 23, 127–53.

Hendry, S.H.C. and Yoshioka, T. (1994). A neurochemically distinct third channel in the macaque dorsal lateral geniculate nucleus. *Science* 264, 575–7.

Heywood, C.A. and Cowey, A. (1987). On the role of cortical area V4 in the discrimination of hue and pattern in macaque monkeys. *J. Neurosci.* 7 (9), 2601–17.

Heywood, C.A., Cowey, A., and Newcombe, F. (1991). Chromatic discrimination in a cortically colour blind observer. *Eur. J. Neurosci.* 3, 802–12.

Heywood, C.A., Cowey, A., and Newcombe, F. (1994). On the role of parvocellular (P) and magnocellular (M) pathways in cerebral achromatopsia. *Brain* 117, 245–54.

Heywood, C.A., Gadotti, A., and Cowey, A. (1992). Cortical area V4 and its role in the perception of colour. *J. Neurosci.* 12 (10), 4056–65.

Heywood, C.A., Gaffan, D., and Cowey, A. (1995). Cerebral achromatopsia in monkeys. *Eur. J. Neurosci.* 7, 1064–73.

Heywood, C.A., Nicholas, J.J., and Cowey, A. (1996). Behavioural and electrophysiological chromatic and achromatic contrast sensitivity in an achromatopsic patient. *J. Neurol., Neurosurg. Psychiatry* 61, 638–43.

Heywood, C.A., Wilson, B., and Cowey, A. (1987). A case study of cortical colour 'blindness' with relatively intact achromatic discrimination. *J. Neurol., Neurosurg., Psychiatry* 50, 22–9.

Heywood, C.A., Kentridge, R.W., and Cowey, A. (1998). Form and motion from colour in cerebral achromatopsia. *Exp. Brain Res.* 123, 145–53.

Hurlbert, A.C., Bramwell, D.I., Heywood, C.A., and Cowey, A. (1998). Discrimination of cone contrast changes as evidence for colour constancy in cerebral achromatopsia. *Exp. Brain Res.* 123, 136–44.

Kastner, S., DeWeerd, P., Desimone, R., and Ungerleider, L.C. (1988). Mechanisms of directed attention in the human extrastriate cortex revealed by functional MRI. *Science* 282, 108–11.

Kennard, C., Lawden, M., Morland, A.B., and Ruddock, K.H. (1995). Colour identification and colour constancy are impaired in a patient with incomplete achromatopsia associated with a prestriate cortical lesions. *Proc. R. Soc. Lond. B* 260 (1358), 169–75.

Kinsbourne, M. and Warrington, E.K. (1964). Observations on colour agnosia. *J. Neurol., Neurosurg. Psychiatry* 27 296–9.

Kleinschmidt, A., Lee, B.B., Requardt, M., and Frahm, J. (1996). Functional mapping of color processing by magnetic resonance imaging of responses to selective P- and M-pathway stimulation. *Exp. Brain Res.* 110, 279–88.

Kölmel, H.W. (1988). Pure homonymous hemiachromatopsia: findings with neuro-ophthalmologic examination and imaging procedures. *Eur. Arch. Psychiat. Neurol. Sci.* 237, 237–42.

Lewandowsky, M. (1908a). Abspaltung des Farbensinnes durch Herderkrankung des Gehirns. In *Compte Rendu des Travaux du 1er Congrès International de Psychiatrie, de Neurologie, de Psychologie et de l'Assistance des aliénés* (ed. G.A.M. van Weyenberg), 402–7. J.H. de Bussy, Amsterdam.

Lewandowsky, M. (1908b). Ueber Abspaltung des Farbensinnes. *Monatsschr. Psychiatrie Neurol.* 23, 488–510.

Livingstone, M.S. and Hubel, D.H. (1987a). Segregation of form, color and stereopsis in primate area 18. *J. Neurosci.* 7 (11), 3378–415.

Livingstone, M.S. and Hubel, D.H. (1987b). Psychophysical evidence for separate channels for the perception of form, color, movement and depth. *J. Neurosci.* 7 (11), 3416–68.

Luzzatti, C. and Davidoff, J. (1994). Impaired retrieval of object-colour knowledge with preserved colour naming. *Neuropsychologia* 32, 933–50.

Mackay, G. and Dunlop, J.C. (1899). The cerebral lesions in a case of complete acquired colour-blindness. *Scot. Med. Surg. J.* 5, 513–17.

Meadows, J.C. (1974). Disturbed perception of colours associated with localized cerebral lesions. *Brain* 97, 615–32.

Milner, A.D. and Goodale, M.A. (1995). *The visual brain in action.* Oxford University Press, Oxford.

Mollon, J.D. (1989). 'Tho' she kneel'd in that place where they grew . . . ': the uses and origins of primate colour vision. *J. Exp. Biol.* 146, 21–38.

Mollon, J.D., Newcombe, F., Polden, P.G., and Ratcliffe, G. (1980). On the presence of three cone mechanisms in a case of total achromatopsia. In *Colour vision deficiencies* (ed. G. Verriest) vol V, pp. 130–5. Hilger, Bristol.

Oxbury, J.M., Oxbury, S.M., and Humphrey, N.K. (1969). Varieties of colour anomia. *Brain* 92, 847–60.

Pearlman, A.L., Birch, J., and Meadows, J.C. (1979). Cerebral color blindness: an acquired defect in hue discrimination. *Ann. Neurol.* 5, 253–61.

Rizzo, M., Smith, V., Pokorny, J., and Damasio, A.R. (1993). Color perception profiles in central achromatopsia. *Neurology* 43, 995–1001.

Rüttiger, L., Braun, D.I., Gegenfurtner, K.R., Petersen, D., Schönle, P., and Sharpe, L.T. (1999). Selective color constancy deficits after circumscribed unilateral brain lesions. *J. Neurosci.* 19 (8), 3094–106.

Sacks, O., Wasserman, R.L., Zeki, S., and Siegel, R.M. (1988). Sudden color-blindness of cerebral origin. *Soc. Neurosci. Abstracts* 14, 1251.

Saito, H., Tanaka, K., Isono, H., Yasuda, M., and Mikami, A. (1989). Directionally selective response of cells in the middle temporal area (MT) of the macaque monkey to the movement of equiluminous opponent color stimuli. *Exp. Brain Res.* 75, 1–14.

Sakai, K., Watanabe, E., Onodera, Y., Uchida, I., Kato, H., Yamamoto, E., Koizumi, H., and Miyashita, Y. (1995). Functional mapping of the human colour centre with echo-planar magnetic resonance imaging. *Proc. R. Soc. Lond., Biol.* 261, 89–98.

Schein, S.J. and Desimone, R. (1990). Spectral properties of V4 neurons in the macaque. *J. Neurosci.* 10, 3369–89.

Schein, S.J., Marrocco, R.T., and De Monasterio, F.M. (1982). Is there a high concentration of colour-selective cells in area V4 of monkey visual cortex? *J. Neurophysiol.* 47, 193–213.

Schiller, P.H. and Lee, K. (1991). The role of the primate extrastriate area V4 in vision. *Science* 251, 1251–3.

Schiller, P.H., Logothetis, N.K., and Charles, E.R. (1990). Functions of the colour-opponent and broad-band channels of the visual system. *Nature* 343, 16–17.

Shuren, J.E., Brott, T.G., Scheft, B.K., and Houston, W. (1996). Preserved color imagery in an achromatopsic. *Neuropsychologia* 34, 485–9.

Sittig, O. (1921). Stoerungen im Verhalten gegenueber Farben bei Aphasischen. *Monatsschr. Psychiatrie Neurol.* 49, 63–8, 169–87.

Sperling, H.G. and Harwerth, R.S. (1971). Red–green cone interactions in the increment-threshold spectral sensitivity of primates. *Science* 172, 180–4.

Stiles, W.S. (1978). *Mechanisms of colour vision.* Academic Press, London.

Tootell, R.B.H. and Hadjikhani, N. (1998). Reply to 'Has a new color area been discovered'. *Nat. Neurosci.* 1 (5), 335–6.

Turnbull, H.W. (1961). *The correspondence of Isaac Newton* Volume I, 1688–94. Cambridge University Press, Cambridge.

Van Essen, D.C. and Zeki, S.M. (1978). The topographic organization of rhesus monkey prestriate cortex. *J. Physiol., Lond.* 277, 193–226.

Van Essen, D.C., Maunsell, J.H., and Bixby, J.L. (1981). The middle temporal visual area in the macaque—myeloarchitecture, connections, functional-properties and topographic organization. *J. Comp. Neurol.* 199, 293–326.

Verrey, L. (1888). Hemiachromatopsie droite absolue. *Archs. Ophtalmol. (Paris)* 8, 289–301.

Victor, J.D., Maiese, K., Shapley, R., Sidtis, J., and Gazzaniga, M.S. (1989). Acquired central dyschromatopsia: analysis of a case with preservation of color discrimination. *Clin. Vision Sci.* 4, 183–96.

Wachtler, T., Sejnowski, T.J., and Albright, T.D. (1999). Responses of cells in macaque V1 to chromatic stimuli are compatible with human color constancy. *Soc. Neurosci. Abstr.* **25**, 4.

Walsh, V., Butler, S.R., Carden, D., and Kulikowski, J.J. (1993). The effects of V4 lesions on the visual behaviour of macaques: Hue discrimination and colour constancy. *Behav. Brain Res.* **53**, 51–62.

Wilbrand, H. (1884). *Ophthalmiatrische Beiträge zur Diagnostik Gehirnkrankheiten.* J.F. Bergmann, Wiesbaden.

Wild, H.M., Butler, S.R., Carden, D., and Kulikowski, J.J. (1985). Primate cortical area V4 important for colour constancy but not wavelength discrimination. *Nature* **313**, 133.

Williams, L.G. (1966). The effect of target specification on objects fixated during visual search. *Percept. Psychophys.* **1**, 315–18.

Zeki, S. (1990*a*). A century of cerebral achromatopsia. *Brain* **113**, 1721–77.

Zeki, S. (1990*b*). *Colour vision and functional specialisation in the visual cortex,* Discussions in Neuroscience, IV(2). Elsevier, Amsterdam.

Zeki, S. (1993). *A vision of the brain.* Blackwell Scientific Publications, Oxford.

Zeki, S. and Bartels, A. (1999*a*). The clinical and functional measurement of cortical (in-) activity in the visual brain, with special reference to the ywo subdivisions (V4 and V4α) of the human colour centre. *Phil. Trans. R. Soc. Lond. B* **354**, 1371–82.

Zeki, S. and Bartels, A. (1999*b*). Towards a theory of visual consciousness. *Consciousness Cogn.* **8**, 225–59.

Zeki, S. and Marini, L. (1998). Three cortical stages of colour processing in the human brain. *Brain* **121**, 1669–85.

Zeki, S. and Shipp, S. (1988). The functional logic of cortical connections. *Nature* **335**, 311–17.

Zeki, S., Watson, J.D.G., Lueck, C.J., Friston, K.J., Kennard, C., and Frackowiak, R.S.J. (1991). A direct demonstration of functional specialization in human visual cortex. *J. Neurosci.* **11**, 641–9.

Zeki, S., Aglioti, S., McKeefry, D., and Berlucchi, G. (1999). The neurological basis of conscious color perception in a blind patient. *Proc. Natl. Acad. Sci., USA* **96**, 14124–9.

Zeki, S.M. (1973). Colour coding in rhesus monkey prestriate cortex. *Brain Res.* **53**, 422–7.

Zeki, S.M. (1977). Colour coding in the superior temporal sulcus of rhesus monkey visual cortex. *Proc. R. Soc. Lond. B* **197**, 195–223.

Zeki, S.M. (1978). Uniformity and diversity of structure and function in rhesus monkey prestriate visual cortex. *J. Physiol. (Lond.)* **277**, 273–90.

Zeki, S.M. (1983). Colour coding in the cerebral cortex: the reaction of cells in monkey visual cortex to wavelengths and colours. *Neuroscience* **9** (4), 741–65.

Chapter 9

Unconscious perception: blindsight

L. Weiskrantz

Introduction

The definition of 'blindsight' can now be obtained directly from the *Concise Oxford dictionary* (and other dictionaries): 'Medicine: a condition in which the sufferer responds to visual stimuli without consciously perceiving them'. It is associated with damage to V1, primary visual cortex. The historical background to the origin of the oxymoron stems originally from animal work, because it has been known for some decades that monkeys with V1 removal can nevertheless carry out particular visual discriminations with moderate success. *Prima facie*, this is not surprising because V1 is not the only target in the brain for signals originating in the retina, although it is the major one. There are several other pathways from the retina to subcortical targets that remain intact after damage to V1, the largest one being the superior colliculus, from which information can reach a very wide distribution of other cerebral areas, both cortical and subcortical (Cowey and Stoerig 1991; Benevento and Yoshida 1981; Herandez-Gonzales and Reinoso-Suarez 1994; Fries 1981; Yukie and Iwai 1981). In man, in seeming contrast to the animal findings, subjects with V1 damage are said to be densely 'blind' in the corresponding part of the affected visual fields, the field defect having a size and shape to be expected from the classical retinocortical maps (Holmes 1918). And so the question arises: can these disparate patterns of results be reconciled, or are humans and monkeys qualitatively different in this respect despite the similarity of their visual anatomy?

There are some serious difficulties that stand in the way of an answer. The first is topological: the striate cortex of the human is mainly buried in the medial surface in the calcarine fissure, whereas in the monkey the macular projection is on the lateral surface and readily accessible. Therefore, in the human brain, it is rare for any lesion of the striate cortex to occur without damage to overlying tissue, including visual association cortex, whereas it is relatively easy for lesions restricted to striate cortex to be studied in experimental animals. The difference is important for two reasons. First, the effect of enlarging a striate cortex lesion in the monkey so as to include posterior association cortex is reported to lead to a significant reduction in residual visual capacity (Pasik and Pasik 1971). Secondly, it is becoming clear that these closely adjoining more anterior cortical regions are functionally segregated and may have partially specialized capacities of a modular type, e.g. colour, movement, spatial features, form, etc.

(cf. Cowey 1985; Zeki 1978, 1993). As at least some of these regions are likely to be damaged in the human whenever striate cortex is also damaged, the pattern of deficits can differ considerably from patient to patient with relatively slight differences in the disposition of the lesions. This means that comparisons between experimental striate lesions in monkey and clinically occurring lesions in the human are not typically comparisons of like with like and, moreover, there are inherent, but structurally sound, sources of variance in the clinical material. A further difference is that lesions to striate cortex in a clinical population will have variable histories of onset and subsequent course, or may even have been present prenatally. The classical animal studies were based largely on adolescent or mature animals with lesions that had an abrupt onset rather than a developmental history.

A second serious difficulty is methodological. Residual vision in the animal is, of course, studied by behavioural methods, typically by making reward contingent upon a particular response choice between alternative stimuli. For systematic studies of particular dimensions of discrimination, or even of detection *per se*, a long history of prior training and large series of trials are usually necessary. In contrast, human visual assessment is rarely carried out in such a fashion in the clinic. Instead, patients in clinical examination are asked to respond to a verbal instruction to report whether and what they 'see'.

But when patients with field defects caused by occipital lesions are studied psychophysically with 'animal-type' forced-choice methodology—requiring them to make differential responses to the stimuli whether or not they verbally acknowledge 'seeing' them—unsuspected visual capacities may be uncovered that do not necessarily correlate with the patients' reported experiences and that are often radically and surprisingly different. Good discriminative capacity was demonstrated some years ago in well-studied patients despite their claiming to have no visual experience whatever in their blind fields (Pöppel *et al.* 1973; Weiskrantz *et al.* 1974; cf. an early report by Bard 1905), giving rise to the term 'blindsight'—visual discrimination in the absence of acknowledged awareness (Sanders *et al.* 1974; Weiskrantz.*et al.* 1974; Weiskrantz 1986). The history and some of the related background issues are also discussed more fully elsewhere (Weiskrantz 1972, 1980, 1986, 1998, 2001; Stoerig and Cowey 1997; Cowey and Stoerig 1991, 1992). 'Blindsight' originally applied only to human subjects, deriving from the contrast between human and animal results, but, as will be seen, the concept can now be applied both to humans and monkeys.

Categories of residual visual capacities

The evidence regarding blindsight capacities is necessarily based on a relatively small number of intensively studied subjects (the two most exhaustively studied being D.B. and G.Y.), as is often the case in neuropsychology, especially as lengthy testing psychophysical sessions are required. Taking the evidence collectively, not all necessarily found in all subjects, the findings are as follows.

Localizing

Several subjects investigated by a number of investigators have demonstrated a capacity to localize stimuli within their 'blind' fields, either by making a saccade to the supposed locus of the stimulus, typically a briefly flashed spot (Pöppel *et al.* 1973), or by pointing or touching the locus of a target on a perimeter screen (Weiskrantz *et al.* 1974). In yet another study, G.Y. was trained to give a numerical score on a ruled scale to successfully describe the locus (Barbur *et al.* 1980). The accuracy is typically not as high as in the intact visual field, but nevertheless can be very impressive. Successful detection is obviously a necessary prerequisite for localization, but detection has also been studied independently of localizing (Barbur *et al.* 1980; Stoerig 1987; Stoerig *et al.* 1985; Stoerig and Pöppel 1986; Weiskrantz 1986; Azzopardi and Cowey 1997).

Acuity

There is not much systematic evidence, but D.B.'s acuity has been measured with Moirè fringe interference gratings (approximating to sine-wave gratings). The reduction in acuity for the region 16–20° eccentric is about 2 octaves as compared to the mirror-symmetric region of the intact field (2.5 cycles/° compared with 10 cycles/°; Weiskrantz 1986). G.Y.'s acuity has not been measured directly, but the contrast sensitivity function in his scotoma (using a grating of 12° × 12°, with its centre 9° from the fixation point) falls to zero at approximately 7 cycles/°, which also is approximately a drop of about 2 octaves compared to his intact field with this stimulus situation (Barbur *et al.* 1994*a*; Weiskrantz *et al.* 1998).

Orientation

D.B. is unusual in repeatedly demonstrating a good discriminative capacity for orientation in the frontal plane. Although impaired relative to his good field, he could nevertheless discriminate a difference in orientation of 10° between two gratings presented successively and briefly, even at an eccentricity of 45° in the impaired field, with no acknowledged experience of the gratings or even of a flash. Most other subjects who have been tested have shown rather less residual capacity for orientation (e.g. Barbur *et al.* 1980). G.Y. does not show orientation discrimination using gratings, but positive evidence has been obtained using single lines (Morland *et al.* 1996).

Colour

Initial evidence for wavelength discrimination in D.B. was at best marginal and slim, although he was not studied extensively (Weiskrantz *et al.* 1974, but recent unpublished evidence reveals substantial colour discrimination in him). The situation has been advanced considerably in more recent studies. Stoerig and Cowey (1989, 1991, 1992; Cowey and Stoerig 1999) measured the spectral sensitivity functions of the blind fields of a number of hemianopes and found them to be qualitatively normal, although with quantitatively reduced sensitivity. The spectral sensitivity profiles include the humps and troughs thought to reflect colour opponency. They also show the characteristic loss of long wavelength sensitivity following dark adaptation, the 'Purkinje shift'. Moreover, wavelength *discrimination*, e.g. red versus green, but even of more closely spaced wavelengths, is possible in some subjects (Stoerig and Cowey 1992), using forced-choice guessing. Barbur *et al.* (1994*b*) demonstrated good discrimination between 'coloured' patches and achromatic patches matched in luminance, using a two-alternative forced-choice paradigm in G.Y. Ruddock and his colleagues (Brent *et al.* 1994) have also found good discrimination between red and achromatic stimuli in G.Y. In this connection it would appear that the discriminative sensitivity of the blind field is biased towards the red end of the spectrum. Using pupillometry (see below) a strong inference can be made that *successive colour contrast* is intact in G.Y. and another hemianopic blindsight subject (Barbur *et al.* 1999, and recently confirmed in unpublished data with D.B. by Barbur and Weiskrantz).

It should be stressed that in all of these studies, the subjects *never* reported any experience of colour *per se*. Here is Stoerig and Cowey's comment about the subjects' commentaries in their spectral sensitivity study, which involved repeated measures of thresholds of chosen wavelengths, revealing qualitatively normal sensitivity functions:

> ... the patients were often asked whether they could perceive anything when the blind field was tested. Throughout the experiments, which involved from 2 to 4 three-hour sessions per month for approximately six months, they consistently claimed that this was not the case and that they never saw or felt anything that was related to stimulus presentation (1991, p. 1496).

Movement and transient stimuli

There are a number of reports of detection of moving stimuli by subjects in their impaired fields (Brindley *et al.* 1969; Barbur *et al.* 1980; Perenin 1978). The subject has long antecedents given the classical evidence of Riddoch (1917) and Poppelreuter (1917) who described gunshot-wound cases who reported seeing moving but not stationary stimuli. D.B. showed a good ability to detect moving targets, although with a reduced sensitivity depending on the location in the blind field (Weiskrantz 1986). A number of parametric psychophysical studies of *directional* discrimination of moving spots or bars have been carried out by Barbur and his colleagues on G.Y. (Barbur *et al.* 1993; Sahraie *et al.* 1997, 1998; Weiskrantz *et al.* 1995), measuring the limits of velocity and contrast for successful directional discrimination in the blind field. A clear capacity remains but with reduced sensitivity. It was some of these studies that led to the experimental exploration of the distinction between 'awareness' and 'unawareness' modes, and also to brain imaging (see below).

While there is no doubt that blindsight subjects can detect moving bars or spots and discriminate their direction of movement, other modes of movement discrimination, viz. the discrimination of direction of movement of random dot kineograms and plaids has been found lacking, at least in G.Y. (Azzopardi *et al.* 1998; Cowey and Azzopardi in press).

Movement is, of course, one form of a transient stimulus. But it has been clear for some time that the transients exemplified by sharp temporal onset/offset of stationary stimuli are also of particular significance in the blind field. Weiskrantz *et al.* (1991) carried out a systematic study in G.Y. by varying the temporal slope of the Gaussian envelope of the onset and offset of stimuli in a two-alternative forced-choice paradigm for gratings versus homogeneous patches (of equal luminance). Performance improved as the temporal slope increased. In a related study, the manipulation of spatial as well as temporal transients also allowed a specification to be made of both the spatial and the temporal parameters required for good detection. This made it clear that, in G.Y., his blind field possesses a narrowly tuned spatiotemporal visual 'channel', with a peak of about 1 cycle/° and a cut-off ('acuity') of about 7 cycles/° (Barbur *et al.* 1994a). Subsequently, this has been linked to a closely similar channel in monkeys revealed by pupillometry (see below).

A somewhat different approach had been used in an early study of D.B. in which the temporal rate of onset was varied systematically over a wide range in a forced-choice discrimination between a circular, homogeneous luminous disc versus no stimulus. Although the sharper the rate of onset the better the performance, D.B. still performed reliably well above chance, and without acknowledged awareness, even with extremely slow rates of onset (Weiskrantz 1986, chapter 9). Hence, a rapid temporal transient is not a necessary feature for good detection. It also indicates that this mode of blindsight is quite different from the early reports by Riddoch (1917) of conscious reports of vigorous movement in the blind field. A similar point emerges from a pupillometric analysis (see below).

'Form'

Most early reports of evidence for form discrimination have been negative, or weak (cf. Weiskrantz 1986). The situation may be different, however, if the subject is asked to reach for and grasp solid objects in his or her blind field. Both Marcel (1998) and Perenin and Rossetti (1996) have reported that the subject's hand adopts the appropriate arrangement for a shape in advance of grasping it when reaching for an object in the blind field. Such a result would be nicely in accord with the thesis forwarded by Milner and Goodale (1995) that the shape and orientation of objects can be involved in directed visual actions towards the objects even when subjects are unable to perceive the objects correctly.

On the other hand, Milner and Goodale's distinction (between the 'action' mode and the 'perception' mode—linked by them to separate mediation by the dorsal and ventral visual streams) would not easily account for the striking claim by Marcel (1998) that words flashed into the blind field can influence the interpretation of meanings of words subsequently shown in the intact field. He reports, for example, that the word 'money' flashed into the blind field will bias the reported meaning of the ambiguous word 'bank' subsequently shown in the intact field—i.e. bank can either be related to 'money' or to 'river'. This intriguing report is isolated and deserves to be followed up. It would require a considerable expansion of the known capacity for residual processing of stationary shapes in the blind field.

Emotional content

There are claims that conditioned aversive properties of stimuli in normal human subjects can give rise to autonomic responses, even when the subjects have no awareness of them (Øhman and Soares 1998; Esteves *et al.* 1994). Moreover, functional imaging experiments have demonstrated that conditioned fear stimuli rendered invisible by backward masking can nevertheless activate the amygdala via a colliculopulvinar pathway (Morris *et al.* 1999, 2001; Breiter *et al.* 1996). This may or may not lead to an observable behavioural reaction. When a fear-evoking stimulus, such as a strange doll, is presented to the blind hemifield of a monkey with unilateral V1 removal, the animal appears to ignore it completely although it emits loud shrieks of fear and outrage when it is confronted in the normal visual field. Nor does the monkey react, for example, to a highly prized banana in the blind field (Cowey 1967; Cowey and Weiskrantz 1963). On the other hand, no concurrent measures of autonomic activity have been made, and it is possible that emotion-provoking stimuli would produce responses in the absence of overt behavioural responses, just as, for example, galvanic skin responses can be recorded to familiar faces in prosopagnosic patients who in perceptual tests cannot distinguish familiar from unfamiliar faces (Tranel and Damasio 1985).

A recent study of faces with emotional expression projected to G.Y.'s blind field has some direct bearing on this surmise (de Gelder *et al.* 1999). He has been shown to be able to discriminate between different facial expressions in moving video images projected into his blind field, e.g. happy versus sad and angry versus fearful, and he could also identify which of four different expressions were presented on any single exposure. He failed to 'see' the faces as such, and he was also at chance with inverted faces. It remains unknown so far whether his autonomic system would also be sensitive to those emotional stimuli that he can discriminate in the absence of 'seeing'. A recent functional magnetic resonance imaging (fMRI) study using a conditioned-fear paradigm in G.Y. demonstrated that the amygdala is activated by the conditioned stimulus presented to the blind field, and that the amygdala activity correlates with activity levels in the superior colliculus and pulvinar. Thus, a route that bypasses V1 remains intact for activation by events provoking emotion.

Attention in the blind field

It has been demonstrated with G.Y. that attention can confer an advantage in processing stimuli in the blind field either within an attended time interval or at an attended spatial location. A visual cue that provides information about the time window within which the targets will appear in the blind field improves G.Y.'s discrimination of their location (Kentridge *et al.* 1999*a*). Cues in the blind field that provide information about the likely spatial location of a target confer an advantage, strikingly in the complete absence of reported awareness of either the cue or the target. Such cues in his blind field were effective even in directing his attention to a second location remote from that at which the cue was presented, again under conditions when there was no reported awareness of the cue or the target (Kentridge *et al.* 1999*b*). The evidence leads to the conclusion that spatial selection by attention, on the one hand, and conscious awareness of attentional control, on the other, cannot be one and the same process.

Verbal versus non-verbal approaches

Awareness versus unawareness

In most studies, with the exception of those of D.B., details of verbal reports were not garnered. But, in D.B., transient stimuli, e.g. of movement, looming, and recession or abrupt onset and offset, gave rise to a report of 'awareness', a 'feeling' or 'knowing' that an event has occurred. In D.B. these experiences were apt to mislead him as to the identity of the event, and so such transients were avoided by varying contrast and other conditions (see Weiskrantz 1986, chapter 13), and hence most of the studies involved visual discriminations in the absence of any awareness. A similar distinction between performance with and without awareness emerged in studies with G.Y. and other subjects, and has been named as a distinction between blindsight type 1 (no awareness) and type 2 (with awareness but not perceptual 'seeing') (Weiskrantz 1998, 1999).

As performance without awareness can be matched with that with awareness, a unique opportunity arises to study brain activity associated with matched performances of the subject when there is or is not conscious awareness of the discriminative stimuli. But to do so it is necessary and important to have an indication of the subject's reported awareness, and thus a 'commentary key' paradigm has been used. In addition to the usual pair of response keys for discriminating the stimulus events, two other 'commentary keys' were introduced with which the subject could signal awareness or no awareness after each trial (Weiskrantz *et al.* 1995). The application of the paradigm with discrimination of movement direction is shown in Figs 9.1 and 9.2, varying velocity or contrast in a way that affects incidence of awareness reports, and the corresponding discriminative performance. It can be seen that performance can remain high and relatively independent of awareness levels as such. The relationship between commentaries and confidence reports as well as the use of multivalues versus binary scales (Sahraie *et al.* 1998) has also been examined in a further extension. The paradigm was applied in an imaging study of the two blindsight modes (Sahraie *et al.* 1997; see below).

Non-verbal, indirect methods of revealing residual visual function

Parametric psychophysics, carried out by forced-choice guessing or reaching, requires multiple and lengthy sessions, often totalling thousands of trials. Aside from that,

Fig. 9.1 Directional movement discrimination performance for a moving spot presented to G.Y.'s 'blind' hemifield, as a function of stimulus speed. The subject had to discriminate (by guessing, if necessary) whether the stimulus moved horizontally or vertically. He also had to indicate whether he had any experience whatever of the stimulus event. 'Awareness' refers to the percentage of trials on which he pressed the 'yes, had experience' key. 'Correct when unaware' refers to performance during those trials when he pressed the 'no, I had no experience at all' key. Performance was high even without reported awareness. (From Weiskrantz *et al.* 1995, with permission. Copyright National Academy of Sciences, USA.)

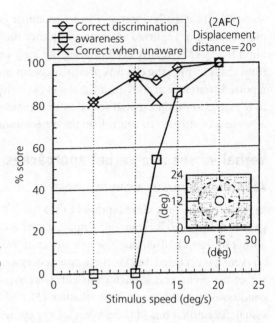

Fig. 9.2 Conditions as in Fig.9.1 but with stimulus contrast varied instead of speed. The luminance of the test spot was constant, at 131 cd/m², and background luminance changed systematically. Awareness declined steeply as background luminance increased, but performance remained relatively stable. (From Weiskrantz *et al.* 1995, with permission. Copyright National Academy of Sciences, USA.)

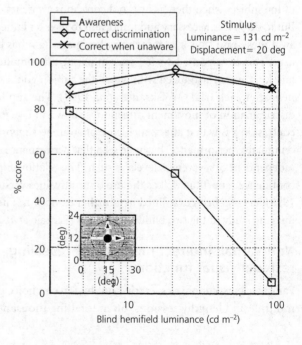

particular problems arise in terms of the subject's confidence in making counterintuitive judgements about stimuli he or she cannot 'see', or in the commentaries that accompany their choices. In other areas of cognitive neuropsychology, residual function can be tested quite readily by methods that do not directly assault credibility. For example, the amnesic patient can be asked to try to identify a word when presented with its first three letters, to enable the experimenter to infer that an earlier 'prime' by the word has facilitated its identification, without requiring the subject to 'remember' as such.

There are two general approaches to indirect methods of testing for residual visual function that allow an inference without requiring the subject to guess 'without seeing': (1) reflexes to visual stimuli in the blind hemifield; (2) interactions between the intact and impaired hemifields. The field has been surveyed by Weiskrantz (1990) and Stoerig and Cowey (1997).

Reflexes

Electrodermal responses to visual stimuli in the blind field (as compared with control 'blanks') were used by Zihl *et al.* (1980) to demonstrate a positive response to light, but they are difficult to relate in a directly quantitative way to the visual events. Pupillometry, in contrast, provides a direct and incisive quantitative measure, given that the pupil constricts differentially in response to visual stimuli depending on their spatial frequency, wavelength, and movement, when there is no change in the total luminance of the stimuli (Barbur and Forsyth 1986; Barbur and Thomson 1987). In this way, the pupil can be used to measure the profile of sensitivity to gratings in the blind field as a function of spatial frequency, and also to obtain the visual acuity, and these have been validated by psychophysical comparisons of the same values. Sensitivity to colour and movement can also be measured. Given that pupillometry does not depend on the subject's verbal report, it can be used to assess the blind fields of human patients, of animals, and also of human infants (cf. Cocker *et al.* 1994).

The method has been used (Weiskrantz *et al.* 1998) to examine the spatial frequency profiles of the affected hemifields of G.Y. and also of two monkeys with unilateral removal of striate cortex (V1), using the P_Scan apparatus (Barbur *et al.* 1987). The results are very clear (Fig. 9.3). In both the human and the monkeys there is a narrowly tuned response of the pupil to different spatial frequencies of an achromatic grating, with a peak at approximately 1 cycle/°. The acuity (the point at which the response falls to zero as spatial frequency increases) is at about 7 cycles/°, which is a reduction of about 2 octaves compared with the intact hemifields under these conditions. G.Y.'s pupillary response could be validated by psychophysical methods because a spatial temporal tuning curve was obtained in an earlier study (Barbur *et al.* 1994a). The psychophysical function and the pupillary profile map on to each other quite closely (see Fig. 9.3), and confirm the potential usefulness of pupillometry as a clinical screening device. Recently, it has been possible to make the same comparison for D.B. (Weiskrantz and Cowey, unpublished), with a similar close agreement between psychophysical and pupillometric determinations (Fig. 9.4).

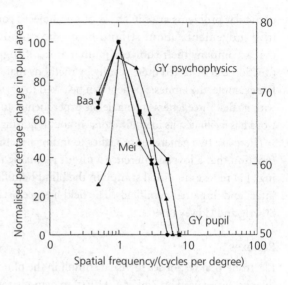

Fig. 9.3 Relative normalized size (peak at 100) of pupil constriction (solid lines) as a function of spatial frequency of an equiluminant grating presented to the 'blind' hemifields of a human subject (G.Y.) and two monkeys ('Baa' and 'Mei'). Also shown is the psychophysical performance for G.Y. from an earlier study (Barbur *et al.* 1994*a*) for gratings versus equiluminant featureless stimulus. (From Weiskrantz *et al.* 1998, with permission. Copyright Oxford University Press.)

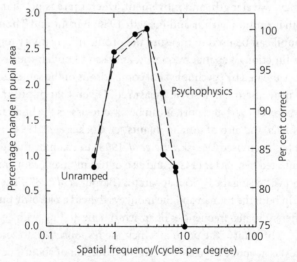

Fig. 9.4 Change in pupillary area (solid line) for subject D.B. as a function of spatial frequency, and percentage correct discrimination performance for gratings versus equiluminant featureless stimulus, with forced-choice guessing (dashed line). Subject's commentaries for each of the spatial frequencies tested are as follows (percentage correct in brackets). 0.5 cycles/°, 'All guess work' (84%); 1 cycle/°, 'Not aware of anything at all, guessed all the time' (96%); 3 cycles/°, 'All guess work' (100%); 5 cycles/°, 'All guesswork, nothing there' (92%); 7.5 cycles/°, 'All guess work, did not do very well 50/50' (82%). (From Weiskrantz and Cowey, unpublished.)

The occurrence of the pupillary response does not depend on the subject's having blindsight type 2—the pupil still constricts to a 1 cycle/° isoluminant grating even when the onset and offset of the grating are smoothed so as to eliminate G.Y.'s reported awareness of the event, although its size is reduced under some, but not all, conditions (Weiskrantz *et al.* 1999). The fact that pupillometric acuity changes with V1 removal means that there must be a direct downstream influence of cortex reaching the midbrain mechanism that provides the final efferent to the pupillary musculature. The strikingly close similarity of the monkey and human results is another piece of evidence that we are dealing with similar mechanisms involved in V1 removal in both species, and also speaks against the view that, in residual function, the human must depend upon fragments of intact visual cortex, given that there are demonstrably no such fragments in the monkey.

Interactions between intact and blind hemifields

Torjussen's studies (1976, 1978) provide the seminal example that demonstrates 'completion' of shapes shown to both the blind and intact hemifields simultaneously. The subject reports seeing nothing when a stimulus is presented to the blind field, but sees a normally completed stimulus that bridges both the intact and the impaired field. More recently, the method has been used by Marcel in two hemianopes, one of whom was G.Y. (Marcel 1998), and also by Perenin *et al.* (1985). This technique is also used in tests with hemispherectomized subjects.

A related approach is that designed by Marzi and his colleagues (Corbetta *et al.* 1990), in which the reaction time of a key-press response to a light in the intact field could be lengthened by a light presented just earlier in the impaired field of human subjects. A similar finding has been reported for the monkey—an unseen target slows the reaction time to the seen target, especially at delays of the order of 400–500 ms (Stoerig and Cowey 1997). In another approach, Marzi *et al.* (1986) exploited the fact that the reaction time to two flashes presented simultaneously is consistently faster than the reaction time to a single flash, whether the two flashes appear in the same hemifield or in opposite fields. The reaction time of hemianopes can be speeded up when the two flashes are presented across the vertical meridian, even though the subject only reports seeing a single stimulus, i.e. the one in the intact hemifield. Recently, the same approach was used by Tomaiuolo *et al.* (1997) to demonstrate visual spatial summation in hemispherectomized subjects.

Another striking example of cross-hemifield interaction in G.Y. was reported by Ruddock and his co-workers (Finlay *et al.* 1997), who found that particular values of moving visual stimuli in the *intact* hemifield actually produce an experience of phenomenal 'seeing' of motion in G.Y.'s *blind* hemifield. This obviously opens up fresh possibilities of exploration in other hemianopes. The phenomenon may be related to cross-field activations found in brain imaging of G.Y. (see above).

Morland *et al.* (1999) studied G.Y.'s ability to match the values of stimuli between the intact and blind hemifields, with variations in luminance, movement, or colour. They found that between-field matches could be made for movement or colour, but not for luminance, although commentaries as such were not recorded, and interpret the findings in terms of the distinction between blindsight types 1 and 2 (see above). This was not a study of between-field interactive effects as such, which might well have been present, but is an interesting use of the good field as an 'assay' of the impaired field.

Functional brain imaging

G.Y. has been the subject both of positron emission tomography (PET) and fMRI investigations. Barbur *et al.* (1993) studied the difference between moving and stationary bars with PET. The results focused on the activation found in area V5 in association with moving stimuli. In this situation G.Y. was typically aware of the movement, i.e. it was blindsight type 2. Indeed, the authors drew the conclusion that there can be conscious awareness of movement in the absence of V1. Blindsight type 1 was not investigated.

The distinction between directional movement discrimination *with and without awareness* (e.g. type 2 versus type 1) was the explicit focus of a subsequent fMRI study of G.Y. (Sahraie *et al.* 1997). The parameters that had previously been used to establish this difference psychophysically (Weiskrantz *et al.* 1995; see above) served as the basis of the stimuli in the imaging study, using stimulus contrast and velocity as the variables. There was an association between the 'awareness' mode and activity in dorsolateral prefrontal activity (areas 46 and 47 (see Fig. 7.5)), both when the subject was 'aware without seeing' in the blind hemifield, as well as when he was 'aware with seeing' in the intact hemifield. In the 'unaware' mode but associated with good discrimination, and only in this mode, there was activation in the superior colliculus. Activations of particular structures were found that were uniquely associated with 'awareness' and 'unawareness' modes, respectively, but the main conclusion of the paper stressed the change in general pattern between the two modes—from dorsolateral structures in the former, to medial and subcortical structures in the latter.

Coloured stimuli, specifically red and green, were the subject of another fMRI study of G.Y.'s blind hemifield. It had previously been established that there was a response both psychophysically as well as by pupillometry in G.Y. to red but not to green colours, with variable background luminance as a control, demonstrating that the response to red was genuinely chromatic (although it must be stressed, again, that the subject did not report any experience of colour, as such). Here, too, there was an activation of the superior colliculus when the red, but not the green stimulus, was presented to the blind hemifield. No such midbrain activation was found in the sighted hemifield (Barbur *et al.* 1998).

Animal homologues

The origin of blindsight, as mentioned, stemmed from the longstanding evidence that infrahuman primates could still make visual discriminations in the absence of striate cortex, while humans with such damage describe themselves as being blind to experience in the relevant parts of the visual fields. While the quantitative effects of visual cortex damage in monkeys and human 'blindsight' subjects are similar in many respects, an important and much deeper qualitative question remains: does the monkey without striate cortex, who can localize and discriminate visual stimuli so impressively, actually have visual *experience* of those stimuli that it can localize and discriminate so impressively in its affected hemifield? Seminal experiments addressing this question were carried out by Cowey and Stoerig in 1995. They confirmed, as had long been known, that monkeys could accurately localize and reach for a briefly presented visual stimulus in their 'blind' hemifields. But, after this, they proceeded to an important second experiment with the same animals: the monkeys were trained to discriminate between randomly presented 'lights' and 'no lights' (i.e. blanks) in their intact hemifields, and rewarded for correct responses (reaching for a light, or pressing a blank panel for a non-light). The crucial question, after this training was completed, was: how would the animals respond to a visual stimulus in their 'blind' field? The answer was clear and robust: the monkeys pressed the 'non-light' panel. Even though the animals had just demonstrated that they could detect the lights at virtually perfect performance, they nevertheless did not treat them as *lights*. This is just what a human blindsight subject would do, of course. Some further experimental extensions of this paradigm are discussed by Cowey and Stoerig (1997). Their discussion also provides an excellent review of comparative blindsight research on humans and monkeys. (The matter is also discussed, at a more general level, in Weiskrantz 1997, Chapter 4.)

Charles Gross and his colleagues have carried out two important experiments that are also relevant to the animal–human parallel. Monkeys were trained to make a rapid ('saccadic') eye movement from the point of fixation to a visual target in their blind hemifields (Moore *et al.* 1995). The monkeys could do this very effectively when they had a warning signal (the turning off of the fixation point). But, without this warning, they failed to initiate the eye movement to the target. The authors draw the parallel with clinical testing of human patients with field defects caused by visual cortex damage: typically in clinical perimetric testing, subjects are not given warning signals and are 'blind' to visual events in their field defects. In blindsight experiments carried out in the laboratory, however, warning signals are routinely used.

But, significantly, even the need for a warning signal disappears if the unilateral V1 damage is imposed in infancy (Moore *et al.* 1996). Other animal work (Payne 1994) also strongly supports the conclusion that greater recovery is possible after early rather than late damage to the visual system, accompanied by anatomical reorganization. In this connection, it may be relevant that the two most thoroughly studied human patients, D.B. and G.Y., both had visual defects in childhood: G.Y. because of head injury at the age of 8, and D.B. because of an incipient occipital tumour that first gave rise to a clinical problem at the age of 14, but the pathology might well have been present much earlier, perhaps even prenatally (see Weiskrantz 1986).

A related issue concerns the role of practice in recovery of residual function. It was demonstrated some time ago (Cowey 1967; Mohler and Wurtz 1977) that, if monkeys with visual cortex lesions are given sustained practice with visual discriminations in their blind fields, their sensitivity increases. The increase can be substantial—as much as 3 log units. The size of the field defect also shrinks. But it depends directly on whether the animal is actually *required* to practise with stimuli directed within the field defect. In fact, Mohler and Wurtz showed that recovery was specific even to practice *within a subpart* of the field defect. The beneficial effect of practice in human patients, using a procedure based on the method of Mohler and Wurtz, was demonstrated by Zihl and colleagues (Zihl 1980, 1981, 2000; Zihl and von Cramon 1979, 1985), which can be seen in greater detail in Chapter 11, this volume. Recently, other investigators (Kasten and Sabel 1995; Kerkhoff *et al.* 1994) have also reported encouraging results with human patients, using similar techniques.

The definition of blindsight cited at the beginning of this article refers to 'the sufferer', but the hemianope is not a sufferer. He or she has a perfectly good hemifield with which to negotiate the world, using intact eye and head movements, and this may have a bearing on whether there is any recovery of function in the blind hemifield. The typical hemianope, whether human or animal, has no particular reason to exercise the affected hemifield, given his intact hemifield. Greater pressure on subcortical pathways would exist when there are bilateral defects, but such patients often have other neuropsychological deficits. Nevertheless, the study of selected patients with bilateral defects would be of special interest because of the pressures necessarily placed upon extrastriate pathways (cf. Perenin *et al.* 1980).

Validation and related issues

Some commentators cannot resist, in referring to blindsight, to precede the term with the adjective 'controversial', so that it becomes almost part of a collective noun, like 'red' is to 'herring' or 'green' is to 'belt'. This no doubt stems from the deeply counterintuitive nature of the phenomenon, as is the case for all implicit neuropsychological syndromes, but is probably strongest in the case of blindsight. Some of the issues of validation and theoretical interpretation are the same throughout the field of implicit processing, and some are unique to blindsight. A fuller treatment of these issues can be found in Weiskrantz (1997, 1998, and 2001*a,b*) but, briefly, some of these are as follows.

Stray light, intraocular diffusion, and other possible artefacts

As the principal subjects of investigation are hemianopic and thus have an intact, normal visual hemifield ipsilateral to the lesion, it is important to rule out the possibility that supposed processing by the blind field is not, in fact, being carried out by stray light or intraocular diffused light reaching the intact hemifield (Campion *et al.* 1983). Suitable controls include the use of comparison cases with scotomas caused by retinal pathology (who show no residual capacity), and the use of stimuli that would be severely degraded by diffusion, such as high spatial frequency gratings for measuring acuity in the impaired field. Stray light has been controlled in a variety of ways, e.g. by flooding the intact visual hemifield with high levels of illumination so that, if there were any stray light, it could not be detected. The stray light function has also been determined experimentally (Barbur *et al.* 1994*a*). The most demanding method to ensure that there can be no effective stray light into intact parts of the field is to use the *genuinely* blind part of the eye as a control—the optic disc, in which there are no receptors. The size of this natural absolutely blind area is fixed and known (about 5° × 7°). One can be certain that, if a small target light projected on to it cannot be detected by the subject, there can be no diffusion of light beyond the edge of the disc, and hence maximum diffusion would be no more than half of the size of the disc. As far as the subject is concerned, all of the lights, whether or not they fall on the disc, are unseen. But on the disc the subject's detection performance is at chance levels, and, when it is on the neighbouring region, it is significantly above chance. Weiskrantz and Warrington (cf. Weiskrantz 1986, chapter 10), Stoerig *et al.* (1985), and Tomaiuolo *et al.* (1997) have used this control effectively. It can be said with assurance that residual visual capacity in the blind field of hemianopes cannot be explained away as a matter of stray light or intraocular diffusion.

Eye movement recordings and monitoring are standard features of many studies, which have ruled out inadvertent fixation shifts, as well as the use of stimuli too brief to survive a saccade. An eye-tracking device has also been used with G.Y., which ensured that even if the eye moved the stimulus would remain fixed on the same retinal location (Kentridge *et al.* 1997). Residual function cannot be explained away in terms of inadvertent fixation shifts.

Incidence

Across a random sample of patients with hemianopias resulting from cortical damage, it is still not known how many would be likely to demonstrate blindsight, but it probably is a minority. Blythe *et al.* (1987) found five patients (one of whom was G.Y.) with evidence of residual function (responses to movement, and localization by reaching or eye movements) out of a studied population of 25. Similarly, Weiskrantz (1980) found in a study of acute hospital cases that 14 hemianopic patients of 69 showed some evidence of residual function. In the remainder either no such evidence was found or remained inconclusive.

Why should this be? Briefly, there are at least four reasons (cf. Weiskrantz 1995, 1996). Probably the most important is the variable extent of the occipital lesions in human subjects, and the unlikelihood of any such lesion being restricted to V1, which itself is buried deep in the medial aspect of the brain. As noted above, animal work has demonstrated that extension of lesions beyond V1 degrades the degree of residual function, and many lesions seen clinically probably lead to the same diminution, especially as the visual association areas are tightly compressed in the proximity of V1. Secondly, the age at which the lesion occurs could be important, as has already been demonstrated in animal work (Moore *et al.* 1996; Payne 1994; see above). A third reason is that the stimulus parameters used in testing for residual function can be critical—parameters that may be suitable or even optimal for testing of normal function may not apply to that of the blind field. Even a slight change in the slope of the temporal onset or offset of the stimulus can transform chance performance into virtually perfect performance. For example, Hess and Pointer (1989), using particular fixed parameters of temporal and spatial Gaussian envelopes of unstructured stimuli, concluded that there was no residual function in G.Y. (and other subjects). This negative result was confirmed (Weiskrantz *et al.* 1991) using the same parameters, but a relatively small change in the parameters led to excellent performance by G.Y. in his blind hemifield. This and another example of an apparently unfortunate choice of parameters are discussed in Weiskrantz (1997, pp. 154–5; 247–8). Finally, another possible reason for variable incidence is the strangeness of the question that the researcher is bound to ask when testing blindsight type 1, when subjects are asked to guess about stimuli of which they have no awareness. Some refuse to do so. No doubt some experimenters share their scepticism in asking such a question, compounded by the need to test subjects extensively over tens of hundreds of trials to obtain parametric families of functions. This, no doubt, is why research has been carried out on a relatively few number of long-suffering subjects with the appropriately delimited lesions, who are willing and able to be make themselves available.

Completeness of the visual cortex lesion and extensions to non-striate cortex

It is a complicating fact that damage in human clinical patients is rarely confined to just striate cortex. A further possible complication is that the damage to striate cortex itself may not be complete. Some have argued—along the lines of the late nineteenth century view that assigns special higher properties to cerebral cortex (cf. Weiskrantz 1961, for a critique)—that intact striate cortex is itself necessary for the capacity for visual discriminations. In particular, Fendrich *et al.* (1992), Gazzaniga *et al.* (1994), and Wessinger *et al.* (1997) have argued that blindsight, when demonstrated, may depend critically not on extrastriate pathways, but on small islands of intact striate cortex. Briefly, small islands of intact visual function were found (65% correct, chance being 50%) in an otherwise dead visual hemifield of occipital patients; it was blindsight because the subject reported no awareness of the stimuli within the island. Brain imaging also revealed a small region of intact striate cortex at the occipital pole (which would be expected, of course, in a subject with macular sparing). Their evidence was found using an eye-tracker, which allows the visual image to be fixed on the retina (within limited eccentricities) and which thus eliminates detection due to inadvertent or uncontrolled fixation shifts (although these have been controlled by other methods in earlier blindsight studies; see above).

It may well be that some cases are amenable to an explanation in terms of intact, tiny islands of striate cortex, but it does not follow that this is the only explanation even in such cases, nor can it be a general explanation of all examples of residual visual function with V1 lesions. First, while D.B.'s and G.Y.'s visual fixation maintenance is excellent, and has been monitored and measured as a matter of routine in several experiments, G.Y. has also been tested with an 'eye-tracker' device as described by Fendrich *et al.* (1992) to control for inadvertent eye movements that might allow brief fixation of an 'island'. The result was that *no* islands were found in G.Y., using the same eye-tracking apparatus and the same parameters as in the Fendrich study (Kentridge *et al.* 1997).

Secondly, of course, such an account cannot apply to the evidence with monkeys, where the completeness of the lesion and the absence of islands can be confirmed with certainty. Moreover, as we have discussed (above), the monkey without V1 classifies those visual events that it can detect in the blind field with almost perfect accuracy as 'non-visual blanks', just as the human blindsight subject does. Also, there is a remarkably close fit between the narrowly tuned visual channel in the blind fields of monkeys and of G.Y., as revealed by pupillometry and by G.Y.'s psychophysics (see above).

Thirdly, there is another possible explanation of 'patchiness', when it is found, at the level of the retina itself. Following V1 damage there is, of course, retrograde degeneration of the large majority of cells in the lateral geniculate nucleus. However, the matter does not stop there—there can be patchy transneuronal degeneration of ganglion cells in the retina (Van Buren 1963; Cowey *et al.* 1989, 1999), and especially the p-beta class of cells. This class of cells, depleted after V1 lesions, is distributed heavily in the macular region of the retina (the region, as it happens, to which the eye-tracker is restricted for technical reasons). The cells are small, have colour-opponency properties, and project only to the lateral geniculate nucleus. The retina itself can be patchy.

Fourthly, high-resolution MRI scans of the most highly studied subject do not reveal intact islands of tissue (aside from at the pole, corresponding to his region of macular sparing), nor do PET or fMRI scans reveal any functioning visual cortex when he is stimulated in his 'blind field' (Barbur *et al.* 1993, 1998; Sahraie *et al.* 1997; and A. Morland, personal communication).

The assessment of blindsight in relation to response assessment and response criteria

The demonstration of discriminative performance in blindsight, when it is good, can be assessed in standard statistical terms without any reference to signal detection theory. For example, excellent levels of performance can be matched in the 'blind' and sighted hemifields and yet the blindsight subject says he is aware of the latter but not of the former. Also, Stoerig *et al.* (1985) deliberately varied response criteria without this affecting detection thresholds with blindsight subjects, although performance levels were admittedly relatively weak.

In contrast, the region of theoretical concern lies more with the much lower levels of performance, usually at chance or near chance levels. The procedures typically involve a 'yes, I see' or 'no, I do not see' response to stimuli in the blind field, which is typically the evidence upon which a claim of 'blindness' is based. In signal detection terms,

however, a subject may have a high sensitivity (d') even though the measured performance level is at 50% because of response criterion bias (e.g. if the subject is very cautious
and responds 'no' on every trial). Experimental studies of the capacity of the 'blind'
field, on the other hand, are often carried out with a more rigorous procedure, such as a
two-alternative forced-choice paradigm (2AFC), which tends to be free of response bias.
Therefore, the question is whether the dissociation between the reported 'blindness' of
the affected field versus its positive residual 'blindsight' function merely reflects different
response criteria in the 'yes/no' versus the 2AFC discriminating modes.

Azzopardi and Cowey (1997) have carried out a signal detection comparison of these
two modes of responding, 2AFC versus yes/no, in G.Y. using a grating stimulus versus
an equiluminant uniform patch, with a range of stimulus contrasts. For both paradigms ('was the grating in the first or the second temporal interval?') and ('was there a
stimulus or not?'), they obtained receiver-operating characteristic (ROC) curves, and
hence could derive measures of sensitivity (d') that were independent of response
criteria. The result was that, in normal subjects, the two measures of sensitivity were
identical—saying 'yes' or 'no' yields the same outcome as judging in which of two
intervals the stimulus occurred in the 2AFC. But for G.Y. the result was quite different:
he was much more sensitive in the 2AFC paradigm than in the 'yes/no' paradigm. This
is, of course, exactly the difference implied in the meaning of blindsight itself: there is
good performance when the subject is forced to make a response to a stimulus as
opposed to making a 'see/not see' judgement, as in clinical perimetry.

Does blindsight differ qualitatively or just quantitatively from normal vision?

Azzopardi and Cowey take their results to imply 'that blindsight is not just normal, near-
threshold vision and that information about the stimulus is processed in blindsighted
patients in an unusual way' (1997, p. 14190), which is the view originally advanced for
blindsight (cf. Weiskrantz 1986). However, even if criterion-free measures of d' for 'yes/no'
and 2AFC procedures yielded identical values for the blind field, it would not follow that
the existence of qualitative differences would thereby be disproved. The reason is that the
subjects can be encouraged to give 'yes/no' responses in a 'guessing' mode, even though
they continue to say that they do not 'see', as such. This was readily found with D.B.
throughout all of the investigations with him and was how, in fact, the blindsight evidence
was derived. The crux of the matter is not response topography as such but what the subjects take as their task—whether it is to report their experience (or its absence) *in relation
to* the ongoing discrimination. The critical difference is between 'on-line' discriminative
processes and 'off-line' commentaries or judgements about them. It might be more meaningful simply to continue to scale each separately, and to plot their correlations or dissociations. The question concerns the disjunction or the correlation between the two scales.

For example, Kentridge *et al.* (1999a) examined correlations in G.Y. between
commentary-key responses ('aware' or 'not aware') and 2AFC spatial localization

discriminations in the good and bad fields, selecting approximately similar levels of discrimination for both fields. In fact, a double dissociation emerged: even though G.Y.'s 2AFC performance happened to be poorer in his good field than in his blind field, he had a higher level of awareness responses in the good field than in the blind. Warrington and Weiskrantz also reported a double dissociation between the intact and impaired fields of D.B. The conditions were arranged so that the impaired field was poorer than the intact for form discrimination, but better for forced-choice detection of a sine wave grating, leading to the suggestion of a qualitative dissociation between form discrimination and detection between the intact and impaired fields (Weiskrantz 1986, chapter 16).

Other considerations speak against the properties of the blind field being simply a weaker version of normal vision. Briefly, there is a retrograde transneuronal degeneration in the human (Van Buren 1963), which in the monkey leads to a shift from a predominance of p-beta ganglion cells of the affected retina towards p-alpha and p-gamma cells, which have different structures, different projections in the brain and different functional properties from p-beta: the hemiretina corresponding to the field defect is qualitatively different from the normal hemiretina (Cowey *et al.* 1989). The levels of performance in the blind field can also be very high, approaching 100%, even when the subject reports complete absence of awareness (Weiskrantz 1986, 1995), unlike the 'degraded' levels characteristic of parathreshold levels in normal vision.

Other differences (see above) include the finding that colour discrimination and detection, measured psychophysically or by pupillometry in the blind field, appear to favour the red end of the spectrum, unlike that of a normal field, and the fMRI evidence shows a different pattern of activation in the fMRI brain images when G.Y. reports awareness and when he does not, despite comparable levels of performance psychophysically under these contrasting conditions.

Concluding comment

There can be no doubt that parallel extrastriate visual pathways can mediate visual discriminations, in humans as well as in other primates, but it is the dissociations that emerge suggesting a segregation of functions that we are only beginning to characterize. The most surprising aspect to emerge has been the dissociation between subjects' reported lack of experience of visual stimuli, whether registered verbally or by 'commentary keys', and the contrast with their objectively measured capacity. Or, in the case of monkeys, their classification of the visual stimuli that they objectively can detect with impressive sensitivity as being 'blanks'. But this same disjunction is found right across the entire neuropsychological research spectrum, e.g. commissurotomy, amnesia, aphasia, prosopagnosia, dyslexia (cf. Schacter *et al.* 1988; Weiskrantz 1991, 1997 for reviews). Indeed, even in normal function, it could be argued that much, perhaps even most, neural processing proceeds without any associated awareness or other 'off-line' measure. If blindsight research has helped to elucidate such a class of disjunctions more precisely, and to open up a route by which their neural underpinnings can be explored, that would be a welcome bonus.

References

Azzopardi, P. and Cowey A. (1997). Is blindsight like normal, near-threshold vision? *Proc. Natl. Acad. Sci., USA* **94**, 14190–4.

Azzopardi, P., Fallah, M., Gross, C.G., and Rodman, H.T. (1998). Responses of neurons in visual areas MT and MTS offer lesions of striate cortex in macaque monkeys. *Society for Neuroscience Abstracts* **24**, 648.

Barbur, J.L. and Forsyth, P.M. (1986). Can the pupil response be used as a measure of the visual input associated with the geniculo-striate pathway? *Clin. Vis. Sci.* **1**, 107–11.

Barbur, J.L. and Thomson, W.D. (1987). Pupil response as an objective measure of visual acuity. *Ophthalm. Physiol. Optics* **7**, 425–9.

Barbur, J.L., Ruddock, K.H., and Waterfield, V.A. (1980). Human visual responses in the absence of the geniculostriate projection. *Brain* **102**, 905–27.

Barbur, J.L., Thomson, W.D., and Forsyth, P.M. (1987). A new system for the simultaneous measurement of pupil size and two-dimensional eye movements. *Clin. Vis. Sci.* **2**, 131–42.

Barbur, J.L., Watson,.J.A.G., Frackowiak, R.A.J., and Zeki, S. (1993). Conscious visual perception without V1. *Brain* **116**, 1293–302.

Barbur, J.L., Harlow, J.A., and Weiskrantz, L. (1994*a*). Spatial and temporal response properties of residual vision in a case of hemianopia. *Philo. Trans. R. Soc. B* **343**, 157–66.

Barbur, J.L, Harlow, J.A., Sahraie, A., Stoerig, P., and Weiskrantz, L. (1994*b*). Responses to chromatic stimuli in the absence of V1: pupillometric and psychophysical studies. In *Vision science and its applications. Opt. Soc. Am. Techn. Digest* **2**, 312–15.

Barbur, J.L., Sahraie, A., Simmons, A., Weiskrantz, L., and Williams, S.C.R. (1998). Processing of chromatic signals in the absence of a geniculostriate projection. *Vision Res.* **38**, 3447–53.

Barbur, J.L., Weiskrantz, L., and Harlow, J.A. (1999). The unseen color after-effect of an unseen stimulus: insight from blindsight into mechanisms of color afterimages. *Proc. Natl Acad. Sci., USA* **96**, 11637–41.

Bard, L. (1905). De la persistence des sensations luminesces dans le champ avenge des hemianopsiques. *La Semaine Medi.* **22**, 3–25.

Benevento, L.A. and Yoshida, K. (1981). The afferent and efferent organization of the lateral geniculo-striate pathways in the macaque monkey. *J. Comp. Neurol.* **203**, 455–74.

Blythe, I.M., Kennard, C., and Ruddock, K.H. (1987). Residual vision in patients with retrogeniculate lesions of the visual pathways. *Brain* **110**, 887–905.

Breiter, H.C., Etcoff, N.L., Whalen, P.J., Kennedy, W.A., Rauch, S.L., Buckner, R.L., Strauss, M.M., Hyman, S.E., and Rosen, B.R. (1996). Response and habituation of the human amygdala during visual processing of facial expression. *Neuron* **17**, 875–87.

Brent, P.J., Kennard, C., and Ruddock, K.H. (1994). Residual colour vision in a human hemianope: spectral responses and colour discrimination. *Proc. R. Soc. Lond. B* **256**, 219–25.

Brindley, O.S., Gautier-Smith, P.C., and Lewin, W. (1969). Cortical blindness and the functions of the non-geniculate fibres of the optic tracts. *J. Neurol. Neurosurg. Psychiatry* **32**, 259–64.

Campion, J., Latto, R., and Smith, Y.M. (1983). Is blindsight an effect of scattered light, spared cortex, and near-threshold vision? *Behav. Brain Sci.* **6**, 423–48.

Cocker, D., Moseley, M.J., Bissenden, J.G., and Fielder, A.R. (1994). Visual acuity and pupillary responses to spatial structure in infants. *Invest. Ophthalmol. Vis. Sci.* **35**, 2620–5.

Corbetta, M., Marzi, C.A., Tassinari, G., and Aglioti, S. (1990). Effectiveness of different task paradigms in revealing blindsight. *Brain* 113, 603–16.

Cowey, A. (1967). Perimetric study of field defects in monkeys after cortical and retinal ablations. *Quart. J. Exp. Psychol.* 19, 232–45.

Cowey, A. (1985). Aspects of cortical organization related to selective attention and selective impairments of visual perception. In *Attention and performance*, Vol. 11 (ed. M.I. Posner and O.S.M. Marin), pp. 41–62. Lawrence Erlbaum, Hillsdale, New Jersey.

Cowey, A. and Azzopardi, P. (2001). Is blindsight motion blind? In *Out of mind* (ed. B. de Gelder, E. de Haan, and C. Heywood), pp. 87–103. Oxford University Press, Oxford.

Cowey, A. and Stoerig, P. (1991). The neurobiology of blindsight. *Trends Neurosci.* 29, 65–80.

Cowey, A. and Stoerig, P. (1992). Reflections on blindsight. In *The neuropsychology of consciousness* (ed. D. Milner and M.O. Rugg), pp. 11–37. Academic Press, London.

Cowey, A. and Stoerig, P. (1995). Blindsight in monkeys. *Nature, Lond.* 373, 247–9.

Cowey, A. and stoerig, P. (1997). Visual detection in monkeys with blindsight. *Neuropsychologia* 35, 929–37.

Cowey, A. and Stoerig, P. (1999). Spectral sensitivity of hemianopic macaque monkeys. *Eur. J. Neurosci.* 11, 2114–20.

Cowey, A. and Weiskrantz, L. (1963). A perimetric study of visual field defects in monkeys. *Quart. J. Exp. Psychol.* 15, 91–115.

Cowey, A., Stoerig, P., and Perry, V.H. (1989). Transneuronal retrograde degeneration of retinal ganglion cells after damage to striate cortex in macaque monkeys: selective loss of P-beta cells. *Neuroscience* 29, 65–80.

Cowey, A., Stoerig, P., and Williams C. (1999). Variance in transneuronal retrograde ganglion cell degeneration in monkeys after removal of striate cortex: effects of size of the cortical lesion. *Vision Res.* 39, 3642–52.

de Gelder, B., Vrooman, J., Pourtois, G., and Weiskrantz, L. (1999). Non-conscious recognition of affect in the absence of striate cortex. *NeuroReport* 10, 3759–63.

Esteves, F., Parra, C., Dimberg, U., and Øhman, A. (1994). Nonconscious associative learning: Pavlovian conditioning of skin conductance responses to masked fear-relevant facial stimuli. *Psychophysiology* 31, 375–85.

Fendrich, R., Wessinger, C.M., and Gazzaniga, M.S. (1992). Residual vision in a scotoma; implications for blindsight. *Science* 258, 1489–91.

Finlay, A.R., Jones, S.R., Morland, A.B., Ogilvie, J.A., and Ruddock, K.H. (1997). Movement elicits ipsilateral activity in the damaged hemisphere of a human hemianope. *Proc. R. Soc. Lond. B* 264, 267–97.

Fries, W. (1981). The projection from the lateral geniculate nucleus to the prestriate cortex of the macaque monkey. *Proc. Natl. Acad. Sci., USA* 213, 73–80.

Gazzaniga, M.S., Fendrich, R., and Wessinger, C.M. (1994). Blindsight reconsidered. *Curr. Directions Psychol. Sci.* 3, 93–6.

Hernandez-Gonzalez, C.C. and Reinoso-Suarez, F. (1994). The lateral geniculate nucleus projects to the inferior temporal cortex in the macaque monkey. *NeuroReport* 5, 2692–6.

Hess, R.F. and Pointer, J.S. (1989). Spatial and temporal contrast sensitivity in hemianopia. A comparative study of the sighted and blind hemifields. *Brain* 112, 871–94.

Holmes, G. (1918). Disturbances of vision by cerebral lesions. *Br. J. Ophthalmol.* 2, 353–84.

Kasten, E. and Sabel, B.A. (1995). Visual field enlargement after computer training in brain-damaged patients with homonymous deficits: an open pilot trial. *Restor. Neurol. Neurosci.* 8, 113–27.

Kentridge, R.W., Heywood, C.A., and Weiskrantz, L. (1997). Residual vision in multiple retinal locations within a scotoma: implications for blindsight. *J. Cogn. Neurosci.* **9**, 191–202.

Kentridge, R.W., Heywood, C.A., and Weiskrantz, L. (1999*a*). Effects of temporal cueing on residual discrimination in blindsight. *Neuropsychologia* **37**, 479–83.

Kentridge, R.W., Heywood, C.A., and Weiskrantz, L. (1999*b*). Attention without awareness in blindsight. *Proc. R. Soc. B* **266**, 1805–11.

Kerkhoff, G., Munsinger, U., and Meier, E. (1994). Neurovisual rehabilitation in cerebral blindness. *Arch. Neurol.* **51**, 474–81.

Marcel, A.J. (1998). Blindsight and shape perception: deficit of visual consciousness or of visual function? *Brain* **121**, 1565–88.

Marzi, C.A., Tassinari, G., Lutzemberger, L., and Aglioti, A. (1986). Spatial summation across the vertical meridian in hemianopics. *Neuropsychologia* **24**, 749–58.

Milner, A.D. and Goodale, M.A. (1995). *The Visual brain in action.* Oxford University Press, Oxford.

Mohler, C.W. and Wurtz, R.H. (1977). Role of striate cortex and superior colliculus in visual guidance of saccadic eye movements in monkeys. *J. Neurophysiol.* **40**, 74–94.

Moore, T., Rodman, H.R., Repp, A.B., and Gross, C.G. (1995). Localization of visual stimuli after striate cortex damage in monkeys: parallels with human blindsight. *Proc. Natl. Acad. Sci., USA* **92**, 8215–8.

Moore, T., Rodman, H.R., Repp, A.B., and Gross, C.G. (1996). Greater residual vision in monkeys after striate cortex damage in infancy. *J. Neurophysiol.* **76**, 3928–33.

Morland, A.J., Ogilvie, J.A., Ruddock, K.H., and Wright, J.R. (1996). Orientation discrimination is impaired in the absence of the striate cortical contribution to human vision. *Proc. R. Soc. B* **263**, 633–40.

Morland, A.J., Jones, S.R., Finlay, A.L., Deyzac, E., Lê, S., and Kemp S. (1999). Visual perception of motion, luminance, and colour in a human hemianope. *Brain* **122**, 1183–98.

Morris, J.S.,Øhman, A., and Doland, R.J. (1999). A subcortical pathway to the right amygdala mediating 'unseen' fear. *Proc. Natl. Acad. Sci., USA* **96**, 1680–5.

Morris, J.S., de Gelder, B., Weiskrantz, L., and Dolan, R.J. (2001). Differential extrageniculostriate and amygdala responses to presentation of emotional faces in a cortically blind field. *Brain* **124**, 1241–52.

Øhman, A. and Soares, J.J.F. (1998). Emotional conditioning to masked stimuli: expectancies for aversive outcomes following non-recognized fear-relevant stimuli. *J. Exp. Psychol. Gen.* **127**, 69–82.

Pasik, T. and Pasik, P. (1971). The visual world of monkeys deprived of striate cortex: effective stimulus parameters and the importance of the accessory optic system. In *Visual processes in vertebrates*, Vision Research Supplement No. 3 (ed. T. Shipley and J.E. Dowling), pp. 419–35. Pergamon Press, Oxford.

Payne, B.R. (1994). System-wide repercussions of damage to the immature visual cortex. *Trends Neurosci.* **17**, 126–30.

Perenin, M.T. (1978). Discrimination of motion direction in perimetrically blind fields. *NeuroReport* **2**, 397–400.

Perenin, M.T. and Rossetti, Y. (1996). Grasping without form discrimination in a hemianopic field. *NeuroReport* **7**, 793–7.

Perenin, M.T., Ruel, J., and Hécaen, H. (1980). Residual visual capacities in a case of cortical blindness. *Cortex* **16**, 605–12.

Perenin, M.T., Girard-Madoux, Ph., and Jeannerod, M. (1985). From completion to residual vision in hemianopic patients. Paper delivered at meeting of European Brain and Behaviour Society, Oxford.

Pöppel, F., Held, R., and Frost, D. (1973). Residual visual function after brain wounds involving the central visual pathways in man. *Nature Lond.* **243**, 295–6.

Poppelreuter, W. (1917). *Die psychischen Schädigungen durch Kopfschuss im Kriege 1914–16; die Störungen der niederen und höherer Sehleistungen durch Verletzungen des Okzipitalhirns,* Vol. L. Voss, Leipzig.

Riddoch, G. (1917). Dissociation of visual perceptions due to occipital injuries, with especial reference to appreciation of movement. *Brain* **40**, 15–17.

Sahraie, A., Weiskrantz, L., Barbur, J.L., Simmons, A., Williams, S.C.R., and Brammer, M.L. (1997). Pattern of neuronal activity associated with conscious and unconscious processing of visual signals. *Proc. Natl. Acad. Sci. USA* **94**, 9406–11.

Sahraie, A., Weiskrantz, L., and Barbur, J.L. (1998) Awareness and confidence ratings in motion perception without geniculo-striate projection. *Behav. Brain Res.* **96**, 71–7.

Sanders, M.D., Warrington, E.K., Marshall, J., and Weiskrantz, L. (1974). 'Blindsight': vision in a field defect. *Lancet* April 20, 707–8.

Schacter, D.L., McAndrews, M.P., and Moscovitch, M. (1998). Access to consciousness: dissociations between implicit and explicit knowledge in neuropsychological syndromes. In *Thought without language* (ed. L. Weiskrantz), pp. 242–78. Oxford University Press, Oxford.

Stoerig, P. (1987). Chromaticity and achromaticity: evidence for a functional differentiation in visual field defects. *Brain* **110**, 869–86.

Stoerig, P. and Cowey, A. (1989). Wavelength sensitivity in blindsight. *Nature Lond.* **342**, 916–18.

Stoerig, P. and Cowey, A. (1991). Increment threshold spectral sensitivity in blindsight: evidence for colour opponency. *Brain* **114**, 1487–12.

Stoerig, P. and Cowey, A. (1992). Wavelength sensitivity in blindsight. *Brain* **115**, 425–44.

Stoerig, P. and Cowey, A. (1997). Blindsight in man and monkey. *Brain* **120**, 535–59.

Stoerig, P. and Pöppel, F. (1986). Eccentricity-dependent residual target detection in visual defects. *Exp. Brain Res.* **64**, 469–75.

Stoerig, P., Hubner, M. and Pöppel, E. (1985). Signal detection analysis of residual vision in a field defect due to a post-geniculate lesion. *Neuropsychologia* **23**, 589–99.

Tomaiuolo, F., Ptito, M., Marzi, C.A., Paus, T., and Ptito, A. (1997). Blindsight in hemispherectomized patients as revealed by spatial summation across the vertical meridian. *Brain* **120**, 795–803.

Torjussen, T. (1976). Residual function in cortically blind hemifields. *Scand. J. Psychol.* **17**, 320–2.

Torjussen, T. (1978). Visual processing in cortically blind hemifields. *Neuropsychologia* **16**, 15–21.

Tranel, D. and Damasio, A.R. (1985). Knowledge without awareness: an autonomic index of facial recognition by prosopagnosics. *Science* **228**, 1453–5.

Van Buren, K.M. (1963). *The retinal ganglion cell layer.* Charles Thomas, Spring field, Illinois.

Weiskrantz, L. (1961). Encephalisation and the scotoma. In *Current problems in animal behaviour* (ed. W.H. Thorpe and O.L. Zangwill), pp. 30–85. Cambridge University Press, Cambridge.

Weiskrantz, L. (1972). Behavioural analysis of the monkey's visual nervous system [review lecture]. *Proc. R. Soc. B* **182**, 427–55.

Weiskrantz, L. (1980). Varieties of residual experience. *Quart. J. Exp. Psychol.* **32**, 365–86.

Weiskrantz, L. (1986). *Blindsight. A case study and implications.* Oxford University Press, Oxford.

Weiskrantz, L. (1987). Residual vision in a scotoma: a follow-up study of 'form' discrimination. *Brain* **110**, 77–92.

Weiskrantz, L. (1990). Outlooks for blindsight: explicit methodologies for implicit processes. The Ferrier Lecture. *Proc. R. Soc. B* **239**, 247.

Weiskrantz, L. (1991). Disconnected awareness for detecting, processing, and remembering in neurological patients. The Hughlings Jackson Lecture. *J. R. Soc. Med.* **84**, 466–70.

Weiskrantz, L. (1995). Blindsight: Not an island unto itself. *Current Directions in Psychological Science* **4**, 146–51.

Weiskrantz, L. (1996). Blindsight revisited. *Current opinion in Neurobiology* **6**, 215–20.

Weiskrantz, L. (1997). *Consciousness lost and found. A neuropsychological exploration.* Oxford University Press, Oxford.

Weiskrantz, L. (1998). Consciousness and commentaries. In *Towards a science of consciousness II— The second Tucson discussions and debates* (ed. S.R. Hameroff, A.W. Kaszniak, and A.C. Scott), pp. 371–7. MIT Press, Cambridge, Massachusetts.

Weiskrantz, L. (1999). Blindsight—Implications for the experience of motion. In *Emotion and cognitive neuroscience* (ed. R. Lane, G. Ahem, J. Allen, L. Nadel, A. Kaszniak, S. Rapcsak, and G. Schwartz), pp. 277–95. MIT Press, Boston.

Weiskrantz, L. (2001*a*). Putting beta (β) on the back burner. In De Gelder B., De Haan E., and Heywood C (Eds.) *Out of mind* (ed. B. De Gelder, E. De Haan, and C. Heywood), pp. 20–31. Oxford University Press, Oxford.

Weiskrantz, L. (2001*b*). Blindsight. In *Handbook of Neuropsychology*, 2nd edn, Vol. 4 (ed. M. Behrmann), pp. 215–37. Elsevier, Amsterdam.

Weiskrantz, L. and Cowey, A. (1970). Filling in the scotoma: a study of residual vision after striate cortex lesions in monkeys. In *Progress in physiological psychology*, Vol. 3 (ed. F. Stellar and V.M. Sprague), pp. 237–60. Academic Press, New York.

Weiskrantz, L., Warrington, E.K., Sanders, M.D., and Marshall, J. (1974). Visual capacity in the hemianopic field following a restricted occipital ablation. *Brain* **97**, 709–28.

Weiskrantz, L., Harlow, A., and Barbur, J.L., (1991). Factors affecting visual sensitivity in a hemianopic subject. *Brain* **114**, 2269–82.

Weiskrantz, L., Barbur, J.L., and Sahraie, A. (1995). Parameters affecting conscious versus unconscious visual discrimination without V1. *Proc. Nat. Acad. Sci., USA* **92**, 6122–6.

Weiskrantz, L., Cowey, A., and Le Mare, C. (1998). Learning from the pupil: a spatial visual channel in the absence of V1 in monkey and human, *Brain* **121**, 1065–72.

Weiskrantz, L., Cowey, A., and Barbur J.L. (1999). Differential pupillary constriction and awareness in the absence of striate cortex. *Brain* **122**, 1533–8.

Wessinger, C.M., Fendrich, R., and Gazzaniga, M.S. (1997). Islands of residual vision in hemianopic patients. *J. Cogn. Neurosci.* **9**, 203–21.

Yukie, M. and Iwai, E. (1981). Direct projection from dorsal lateral geniculate nucleus to the prestriate cortex in macaque monkeys. *J. Comp. Neurol.* **201**, 81–97.

Zeki, S. (1978). Functional specialization in the visual cortex of the rhesus monkey. *Nature Lond.* **274**, 423–8.

Zeki, S. (1993). *A vision of the brain.* Blackwell Scientific Publications, Oxford.

Zihl, J. (1980). 'Blindsight': improvement of visually guided eye movements by systematic practice in patients with cerebral blindness. *Neuropsychologia* **18**, 71–7.

Zihl, J. (1981). Recovery of visual functions in patients with cerebral blindness. *Exp. Brain Res.* **44**, 159–69.

Zihl, J. (2000). *Rehabilitation of visual disorders after brain injury.* Psychology Press, Hove, East Sussex.

Zihl, J. and von Cramon, D. (1979). Restitution of visual function in patients with cerebral blindness. *J. Neurol. Neurosurg. Psychiatry* **42**, 312–22.

Zihl, J. and von Cramon, D. (1985). Visual field recovery from scotoma in patients with postgeniculate damage: a review of 55 cases. *Brain* **108**, 313–40.

Zihl, J., Tretter, F., and singer, W. (1980). Phasic electrodermal responses after visual stimulation in the cortically blind hemifield. *Behav. Brain Res.* **1**, 197–203.

Chapter 10

Perception, memory, and agnosia

Martha J. Farah

Introduction

Alongside such syndromes as amnesia, aphasia, and apraxia, agnosia is one of the startlingly selective impairments of mental capacity that can follow damage to the brain. Typical textbook treatments of agnosia classify it with other perceptual impairments. Yet, for much of the history of neuropsychology, the role of perception in agnosia has been debated. How should the inability to recognize objects through vision, in the absence of obvious memory, visuoperceptual, or general intellectual impairments, be classified? In more theoretical terms, is the underlying problem one of visual perception, memory knowledge, or some other mental capacity? To this day, controversy and confusion persist over the relation of agnosia to perception on the one hand, and to memory on the other. The goal of this chapter is to review the evidence on perception, memory, and agnosia, and suggest a *rapprochement* among the different positions that have been taken on the issue.

Any discussion of agnosia must begin by distinguishing among the many different syndromes that have been labelled with the blanket term agnosia, and specifying which form of agnosia is under discussion. The visual agnosias include a wide array of disorders affecting object recognition. The term has been applied to conditions ranging from a progressive loss of knowledge about objects' uses and associated information (e.g. Warrington 1985) and problems with name retrieval (e.g. Ferro and Santos 1984) to visual impairment so basic that an X and an O are indistinguishable (e.g. Benson and Greenberg 1969) or perception is inadequate to allow independent ambulation (e.g. Williams 1970). For present purposes, I will focus on a form of agnosia called, by most authors, associative visual agnosia.

Associative visual agnosia

The term 'associative agnosia' was first coined by Lissauer (1890), who contrasted this disorder of object recognition with another, termed by him 'apperceptive agnosia'. Apperceptive agnosia was, by definition, a disorder of object recognition that was accompanied by, and therefore attributable to, obvious visual perceptual disturbance. Following Lissauer, many subsequent neuropsychologists have assumed that agnosias without obvious perceptual disturbance are not attributable to an impairment of visual perception. The alternative interpretation was an impairment in associative processes by which a percept addresses relevant knowledge stored in memory. Before reassessing this view of associative agnosia, let us review the defining criteria for this puzzling syndrome.

To be considered an associative agnosic, a patient must demonstrate the following features.

1. He or she must have difficulty recognizing visually presented objects. This must be evident in ways other than just naming, such as sorting objects by category (e.g. putting kitchen utensils together, separate from sports equipment) or pantomiming the objects' functions. If the trouble is confined to naming objects, and is not manifest in nonverbal tests of recognition, then the problem is either anomia or, if confined to the naming of visual stimuli, optic aphasia.

2. The patient must demonstrate that Knowledge of the objects is available through modalities other than vision, e.g. by tactile or auditory recognition, or by verbal questioning (e.g. what is an egg beater?). Some dementias may result in a loss of knowledge about objects regardless of the modality of access, and this is distinct from a visual agnosia (e.g. Hodges *et al.* 1992; Martin and Fedio 1983; Warrington 1985).

3. The patient must be able to see the object clearly enough to describe its appearance, draw it, or answer whether it is the same or different in appearance compared with a second stimulus. Examples of drawings by patients with associative visual agnosia are shown in Fig. 10.1.

Patients who meet these criteria are rare, but are the subjects of a large literature because of what they can tell us about the nature of visual object recognition. What sort of mechanism could, when damaged, allow us to see well enough to draw copies as recognizable as those in Fig. 10.1, but not recognize them?

Empirical evidence on memory and perception in associative agnosia

Although associative agnosics do not have clinically obvious problems with perception or memory, careful investigations in some cases have demonstrated impairments in both. Some associative agnosics appear to suffer from a loss of memory knowledge about the visual appearances of objects. For this reason associative agnosia has sometimes been equated with a form of modality-specific amnesia (Albert *et al.* 1979). The analogy of a library has been used to convey the loss of stored information as distinct from any impairment in the processing of input (Humphreys and Riddoch 1987).

The most persuasive evidence of a memory impairment in agnosia comes from mental imagery tasks. Many associative agnosics complain of a loss of mental imagery, i.e. the ability to represent the visual appearances of objects from memory. Their drawings from memory and imagery-based descriptions of objects from memory are often

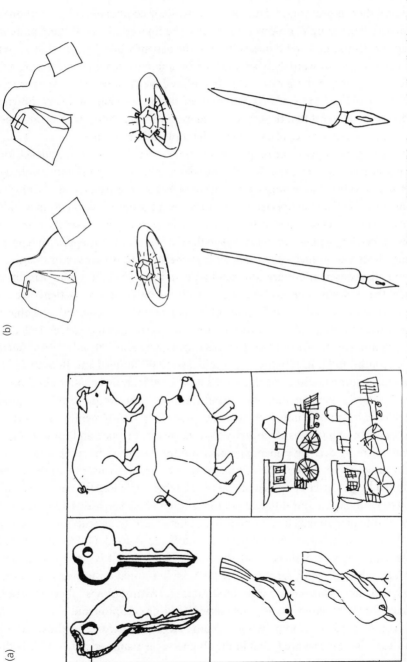

Fig. 10.1 Original drawings and copies made by (a) the agnosic described by Rubens and Benson (1971); (b) the agnosic described by Farah et al. (1988). All drawings were copied without being recognized.

described as poor or lacking in visual detail. The association of mental imagery impairment with agnosia is consistent with a problem that goes beyond perception, at least in the sense of processing retinal inputs.

However, there is growing evidence that at least some components of perception are not normal. For example, however impressive the final products of these patients' copying efforts may be, careful observation of the patient while drawing shows a very abnormal process. The words 'slavish' and 'line-by-line' are often used in describing the manner of copying in these cases (e.g. Ratcliff and Newcombe 1982; Wapner *et al.* 1978; Brown 1972). I watched as a patient drew the pen, tea bag, and ring shown in Fig. 10.1, and can report that they were indeed executed very slowly, with many pauses to check the correspondence of each line of the copy and the original.

In evaluating the copying techniques of associative visual agnosics as evidence for a visual perceptual impairment, we should consider an alternative possibility involving a loss or disconnection of memory knowledge of objects. A normal person's memory of what an object is might be expected to help in keeping the object's elements in working memory while it is being copied. Although a possible contributing factor, the absence of top–down memory support does not explain the slavish line-by-line approach reported in so many cases, as normal subjects do not copy meaningless patterns in this way.

Several other observations are consistent with an impairment in visual perception, although these vary in their decisiveness. Associative visual agnosic patients are also abnormally sensitive to the visual quality of stimuli, performing best with real objects, next best with photographs, and worst with line drawings, an ordering reflecting increasing impoverishment of the stimulus (e.g. Levine and Calvanio 1989; Ratcliff and Newcombe 1982; Riddoch and Humphreys 1987; Rubens and Benson 1971). Tachistoscopic presentation, which also reduces visual stimulus quality, also impairs associative agnosic performance dramatically. Although this would seem to be *prima facie* evidence for a visual impairment, an absence of top–down memory support can also account for an increase in sensitivity to visual factors (Tippett and Farah 1994).

Potentially more decisive evidence comes from the nature of the recognition errors made by associative agnosics. The vast majority of errors are visual in nature, i.e. they correspond to an object of similar shape (e.g. Levine 1978; Ratcliff and Newcombe 1982). For example, on four different occasions when I asked an associative agnosic to name a picture of a baseball bat, he made four different errors, all reflecting shape similarity: paddle, knife, baster, thermometer. Davidoff and Wilson's (1985) subject made some semantic errors as well as visual errors, but she was able to correct her semantic errors later when offered a forced choice between her initial answer and the correct one, whereas her visual errors were less tractable. Although visual errors can be accounted for by impaired access to semantic knowledge (Hinton and Shallice 1991), such accounts predict accompanying semantic errors. Therefore, for those cases in which visual shape errors are found in the absence of semantic errors, it is likely that visual shape perception is at fault.

The matching of unfamiliar faces and complex meaningless designs, in which memory would not play a role, also provides decisive evidence for a visual perceptual impairment. Changing the angle or lighting in the photograph of a face impairs agnosics' ability to match unfamiliar faces (Shuttleworth *et al.* 1982). The matching of abstract geometric forms is even less likely to depend on semantic knowledge than the matching of unfamiliar faces. A patient described by Rubens and Benson (1971) occasionally mistook flaws in the paper or printer's ink for a part of the design. Levine (1978) administered a visual discrimination learning task to an associative agnosic, and found her unable to learn a subtle discrimination between two patterns after 30 trials.

Perception as a multilevel process

Advances in our understanding of perception have widened the range of possible explanations of agnosia. With the development of cognitive science, neuropsychologists realized that perception is not accomplished in a single step. The best known vision theory of cognitive science, that of David Marr (1982), offered the fundamental insight that visual perception is a process of representing and re-representing the retinal inputs in a succession of formats that make different features of the input explicit. In his theory, there were three qualitatively different types of representation: (1) the primal sketch, in which edges and boundaries were made explicit; (2) the two-and-a-half-dimensional sketch, in which surfaces were made explicit; and (3) the three-dimensional models, in which the intrinsic shapes of objects were made explicit, allowing recognition.

Ratcliffe and Newcombe (1982) first made the connection between Marr's theory of vision and associative visual agnosia. They pointed out that the seeming paradox of good perception and memory with poor object recognition could be resolved by supposing that some levels of perception are intact and others impaired. If only the three-dimensional models were damaged, perhaps the two earlier forms of representation could support copying, matching, navigation, and the other preserved perceptual abilities. Of course, without the three-dimensional models, recognition would be impaired.

In the ensuing years, a number of different authors have interpreted and reinterpreted associative agnosia in terms of contemporary theories of vision. In each case, impairments in particular aspects of perception were hypothesized to underlie the agnosia. For example, feature integration (Riddoch and Humphreys 1987), principal axis derivation (Warrington 1985), and part decomposition (Farah 1990) were all suggested as candidate perceptual processes for the underlying perceptual impairment in associative agnosia. These hypotheses are of interest partly for what they tell us about agnosia, and also for what they tell us about the organization of visual perception. By discovering what visual abilities can be selectively impaired, we learn about the dividing lines between the different components of vision. By exploring the impact of these impairments on object recognition and other visual tasks, we learn about the role of different components in different tasks.

Although much remains to be learned about the nature of the perceptual impairments in agnosia, and the current crop of theories may all miss the mark, one important idea has been established. Vision is not a singular entity, but instead it has dissociable components, and different visual tasks used in evaluating agnosia, such as object recognition, copying, and matching, make different demands on these components. Thus, there is nothing patently contradictory about hypothesizing a perceptual impairment in an agnosic patient who performs well in certain perceptual tasks.

Can we reconcile this view of agnosia with evidence for a memory impairment? The apparent contradiction between hypothesizing a perceptual and a memory impairment only arises if we assume that perception and memory are singular and distinct. However, as we will see in the next section, this is true only in certain kinds of computational systems, and there is no reason to assume that it will be true of the human brain.

Where does perception end and memory begin?

Visual recognition requires that memory be searched for a representation that resembles the current stimulus input. In a conventional computer, an input is recognized by comparing a symbolic representation of that input to symbolic representations stored in memory, using an explicit comparison process that is itself part of a stored program in the computer. The process is analogous to taking the title of a book that you have written on a piece of paper, and searching the library shelves to find the same title written on the spine of the book. The slip of paper is the perceptual representation, and the shelved book is the memory representation. In principle, it is possible that visual recognition also works in this way, with a processor comparing a high-level representation of the appearance of the stimulus to stored representations. When a match is found, the associated semantic knowledge of the object is then available, just as the contents of the book become available once the title has been located on the shelf.

However, there is another way of implementing such a search that does not involve distinct perceptual and memory representations. In neural network computation, representations correspond to the activation of certain neuron-like units, which are interconnected. The extent to which the activation of one unit causes an increase or decrease in the activation of a neighbouring unit depends on the 'weight' of the connection between them. Positive weights cause units to excite each other and negative weights cause units to inhibit each other. Upon presentation of the input pattern to the input units, all of the units connected with those input units will begin to change their activation under the influence of two kinds of constraints: the activation value of the units to which they are connected and the weights on the connections. These units might in turn connect to others, and influence their activation levels in the same way. In recurrent, or attractor, networks the units downstream will also begin to influence the activation levels of the earlier units. Eventually, these shifting activation levels across the units of the network settle into a stable pattern of activation, which is the representation that corresponds to the recognized object. That pattern is determined jointly by the input activation (the stimulus input) and the weights of the network (the system's knowledge of all objects).

The two ways of implementing search are so different that it is difficult to compare them except at a very abstract level. For instance, one can say that the system's knowledge in a symbolic implementation of memory search consists of separate stored representations of the stimulus and the comparison procedure, whereas in a neural network it consists just of the connection weights, which store knowledge of object appearance and carry out the search process. In both types of system there is a distinction between the early representations of the stimulus closer to the input level and the high-level object representations that underlie object recognition. However, only the symbolic search involves two tokens of the high-level representation, one 'perceptual' (derived from the stimulus) and the other 'memory' (previously stored). In a neural network search there is only one token. Distinctions such as 'perception' versus 'memory', which seem almost logically necessary when one is thinking in terms of symbol manipulation, dissolve when one considers the neural network implementation of memory search.

On this view of visual object recognition, there is a continuum of types of representation, going from early visual areas, in which the representation is determined largely by the innate structure of the visual system, and ending with higher-level areas, in which the representation is determined in large part by learning. *When activated, these high-level visual representations are perceptual, in the sense that their activation comes from retinal input, and they are mnemonic in the sense that the pattern of weights responsible for their derivation is determined by experience* (in contrast to the smaller role of experience in setting the weights at earlier stages of visual processing). These same representations can also function in a purely mnemonic role when activated by internal means rather than retinal input, as is the case in mental imagery (Farah 1988, 2000). Thus, one could refer to a more perceptual end and a more mnemonic end of the sequence of representations supporting object recognition, but there is no dividing line where processing goes from perceptual to mnemonic.

Conclusions

Normal visual perception encompasses a series of encodings and re-encodings of the input, through different representations that make different aspects of the stimulus explicit. At the early stages, the nature of the representations is affected only minimally by learning and experience. At progressively later stages, learning plays a more important role in determining what is explicitly represented. The experience of having seen particular objects will shape what the later representations are most useful for representing. For example, having seen many faces of a given race equips these higher-level representations to represent these faces accurately. In that sense these representations embody memory. Yet they are also perceptual representations, in that a new and unfamiliar face of the same race will be processed by them.

The hypothesis being put forth here is that associative agnosia arises with damage to the later end of this continuum. This is broadly consistent with the reports of perceptual impairment reviewed earlier, although more directed attempts to test this hypothesis would be helpful. It is also consistent with the impairment of imagery, an ostensibly memory-based form of thought, in associative agnosia. Higher-level perceptual representations are not just active during perception, but also play a role in imagery (e.g. Farah 2000). So, in answer to the question 'Is associative visual agnosia an impairment of perception or memory?' one might well answer 'Yes!'

References

Albert, M.L., Soffer, D., Silverberg, R., and Reches, A. (1979). The anatomic basis of visual agnosia. *Neurology* 29, 876–9.

Benson, D.F. and Greenberg, J.P. (1969). Visual form agnosia. *Arch. Neurol.* 20, 82–9.

Brown, J.W. (1972). *Aphasia, apraxia and agnosia: clinical and theoretical aspects.* Charles C. Thomas, Springfield, Illinois.

Davidoff, J. and Wilson, B. (1985). A case of visual agnosia showing a disorder of pre-semantic visual classification. *Cortex* 21, 121–34.

Farah, M.J. (1988). Is visual imagery really visual? Overlooked evidence from neuropsychology. *Psychol. Rev.* 95, 307–17.

Farah, M.J. (1990). *Visual agnosia: disorders of object recognition and what they tell us about normal vision.* MIT Press/Bradford Books, Cambridge, Massachusetts.

Farah, M.J. (2000). *The cognitive neuroscience of vision.* Blackwell Publishers, Oxford.

Farah, M.J., Hammond, K.H., Levine, D.N., and Calvanio, R. (1988). Visual and spatial mental imagery: dissociable systems of representation. *Cogn. Psychol.* 20, 439–62.

Ferro, J.M. and Santos, M.E. (1984). Associative visual agnosia: a case study. *Cortex* 20, 121–34.

Hinton, G.E. and Shallice, T. (1991). Lesioning an attractor network: investigations of acquired dyslexia. *Psychol. Rev.* 98, 74–95.

Hodges, J.R., Patterson, K., Oxbury, S., and Funnell, E. (1992). Semantic dementia. *Brain* 115, 1783–806.

Humphreys, G.W. and Riddoch, M.J. (1987). *To see but not to see: a case study of visual agnosia.* Lawrence Erlbaum Associates, Hillsdale, New Jersey.

Levine, D.N. (1978). Prosopagnosia and visual object agnosia: a behavioral study. *Neuropsychologia* 5, 341–65.

Levine, D. and Calvanio, R. (1989). Prosopagnosia: a defect in visual configural processing. *Brain Cogn.* 10, 149–70.

Lissauer, H. (1890). Ein Fall von Seelenblindheit nebst einem Beitrage zur Theorie derselben. *Arch. Psychiatrie Nervenkrankh.* 21, 222–70.

Marr, D. (1982). *Vision.* San Fransisco: Freeman.

Martin, A. and Fedio, P. (1983). Word production and comprehension in Alzheimer's disease: the breakdown of semantic knowledge. *Brain Lang.* 19, 124–41.

Ratcliff, G. and Newcombe, F. (1982). Object recognition: some deductions from the clinical evidence. In *Normality and pathology in cognitive functions* (ed. A.W. Ellis). Academic Press, New York.

Riddoch, M.J. and Humphreys, G.W. (1987). Visual object processing in optic aphasia: a case of semantic access agnosia. *Cognitive Neuropsychology* 4, 131–85.

Rubens, A.B. and Benson, D.F. (1971). Associative visual agnosia. *Arch. Neurol.* 24, 305–16.

Shuttleworth, E.C., Syring, V., and Allen, N. (1982). Further observations on the nature of prosopagnosia. *Brain Cogn.* 1, 307–22.

Tippett, L.J. and Farah, M.J. (1994). A computational model of naming in Alzheimer's disease: unitary or multiple impairments? *Neuropsychology* 8, 3–13.

Wapner, W., Judd, T., and Gardner, H. (1978). Visual agnosia in an artist. *Cortex* 14, 343–64.

Warrington, E.K. (1985). Agnosia: the impairment of object recognition. In *Handbook of clinical neurology*, Vol. 45 (ed. P.J. Vinken, G.W. Bruyn, and H.L. Klawans), pp. 333–49. Elsevier, Amsterdam.

Williams, M. (1970). *Brain damage and the mind*. Penguin Books, Baltimore.

Part 6

Rehabilitation and recovery

Chapter 11

Recovery and rehabilitation of cerebral visual disorders

Josef Zihl

Introduction

About 30% of patients with acquired brain injury demonstrate deficits in vision (e.g. Hier *et al.* 1983*a*; Uzzell *et al.* 1988). In the majority of cases, the visual field is affected, but spatial contrast sensitivity and visual acuity, colour vision, visual space perception, visual object and face identification as well as recognition may also be impaired. In addition, specific impairments in visual spatial attention may result in the loss of visual perception in one hemispace, or in both, because of uni- or bilateral visual inattention.

The posterior brain is a patchwork of probably more than 30 functionally specialized visual areas with flexible networks to subserve complex visual abilities, e.g. visual spatial orientation and visual recognition. Despite this modular organization, selective visual disorders are rare because focal brain injury is only rarely limited to one single visual cortical area (for reviews, see Zeki 1993; Cowey 1994). Since cerebrovascular disorders (stroke, haemorrhage), trauma, and tumours are the most frequent underlying aetiologies, the resulting functional impairment as a rule is not restricted to just one visual deficit. Depending on the site and extent of brain injury, patients typically show a combination of several visual deficits. In accordance with the functional organization of the visual cortex (Ungerleider and Haxby 1998), it can be expected that occipitotemporal injuries affect the processing and thus perception of the 'what' properties (e.g. shape, colour) of visual stimuli and thus impair visual identification and recognition. Occipitoparietal injuries, on the other hand, affect the processing and thus perception of the 'where' properties (e.g. position, distance, spatial relationships between stimuli), and thus may impair the visual guidance of oculomotor and hand-motor activities as well as visual navigation.

Adequate vision is a crucial prerequisite for performance in many domains of behaviour, e.g. spatial orientation and navigation, learning and memory, and visual guidance of motor activities. Furthermore, rehabilitation outcome and vocational success depend critically on visual capacities (Reding and Potes 1988). For example, hemianopia, the most frequent visual deficit after brain injury, has been found to significantly affect the time and likelihood of achieving a level of functional outcome adequate for effective activities of daily living (Patel *et al.* 2000). Therefore, the diagnosis and treatment of cerebral visual deficits represent important components in neuropsychological rehabilitation settings. In the last few years there has been growing interest in research devoted to the rehabilitation of visual deficits. Concerning their effectiveness, procedures of treatment not only have to fulfil methodological criteria, but also criteria concerning the resulting benefits for the patient, i.e. a reduction of the degree of a patient's visual handicap (ecological validity) and cost-effectiveness.

This chapter is divided into four parts. The first contains a brief description of visual deficits after brain injury and the second describes observations on spontaneous recovery of vision. In the third and fourth parts the return of visual function using systematic practice and the improvement of visual efficiency by compensation strategies are presented and discussed.

Visual disorders after brain injury

The main visual disorders after acquired brain injury and their frequency of occurrence are summarized in Table 11.1.

Visual field disorders

These undoubtedly represent the largest group of visual disorders. Loss of vision in corresponding parts of both visual fields is called anopia, which signifies total loss of visual perception. Unilateral anopia results from contralateral injury to the retrogeniculate visual pathway including the striate cortex. It can be present in one hemifield (hemianopia), in one quadrant (quadranopia), or in a small part mainly in the paracentral visual field (paracentral scotoma). After bilateral retrogeniculate injury corresponding portions in either visual hemifield are affected. Typical forms are bilateral hemianopia ('tunnel vision'), bilateral upper or lower quadranopia, and bilateral paracentral scotomata. Loss of vision in the central region of the visual field (central scotoma) results from bilateral injury to the occipital pole, where the central visual field is represented, or to the portion

Table 11.1 Incidence of visual deficits after acquired brain injury (modified from Zihl 1994)

Deficit	Incidence (%)
Visual field	74.6
Spatial contrast sensitivity	26.0
Colour vision	6.5
Spatial vision	30–50
Visual recognition	< 5
Visual neglect	23
Balint's syndrome	< 5

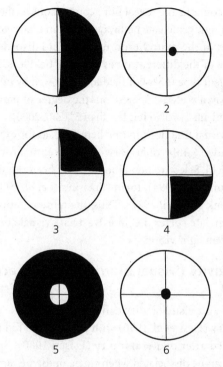

Fig. 11.1 Unilateral injury to the postchiasmatic visual pathways results in contralateral homonymous visual field defects (1–4). Bilateral injury causes bilateral homonymous field defects (5, 6). Regions of binocular visual loss are shown in black. 1, Hemianopia; 2, paracentral scotoma; 3, upper quadranopia; 4, lower quadranopia; 5, bilateral hemianopia (tunnel vision); 6, central scotoma.

Table 11.2 Incidence of homonymous visual field defects and of the underlying aetiology ($N = 636$; modified after Zihl 2000)

	Incidence (%)
Type of defect	
Unilateral ($n = 564$)	88.7
Hemianopia	73.2*
Quadranopia	18.1*
Paracentral scotoma	8.7*
Bilateral ($n = 72$)	11.3
Hemianopia	59.7[†]
Quadranopia	11.1[†]
Paracentral scotoma	15.3[†]
Central scotoma	13.9[†]
Aetiology	
Occipital cerebrovascular disease	76.1
Closed head trauma	11.3
Tumour (operated)	5.5
Hypoxia	3.9
Others	3.2

* Incidence among those with unilateral homonymous visual field defects.

† Incidence among those with bilateral homonymous visual field defects.

of the visual pathway which contains the foveal fibre connections to the striate cortex. Complete destruction of both retrogeniculate pathways results in total cerebral blindness. Figure 11.1 shows examples of the main homonymous field disorders. Table 11.2 gives details on the incidence of the different types of visual field loss. Homonymous hemianopia is the most frequent type (65%) of field loss, followed by quadranopia and paracentral scotomata. The fovea is always spared, but the degree of parafoveal sparing can vary; in the majority of patients (~75%) it is less than 5° (Zihl 2000).

Apart from the loss of all visual functions in one hemifield, as for example in hemianopia, vision may be degraded (amblyopia), or visual perceptual functions may be selectively lost in one hemifield. Selective hemianopias have been reported for colour (hemiachromatopsia; Paulson *et al.* 1994), form (Frassinetti *et al.* 1999), and movement (Plant *et al.* 1993; Schenk and Zihl 1997). Thus, the representation of the visual field exists also beyond the striate cortex, i.e. in extrastriate visual cortical areas, for stimulus dimensions other than light vision.

Spatial contrast sensitivity ('visual blurring'), visual acuity, and visual adaptation

Spatial contrast sensitivity and visual acuity can be impaired after either uni- or bilateral retrogeniculate injury (Hess *et al.* 1990) with pronounced reduction in visual acuity being mainly reported after bilateral injury (Frisén 1980). Spatial contrast sensitivity and visual acuity can be dissociated when single optotypes are used to assess visual acuity. Visual adaptation can also be affected after retrogeniculate injury. Patients may show either reduced light or dark adaptation, or both (Zihl and Kerkhoff 1990).

Colour vision

This can be impaired either in one hemifield (hemiachromatopsia) and partly in the fovea after left- or right-sided injury to the lingual and fusiform gyri, or can be impaired (cerebral dyschromatopsia) or lost (cerebral achromatopsia) in the entire hemifield when these structures are damaged in both hemispheres (Damasio *et al.* 1980; Paulson *et al.* 1994). Some patients also exhibit impaired selective colour constancy (Ruttiger *et al.* 1999).

Disorders in orienting in and exploring of visual space

These refer to impaired visual spatial abilities (e.g. inaccurate visual localization, deviation of visual vertical, horizontal, and straight-ahead axes, defective depth perception and stereopsis, visual spatial orientation), spatial knowledge concerning the actual or virtual (mental) environment, and restriction of spatial attention (visual neglect, Balint's syndrome; see below). Such disorders are common after occipitoparietal and posterior parietal injury, with a right-hemisphere damage more frequently causing deficits (for comprehensive reviews, see De Renzi 1982; Grüsser and Landis 1991; Karnath and Zihl 2001).

Visual agnosic disorders

These refer to the difficulty or inability of patients to visually identify familiar stimuli despite (sufficiently) preserved visual perceptual functions, cognitive capacities, and language. Recognition in another (e.g. auditory or tactile) modality is preserved. Visual *object agnosia* denotes the difficulty in identifying and recognizing objects, *prosopagnosia* refers to the loss of the ability to visually recognize familiar faces (including one's own face), *topographical agnosia* is used to describe various difficulties with geographical orientation, and *letter agnosia* (pure alexia) refers to the impaired identification of individual letters and of building words out of letters ('letter-by-letter reading'). In some cases, category-specific loss of visual recognition has been reported, but usually patients exhibit visual agnosias in more than one visual category (for a comprehensive review, see Grüsser and Landis 1991; see also Chapters 7 and 10, this volume). In its pure form, visual agnosia is a rare condition. Gloning *et al.* (1968) found only three cases (<1%) in a group of 241 patients. Typical sites of injury causing visual agnosia are in the region of the posterior and medial temporooccipital cortex, either bilateral or right-sided, except in the case of pure alexia, where the lesion site is the left-sided angular gyrus.

Visual spatial neglect

This is a lateralized disorder of space-related behaviour resulting mainly from right hemisphere injury predominantly involving the occipitoparietotemporal junction (Vallar and Perani 1986). This syndrome consists of a characteristic failure to explore the side of visual space contralateral to the lesion, and to react or respond to stimuli or subjects located on this side (Karnath *et al.* 1998). In the acute stage, such patients behave as if one side of the surrounding space had ceased to exist. The patients are not aware that they suffer from this disorder.

Balint's syndrome

Patients with Balint's syndrome typically have difficulties in perceiving the visual environment that is normally covered by the binocular field as a whole, because their field of attention is severely restricted, and in perceiving more than one stimulus at a time within the spared field of attention. In addition, they have difficulties in shifting their gaze voluntarily or on command, and in directing the movement of an extremity using visual guidance. As a consequence, visually guided oculomotor and hand motor activities, visuoconstructive abilities, and visual orientation and recognition, including reading, are severely impaired (Ghika *et al.* 1998). Patients with this syndrome may also exhibit severe visual disorientation and defective depth perception, either secondary to the attentional and oculomotor deficits, or as associated visual impairments (Karnath and Zihl 2001).

Summary

Table 11.3 summarizes possible effects of the visual deficits described in this section on various abilities depending crucially on particular visual functions. It becomes evident

Table 11.3 Effects of visual deficits on visual performance

Deficit	Impaired visual capacities
Visual field	Overview, exploration, navigation, reading
Contrast sensitivity, acuity	Depth perception, stereopsis, reading, visual identification and recognition; visually guided motor activities (e.g. drawing, reaching, grasping, walking)
Visual adaptation	Space perception, reading, visual identification and recognition
Colour vision	Visual identification and recognition
Spatial vision	Visual orientation and navigation; visually guided motor activities (e.g. drawing, reaching, grasping, walking)
Visual identification/recognition	Recognition of objects, faces, letters
Visual attention	Detection of stimuli in the contralateral hemispace (unilateral inattention) or the contra- and ipsilateral hemispace (bilateral inattention); visual orientation and navigation; visually guided motor activities (e.g. drawing, reaching, grasping, walking); visual identification, reading

that especially visual overview and visual orientation, visual identification and recognition, and reading can be impaired not only when the underlying visual capacities and abilities are impaired themselves (e.g. visual space perception, visual cognition), but also when crucial prerequisites (e.g. visual field, contrast sensitivity and visual acuity, visual spatial attention) are affected.

Spontaneous recovery of cerebral visual disorders

Visual field disorders

Spontaneous recovery of vision in patients with anopia has been frequently reported; it typically takes place within 2–3 months postinjury. The frequency and amount of recovery appears, however, to be limited. About 15% of patients may show recovery of visual field in the range of 3–24 degrees, with an average of about 5 degrees (Zihl 2000). In only 4 of 225 patients (<2%) was complete recovery observed. Recovery from complete cerebral blindness also may take place within 8–12 weeks after the onset of blindness; however, in some cases it can last for up to 2 years. About 30% of 111 patients reported in the literature showed recovery. In four of them complete return of vision was observed. In the rest recovery ranged from a return of 'crude' light vision to recovery of visual field portions with or without colour and form vision. Typically vision returns first in the

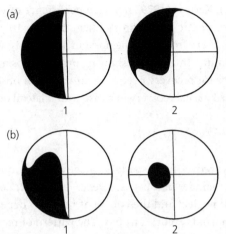

Fig. 11.2 Examples of spontaneous visual field recovery after a right occipital stroke. (a) A 52-year-old patient. Visual fields were taken: 1, 1 week after stroke; 2, 6 months after stroke. (b) A 66-year-old patient. Visual fields were taken: 1, 2 weeks after stroke; 2, 3 weeks after stroke. (a) Note return of vision in left lower quadrant. (b) Vision has returned in the entire hemifield, resulting in a large paracentral scotoma.

central field region. Visual acuity and contrast vision may return to a degree that is sufficient for visual recognition and reading, but may also remain persistently reduced to finger counting and 'blurred vision'. In patients with spontaneous recovery from partial or total blindness, damage to the striate cortex may not have been irreversible, because they show residual striate cortex metabolism and preserved pattern-generated visual evoked potentials (Celesia *et al.* 1980; Bosley *et al.* 1987; Wunderlich *et al.* 2000). Figure 11.2 shows examples of spontaneous visual field recovery.

Contrast vision, visual adaptation, and colour vision

Although recovery of spatial contrast sensitivity has been observed in single cases (e.g. Bodis-Wollner 1972), spontaneous return does not seem to be the rule (Hess *et al.* 1990). Defective visual adaptation persists over years and appears irreversible (Zihl and Kerkhoff 1990). Complete spontaneous recovery of colour vision within 6 months has been reported after carbon monoxide poisoning (Fine and Parker 1996). In cases with cerebral achromatopsia due to bilateral strokes, no recovery of colour vision has been observed over a period of 6 years (Pearlman *et al.* 1979). In a recent study, however, partial recovery of colour vision has been observed after 3 years (Spillmann *et al.* 2000).

Visual spatial capacities

Meerwaldt (1983) found some evidence for the recovery of perception of visual vertical and horizontal axes within 6 months. Hier *et al.* (1983*b*) reported recovery from visuospatial deficits within 15 weeks after stroke in about 70% of 41 patients.

Visual agnosia

Adler (1950) reported only minimal recovery within 5 years in a patient with visual agnosia due to carbon monoxide poisoning. About 40 years later her status was essentially unchanged (Sparr *et al.* 1991). Kertesz (1979) reported persistence of visual agnosia in a patient with bilateral traumatic brain injury for more than 10 years. Wilson and Davidoff (1993) found recovery from visual agnosia in a patient 10 years after she had sustained a severe head injury. In a patient showing prosopagnosia, Bruyer *et al.* (1983) could find no evidence for recovery over a 1-year period of observation, but Spillmann *et al.* (2000) reported partial recovery in a case with bilateral occipital stroke after 3 years.

Visual spatial neglect

About two-thirds of patients recover from spatial neglect within 6 months, but the symptoms of neglect in the remainder may persist (Denes *et al.* 1982; Zoccolotti *et al.* 1989). The severity of spatial neglect and the course of recovery depend on lesion size and the presence of premorbid cerebral atrophy. The pattern of recovery may be different for different behavioural deficits of spatial neglect. In the recovered stage of the disorder, neglect for the contralateral hemispace may still occur in situations in which two stimuli appear simultaneously. In these situations, the patients orient towards the stimulus on the ipsilesional side and neglect that on the contralesional side (for a review, see Karnath and Zihl 2001).

Balint's syndrome

Patients exhibiting this syndrome may show improved visual orientation and oculo-motor scanning of the surroundings within a few months up to some years, while reading and simultaneous processing of multiple stimuli may remain impaired (Allison *et al.* 1969; Trivelli *et al.* 1996).

Summary

Summarizing the reports on spontaneous recovery of visual capacities after brain injury, it can be stated that complete or partial spontaneous recovery does occur. In the majority of patients, however, the disorders persist. It is not entirely clear why spontaneous recovery does not take place more often, but certainly a critical amount of sparing of neurons and of interconnectivity in the affected structure of the visual brain subserving the visual function or capacity in question is required. Possibly, the efficiency of functioning can be supported by systematic practice at least in some cases without spontaneous recovery, thus also leading to recovery of function. Thus, procedures of training are required either to stimulate and support recovery of function or to bypass the irreversibly lost function(s) by substitution using compensatory strategies.

Recovery of visual function by specific training

As was shown in the last section, spontaneous recovery of visual function signifies recovery of the visual function or capacity that was lost or at least impaired by brain injury. Recovery of function by training or practice basically means the same. The function in question, which does not show any recovery at all, or returns only to a limited degree, does return during or after a period of practice specifically addressing this deficit. In the case of elementary and thus rather well defined visual functions, e.g. visual field, spatial contrast sensitivity, visual spatial abilities, or colour vision, training procedures can be developed that may specifically influence these functions. In contrast, in the case of complex visual capacities, e.g. visual orientation, visual identification and recognition, or visual spatial attention, the demonstration of recovery appears more difficult, because the underlying neural network consists of several components. In an individual patient showing a complex visual disorder, it may be impossible to entangle these different components and to decide which one(s) is (are) affected, and which spared, or which component should be improved first. This difficulty is even more pronounced in patients with a combination of elementary and complex visual deficits. This may explain why little experimental evidence is available especially on recovery of complex visual capacities after training. There is no proven golden rule as to how to proceed, but a reasonable and successful guideline may be to compose appropriate methodology and knowledge about the functional organization of the brain in general, and the visual brain in particular. In addition, it appears especially useful to consider basic rules of perceptual learning (Zihl 2000; Fahle and Poggio 2001). In this context a sensible heuristic tool is to predict the outcome on the basis of the known interdependencies and interactions of elementary and complex visual capacities. If, for example, in a patient with paracentral visual field loss or reduced contrast sensitivity, reading is impaired, then this impairment can either be explained by the visual field loss or by the reduction in contrast sensitivity. If the first assumption is correct, then reducing the impairing factor (i.e. the visual field loss) should lead to an improvement in reading without further training. If the second assumption holds true, then training of spatial contrast sensitivity is required. A similar consideration may be helpful when confronted with a complex disorder. For example, a patient's difficulty in visually recognizing objects may result from defective selection of features that characterize certain objects, or defective integration of several object features into a gestalt, or both (which may be difficult to diagnose). The training of selection procedures should lead to recovery of this complex visual ability only if selection is impaired. Otherwise, either feature integration has to be trained, or both selection and integration require specific practice.

Visual field deficits

Visual field loss has attracted the most research interest. One possible reason for this is that highly valid and reliable quantitative methods are available to measure this visual deficit. Another reason is that comparable visual field defects have been produced in primates, and spontaneous recovery as well as recovery by systematic practice have been studied in detail (Cowey and Weiskrantz 1963; Mohler and Wurtz 1977). Thus, there was substantial support for the assumption that vision may also recover in anopic field regions in humans when we (Zihl and von Cramon 1979; Zihl 1981)

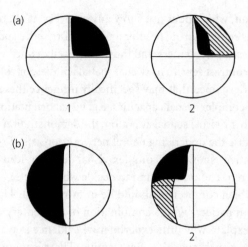

Fig. 11.3 Visual field recovery after systematic practice with saccadic eye movements in two patients showing unilateral occipital stroke. (a) In this 54-year-old patient the visual fields (1) were taken 8 weeks after the stroke; no spontaneous recovery was observed during this period. After 280 trials (2) vision returned (hatched area) in the right upper quadrant. (b) In this 66-year-old patient the visual fields (1) were taken 13 weeks after the stroke; no spontaneous recovery was observed during this period. After 340 trials (2) vision returned (hatched area) in the left lower quadrant. For both patients vision in the peripheral parts remained depressed.

presented the first empirical evidence. The methods of training were based on experimental work in primates, and consisted of a close link between visual attention focused on the field region subjected to practice, and the detection or saccadic localization of a light target presented at the visual field border or within the anopic region. The patient had either to indicate the presence of the target or to shift the gaze to that position in the anopic field region where he guessed that the target may have appeared. In the latter condition, presentation time was always shorter (100 ms) than saccadic latency. Patients were never informed about the correctness of their response. Figure 11.3 shows examples of visual field recovery. Interestingly, visual field recovery was only observed in periods of training and not in intervals without training. Thus recovery was strongly linked to specific practice and did not result, e.g. from delayed spontaneous recovery. In addition, not only light but also colour and form vision returned in many patients indicating that visual information could be conveyed again to exstrastriate visual cortical areas not affected by the lesion.

The explanation that recovery was found in some but not in all patients was based on the assumption that recovery may only take place in patients with reversible neuronal loss and sparing of function—the work of Bosley *et al.* (1987) supports this idea. Since, in our patients, the time elapsed between the onset of the hemianopia and the onset of specific training varied between 1 and 28 months, a further assumption is needed to explain recovery. Visual cortical neurons may have survived at the border zone of the lesion but may still not (fully) be engaged in visual processing. Although this issue has not been studied systematically, there is evidence that this hypothesis might be valid. Spontaneous and training-induced recovery of visual field regions has been reported even 16 and 28 months postonset, respectively (Zihl and von Cramon 1985; Poggel *et al.* 2001). In addition, visual field recovery was only found in patients with some sparing of light vision at the border between the intact field and the blind field. In this zone, thresholds for light detection were found to be particularly sensitive to attention (Zihl and von Cramon 1979). These observations may be taken as evidence that the transition zone may indeed represent residual neuronal function that can be modulated by attentional processes (Zihl and von Cramon 1985). Some authors have confirmed these results using similar methods of practice (Kerkhoff *et al.* 1992*a,b*; van der Wildt and Bergsma 1997; Kasten *et al.* 1998, 2000), but others have not (Balliett *et al.* 1985; Pommerenke and Markowitsch 1989). One main reason for the negative findings lies certainly in the (incorrect) assumption that every patient demonstrating a homonymous visual field defect also shows recovery of vision after training. As pointed out, only patients with spared neuronal activity in the striate cortex can be expected to do so (Zihl and von Cramon 1985). Thus, 'local plasticity' in terms of spared neurons ('silent neurons') surviving the injury does not exist in all patients and, without plasticity, no recovery of vision can be expected (Potthoff 1995; Sabel 1999; Kerkhoff 2000).

Although the results on recovery of visual field from scotoma look very promising, their behavioural significance remains to be examined. Rehabilitation first of all signifies a reduction in the degree of handicap in everyday life. In the case of visual field loss this should imply expanded view over the surroundings, fast and reliable detection of stimuli in all regions of the visual field, and normal reading performance. Thus, visual field enlargement has to reach a certain degree; otherwise it does not reduce the patient's disability. For normal reading performance, at least 5° in the left and 6–7° in the right hemifield are required (Zihl 1995*b*). For a sufficient overview, at least a field extent of 20° on either side is required; otherwise visual orientation and navigation remain impaired (Lovie-Kitchin *et al.* 1990). Admittedly, only a very small number of patients (6 of 44, or 14%) had a visual field with a size of at least 20° after training. The number of patients with at least 5° on the affected side of the fovea was larger (15 of 32, or 47%); these patients showed significantly improved reading after training (Zihl and von Cramon 1985).

Spatial contrast sensitivity

There is preliminary evidence that spatial contrast sensitivity can be improved after systematic training of spatial resolution. Practice with discrimination of spatial frequencies not only increases contrast sensitivity, but is associated with an increase in visual acuity and reading performance (Zihl 2000).

Colour vision

Perception of colour hues in patients with severely impaired foveal colour vision can be improved by systematic practice with hue discrimination (Zihl 2000).

Visual spatial capacities

Specific practice with position and distance estimation, discrimination of line length and line orientation, and discrimination of spatial axes has been reported to represent an effective means for recovery of these spatial abilities at least in some patients (Lütgehetmann and Stäbler 1992).

Visual agnosia

The first evidence of successful treatment of visual agnosic patients was presented by Poppelreuter (1917/1990). In a more recent attempt (Zihl 2000), the essential prerequisites for identifying and recognizing complex visual stimuli were trained in two patients with severe visual agnosia for objects, faces, scenes, and letters. Specific practice procedures included processing and selection of relevant features, and the use of cognitive strategies to supervise and control these processes. After training, both patients showed a significant improvement in visual identification and recognition (including naming) for all stimulus categories used in practice, but one patient still showed prosopagnosia. Thus visual agnosia may also show recovery and patients may regain, at least in part, the ability to visually recognize stimuli.

Visual neglect

Since the main symptom of visual spatial neglect is an absent or at least reduced exploration of contralesional space, the main treatment is based on procedures to direct orientation towards this side. These procedures aim to enlarge the field of attention in the affected hemispace and thus enhance exploration towards this side by training the patient to perform eye or hand movements to the impaired side. In this way, contra-lesional shifts of attention and visual exploration are improved (for a review, see Karnath and Zihl 2001). Because of the widespread neural network subserving visual spatial attention and visually guided activities in space (e.g. Mesulam 2000), it is not entirely clear whether the effect can be interpreted as recovery from visual neglect or as circumvention of the underlying visual-attentional disorder by learning compensatory strategies. In functional terms, the return of attention and of visually guided oculomotor and hand motor activities in the affected hemispace can certainly be understood as recovery.

Balint's syndrome

In three patients suffering from severe Balint's syndrome, specific practice with the initiation and execution of gaze shifts, with shifting attention and fixation to stimuli outside the actual field of attention, and reaching or grasping for them resulted in an enlargement of the field of attention and of the range of oculomotor and handmotor

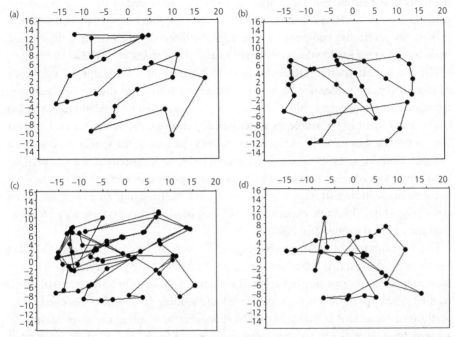

Fig. 11.4 Oculomotor scanning patterns (infrared eye movement recordings) during inspection of a scene. (a) A 42-year-old normal subject (scanning time, 12.8 s). (b) A 53-year-old patient with left-sided hemianopia (field sparing, 3°) and spontaneous adaptation to the field loss (scanning time, 13.4 s). (c), (d) A 47-year-old patient with left-sided homonymous hemianopia (field sparing, 3°) without spontaneous adaptation (c) before (scanning time, 26.5 s) and (d) after (scanning time, 11.4 s) specific practice with visual scanning. x-axis, horizontal extension of stimulus field (40°); y-axis, vertical extension (32°). 0, Centre; negative values, left and down; positive values, right and up. Dots indicate fixation (duration > 100 ms) positions.

activities. This enlargement also led to an improved visual spatial orientation as well as object and scene identification (Zihl 2000).

Substitution of visual capacities by compensatory strategies

Oculomotor compensation of visual field defects

Compensation of visual field defects is mainly based on regaining of effective oculomotor gaze shifts to the visual environment into the region of visual field loss and on improving reading eye movements. Hemianopic patients may show short-term improvements in visual scanning (Zangemeister *et al.* 1995), but this adaptation is typically present in familiar surroundings only. The great majority of patients (about 80%) has difficulty in gaining a quick and complete overview, especially in unfamiliar surroundings. They have problems avoiding obstacles and with reading even several weeks after the onset of the visual field loss. These difficulties are mirrored by their eye movement patterns (Zihl 1995*a*; Pambakian *et al.* 2000; see Fig. 11.4). Interestingly, about 10–15% of patients show effective compensation strategies without any treatment; in these cases, brain injury is restricted to the optic radiation and/or the striate cortex (Zihl 1995*a,b*).

The first stage in training efficient oculomotor behaviour is to enlarge the amplitude of saccadic eye movements, which enables the patient to cover the entire visual surroundings with a few gaze shifts. This information can then be used to visually guide oculomotor scanning movements systematically through the actual scene. The next stage is the adaptation of the oculomotor scanning pattern to the spatial structure of a complex stimulus array using, e.g. visual search tasks. After systematic practice patients used larger saccadic eye movements and a more systematic and spatially organized oculomotor scanning strategy, and required less time to scan even a complex visual scene (Fig. 11.4). This improvement was still present when patients were tested 6 weeks after the end of training (Zihl 2000).

The improvement of reading in patients with less than 5° of field sparing (so-called hemianopic dyslexia) is based on the compensation of the visual field loss by eye movements. As was mentioned earlier, these patients have difficulties especially with reading. Their speed of reading is decreased and reading is often also inaccurate. The method of treatment is basically one of reorganizing reading eye movements. To achieve this goal, patients with left-sided field loss are forced to shift their gaze first of all to the beginning of the line and the first letter of every single word in the line, whereas patients with right-sided field loss have to shift their gaze to the end of the word. Thus, in both instances, patients are instructed to intentionally perceive the whole word before reading it. After systematic training, patients show a significant increase in the speed of reading and a decrease in the number of errors. As shown by eye movement recordings, the improvement can indeed mainly be explained in terms of adaptation of the eye movement pattern, which, after practice, consisted of fewer fixations, larger saccadic jumps, and shorter fixation periods (Fig. 11.5; Zihl 1995*b*). Because of our left-to-right orthography, patients with right-sided field loss require more training sessions than do patients with left-sided field loss. Follow-up testing for up to 2 years revealed either a further improvement or at least the maintenance of the level of reading performance after treatment.

Optical aids

Mirror spectacles or prism systems may have a positive effect in overcoming the field loss (e.g. Rossi *et al.* 1990). Using a high-power prism segment in 12 patients, Peli (2000) reported an improvement in patients' visually guided behaviour. The usefulness of optical aids under defined everyday life conditions has still to be proven.

Visual agnosia

The conventional way of circumventing the inability to visually recognize objects and people is to teach the patient to use context information and to reorganize his/her visual perception with intact kinaesthetic information (e.g. Tanemura 1999).

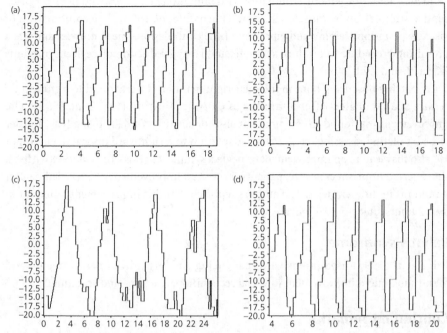

Fig. 11.5 The subjects in parts (a)–(d) of this figure are the same as those in Fig. 11.4 (a)–(d), respectively. Reading eye movements (infrared eye movement recordings): (a) in a normal subject; (b) in a patient with spontaneous adaptation; (c), (d) in a patient without spontaneous adaptation (c) before and (d) after specific practice with reading. Note the typical staircase pattern of fixations and saccadic jumps in (a) and (b), the interruptions in (c) and the improvement in (d). Reading performance (in words per minute, wpm) was: (a) 169 wpm; (b) 132 wpm; (c) 64 wpm; (d) 112 wpm. x-axis, time period of recording (s); y-axis, horizontal position of eye. 0, Centre; negative values, left; −20, beginning of the line.

Visual neglect

While recovery from visual neglect is based on training procedures demanding active orientation of the eyes, head, trunk, and hands towards the contralesional side, motor activation of the left-sided limbs can be used (Robertson and North 1993). In a larger group of acute stroke patients, this technique was found to shorten the length of hospital stay (Kalra *et al.* 1997). Unfortunately, this procedure does not seem to induce lasting effects. It has repeatedly been shown that even forced cueing is only transiently effective. Cueing procedures using visual stimuli (e.g. Antonucci *et al.* 1995), transcutaneous electrical stimulation (Pizzamiglio *et al.* 1996), or the verbal instruction to attend to the neglected side did not reveal lasting reduction of contralesional neglect (for a review, see Karnath and Zihl 2001).

Several studies have demonstrated a substantial, though transient reduction of visual neglect symptoms by different sensory stimulations via the peripheral pathways contributing to higher-order representations of space, such as vestibular stimulation

(Rubens 1985), optokinetic stimulation (Pizzamiglio *et al.* 1990), and neck proprioceptive stimulation by muscle vibration (Karnath *et al.* 1993). The combination of visual exploration training and vibration of the contralesional neck muscles appears a promising procedure to produce a specific and lasting reduction of neglect symptoms (Karnath and Zihl 2001).

Eye patches obscuring both monocular right hemifields were found to significantly reduce spatial neglect after 3 months of daily application (Beis *et al.* 1999). The improvement was found for reading, but also for activities of daily living (e.g. transfer to bed, toileting, dressing, etc.). Prism adaptation to a rightward optical deviation of 10° also may lead to an improvement of neglect symptoms (Rossetti *et al.* 1998). After a short period of prism exposure, patients showed an improvement of left-sided neglect symptoms in different tests. The authors reported that this improvement lasted for at least 2 hours after prism removal.

Balint's syndrome

Perez *et al.* (1996) used intensive verbal cueing and 'organizational strategies' and found subsequent improvement in visual recognition, reaching, and scanning.

Concluding remarks

There is evidence that visual deficits caused by acquired brain injury can spontaneously recover, at least to a certain degree. In a small number of patients spontaneous recovery can also be complete, or can at least reach a level sufficient for reducing the patient's visual handicap. There is further evidence that specific training can support functional recovery, although the underlying mechanisms are not exactly known. Of course, the incidence of a visual deficit as well as the percentage of recovered patients strongly depend on the measures used to diagnose and follow up this deficit. In the case of irreversible functional loss or impairment, the acquisition of compensatory strategies allows the substitution of the affected function or capacity by other means. This typically means the adaptation of either oculomotor or of cognitive activities involved in the particular function or capacity, or both. Many of the procedures described in this chapter still have an experimental character, but they represent a first step in developing more sophisticated procedures to reduce visual deficits or their consequences. What seems important is that training procedures address the deficit as specifically as possible (which also implies its specific assessment), and are carried out in a highly systematic way to enhance the acquisition process. It has to be kept in mind, however, that the use of the term rehabilitation always has to also imply measures beyond the narrow field of training and practice, which may not always be sufficient in reducing the degree of visual handicap (for a review, see Kerkhoff 2000).

References

Adler, A. (1950). Course and outcome of visual agnosia. *J. Nerv. Ment. Dis.* 3, 41–51.

Allison, R.S., Hurwitz, L.J., White, G.J., and Wilmot, T.J. (1969). A follow-up study of a patient with Balint's syndrome. *Neuropsychologia* 7, 319–33.

Antonucci, G., Guariglia, C., Judica, A., Magnotti, L., Poalucci, S., Pizzamiglio, L., and Zoccolotti, P. (1995). Effectiveness of neglect rehabilitation in a randomized group study. *J. Clin. Exp. Neuropsychol.* 17, 383–9.

Balliett, R., Blood, K.M.T., and Bach-y-Rita, P. (1985). Visual field rehabilitation in the cortically blind? *J. Neurol. Neurosurg. Psychiatry* 46, 426–9.

Beis, J.-M., André, J.-M., Baumgarten, A., and Challier, B. (1999). Eye patching in unilateral spatial neglect: efficacy of two methods. *Arch. Phys. Med. Rehabil.* 80, 71–6.

Bodis-Wollner, I. (1972). Visual acuity and contrast sensitivity in patients with cerebral lesions. *Science* 178, 769–71.

Bosley, T.M., Dann, R., Silver, F.L., Alavi, A., Kushner, M., Chawluck, J.B., Savi, P.J., Sergott, R.C., Schatz, N.J., and Raivich, M. (1987). Recovery of vision after ischemic lesions: positron emission tomography. *Ann. Neurol.* 21, 444–50.

Bruyer, R., Laterre, C., Seron, X., Feyereisen, P., Strypstein, E., Pierrard, E., and Rectem, D. (1983). A case of prosopagnosia with some preserved covered remembrance of familiar faces. *Brain Cogn.* 2, 257–84.

Celesia, G.G., Archer, C.R., Kuroiwa, Y., and Goldfader, P.R. (1980). Visual function of the extrageniculo-calcarine system in man: relationship of cortical blindness. *Arch. Neurol.* 37, 704–6.

Cowey, A. (1994). Cortical visual areas and the neurobiology of higher visual processes. In *The neuropsychology of high-level vision* (ed. M. Farah and G. Ratcliff), pp. 3–31. Lawrence Erlbaum Associates, Hillsdale, New Jersey.

Cowey, A. and Weiskrantz, L. (1963). A perimetric study of visual field defects in monkeys. *Quart. J. Exp. Psychol.* 15, 91–115.

Damasio, A.R., Yamada, T., Damasio, H., and McKee, J. (1980). Central achromatopsia: behavioral, anatomic, physiological aspects. *Neurology* 30, 1064–71.

Denes, G., Semenza, C., Stoppa, E., and Lis, A. (1982). Unilateral spatial neglect and recovery from hemiplegia—a follow-up study. *Brain* 105, 543–52.

De Renzi, E. (1982). *Disorders of space exploration and cognition.* Wiley, Chicester.

Fahle, M. and Poggio, T. (2001). *Perceptual learning.* MIT Press, Cambridge, Massachusetts.

Fine, R.D. and Parker, G.D. (1996). Disturbance of central vision after carbon monoxide poisoning. *Aus. NZ J. Ophthalmol.* 24, 137–41.

Frassinetti, F., Nichelli, P., and di Pellegrino, G. (1999). Selective horizontal dysmetropsia following prestriate lesion. *Brain* 122, 339–50.

Frisén, L. (1980). The neurology of visual acuity. *Brain* 103, 639–70.

Ghika, J., Ghika-Schmid, F., and Bogousslavsky, J. (1998). Parietal motor syndrome: a clinical description in 32 patients in the acute phase of pure parietal stroke studied prospectively. *Clin. Neurol. Neurosurg.* 100, 271–82.

Gloning, I., Gloning, K., and Hoff, H. (1968). *Neuropsychological symptoms and syndromes in lesions of the occipital lobe and adjacent areas.* Gauthier-Villars, Paris.

Grüsser, O.-J. and Landis, Th. (1991). *Visual agnosias and other disturbances of visual perception and cognition.* CRC Press, Boca Raton, Florida.

Hess, R.F., Zihl, J., Pointer, S., and Schmid, C. (1990). The contrast sensitivity deficit in cases with cerebral lesions. *Clin. Vision Sci.* 5, 203–15.

Hier, D.B., Mondlock, J., and Caplan, L.R. (1983a). Behavioral abnormalities after right hemisphere stroke. *Neurology* 33, 337–44.

Hier, D.B., Mondlock, J., and Caplan, L.R. (1983b). Recovery of behavioural abnormalities after right hemisphere stroke. *Neurology* 33, 345–50.

Kalra, L., Perez, I., Gupta, S., and Wittink, M. (1997). The influence of visual neglect on stroke rehabilitation. *Stroke* 28, 1386–91.

Karnath, H.-O. and Zihl, J. (2001). Disorders of spatial orientation. In *Therapy and course of neurological disorder* (ed. Th. Brandt, L.R. Caplan, J. Dichgans, H.C. Diener, and C. Kennard). Academic Press, San Diego, in press.

Karnath, H.-O., Christ, K., and Hartje, W. (1993). Decrease of contralateral neglect by neck muscle vibration and spatial orientation of trunk midline. *Brain* 116, 383–96.

Karnath, H.-O., Niemeier, M., and Dichgans, J. (1998). Space exploration in neglect. *Brain* 121, 2357–67.

Kasten, E., Wust, S., Behrensbaumann, W., and Sabel, B.A. (1998). Computer-based training for the treatment of partial blindness. *Nat. Med.* 4, 1083–7.

Kasten, E., Poggel, D.A., and Sabel, B.A. (2000). Computer-based training of stimulus detection improves color and simple pattern recognition in the defective field of hemianopic subjects. *J. Cogn. Neurosci.* 12, 1001–12.

Kerkhoff, G. (2000). Neurovisual rehabilitation: recent developments and future directions. *J. Neurol. Neurosurg. Psychiatry* 68, 691–706.

Kerkhoff, G., Münsinger, U., Haaf, E., Eberle-Strauss, G., and Stögerer, E. (1992a). Rehabilitation of homonymous scotomata in patients with postgeniculate damage of the visual system: Saccadic compensation training. *Restor. Neurol. Neurosci.* 4, 245–54.

Kerkhoff, G., Münsinger, U., Eberle-Strauss, G., and Stögerer, E. (1992b). Rehabilitation of hemi-anopic dyslexia in patients with postgeniculate field disorders. *Neuropsychol. Rehabil.* 2, 21–42.

Kertesz, A. (1979). Visual agnosia: the dual deficit of perception and recognition. *Cortex* 15, 403–19.

Lovie-Kitchin, J., Mainstone, J.M., Riobinson, J., and Brown, B. (1990). What areas of the visual field are important for mobility in low vision patients? *Clin. Vision Sci.* 5, 249–63.

Lütgehetmann, R. and Stäbler, M. (1992). Deficiences of visual spatial orientation: diagnostic and therapy of brain damaged patients [in German]. *Z. Neuropsychol.* 3, 130–42.

Meerwaldt, J.D. (1983). Spatial disorientation in right-hemisphere infarction: a study of the speed of recovery. *J. Neurol. Neurosurg. Psychiatry* 46, 426–9.

Mesulam, M.-M. (2000). Attentional networks, confusional states, and neglect syndromes. In *Principles of behavioral and cognitive neurology* (ed. M.-M. Mesulam), pp. 174–256. Oxford University Press, Oxford.

Mohler, C.W. and Wurtz, R.H. (1977). Role of striate cortex and superior colliculus in visual guidance of saccadic eye movements in monkeys. *J. Neurophysiol.* 40, 74–94.

Pambakian, A.L.M., Wooding, D.S., Patel, N., Morland, A.B., Kennard, C., and Mannan, S.K. (2000). Scanning the visual world: a study of patients with homonymous hemianopia. *J. Neurol. Neurosurg. Psychiatry* 69, 751–9.

Patel, A.T., Duncan, P.W., Lai, S.M., and Studenski, S. (2000). The relation between impairments and functional outcomes poststroke. *Arch. Phys. Med. Rehabil.* 81, 1357–63.

Paulson, H.L, Galetta, S.L., Grossman, M., and Alavi, A. (1994). Hemiachromatopsia of unilateral occipitotemporal infarcts. *Am. J. Ophthalmol.* 118, 518–23.

Pearlman, A.L., Birch, J., and Meadows, J.C. (1979). Cerebral color blindness. An acquired defect in hue discrimination. *Ann. Neurol.* 5, 253–61.

Peli, E. (2000). Field expansion for homonymous hemianopia by optically induced peripheral exotropia. *Optometry Vis. Sci.* 77, 453–64.

Perez, F.M., Tunkel, R.S., Lachmann, E.A., and Nagler, W. (1996). Balint's syndrome arising from bilateral posterior cortical atrophy or infarction—rehabilitation strategies and their limitation. *Disabil. Rehabil.* 18, 300–4.

Pizzamiglio, L., Frasca, R., Guariglia, C., Incoccia, C., and Antonucci, G. (1990). Effect of optokinetic stimulation in patients with visual neglect. *Cortex* 26, 535–40.

Pizzamiglio, L, Vallar, G., and Magnotti, L. (1996). Transcutaneous electrical stimulation of the neck muscles and hemineglect rehabilitation. *Restor. Neurol. Neurosci.* 10, 197–203.

Plant, G.T., Laxer, K.D., Barbaro, N.M., Schiffman, J.S., and Nakayama, K. (1993). Impaired visual motion perception in the contralateral hemifield following unilateral posterior cerebral lesions in humans. *Brain* 116, 1303–35.

Poggel, D.A., Kasten, E., Müller-Oehring, E.M., Sabel, B.A., and Brandt, S.A. (2001). Unusual spontaneous and training induced visual field recovery in a patient with a gunshot lesion. *J. Neurol. Neurosurg. Psychiatry* 70, 236–9.

Pommerenke, K. and Markowitsch, J.H. (1989). Rehabilitation training of homonymous visual field defects in patients with postgeniculate damage to the visual system. *Restor. Neurol. Neurosci.* 1, 47–63.

Poppelreuter, W. (1917/1990). *Disturbances of lower and higher visual capacities caused by occipital damage* [transl. J. Zihl and L. Weiskrantz]. Clarendon Press, Oxford.

Potthoff, R.D. (1995). Regeneration of specific nerve cells in lesioned visual cortex of the human brain—an indirect evidence after constant stimulation with different spots of light. *J. Neurosci. Res.* 40, 787–96.

Reding, M.J. and Potes, E. (1988). Rehabilitation outcome following initial unilateral hemispheric stroke. Life table analysis approach. *Stroke* 19, 1354–8.

Robertson, I.H. and North, N. (1993). Active and passive activation of left limbs: influence on visual and sensory neglect. *Neuropsychologia*, 31, 293–300.

Rossetti, Y., Rode, G., Pisella, L, Farné, A., Ling, L., Boisson, D., and Perenin, M.-T. (1998). Prism adaptation to a rightward optical deviation rehabilitates left hemispatial neglect. *Nature* 395, 166–9.

Rossi, P.W., Kheyfets, S., and Reding, M. (1990). Fresnal lens improve visual perception in stroke patients with homonymous hemianopia or unilateral visual neglect. *Neurology*, 40, 1587–99.

Rubens, A.B. (1985). Caloric stimulation and unilateral visual neglect. *Neurology* 35, 1019–24.

Ruttiger, L., Braun, D.I., Gegenfurtner, K.R., Petersen, D. Sconle, P., and Sharpe L.T. (1999). Selective color constancy deficits after circumscribed unilateral brain lesions. *J. Neurosci.* 19, 3094–106.

Sabel, B.A. (1999). Restoration of vision I: neurobiological mechanisms of restoration and plasticity after brain damage—a review. *Restor. Neurol. Neurosci.* 15, 177–200.

Schenk, T. and Zihl, J. (1997). Visual motion perception after brain damage: I. Deficits in global motion perception. *Neuropsychologia*, 35, 1289–97.

Sparr, S.A., Jay, M., Drislane, F.W., and Venna, N. (1991). A historic case of visual agnosia revisited after 40 years. *Brain* 114, 789–800.

Spillmann, L., Iskowski, W., Lange, K.W., Kasper, E., and Schmidt, D. (2000). Stroke-blind for colors, faces and locations: partial recovery after three years. *Restor. Neurol. Neurosci.* 17, 89–103.

Tanemura, R. (1999). Awareness in apraxia and agnosia. *Topics Stroke Rehabil.* 6, 33–42.

Trivelli, C., Turnbull, O., and della Sala, S. (1996). Recovery of object recognition in a case of simultanagnosia. *Appl. Neuropsychol.* 3, 166–73.

Ungerleider, L.G. and Haxby, J.V. (1998). 'What' and 'where' in the human brain. *Curr. Opin. Neuropiol.* 4, 157–65.

Uzzell, B.P., Dolinskas, C.A., and Langfitt, T.W. (1988). Visual field defects in relation to head injury severity. *Arch. Neurol.* 45, 420–4.

Vallar, G. and Perani, D. (1986). The anatomy of unilateral neglect after right-hemisphere stroke lesions. A clinical/CT-scan correlation study in man. *Neuropsychologia* 24, 609–22.

Van der Wildt, G.J. and Bergsma, D.P. (1997). Visual field enlargement by neuropsychological training of a hemianopsia patient. *Documenta Ophthalmol.* 93, 277–92.

Wilson, B. and Davidoff, J. (1993). Partial recovery from visual object agnosia: a 10 year follow-up study. *Cortex* 29, 529–42.

Wunderlich, G., Suchan, B., Herzog, H., Hömberg, V., and Seitz, R.J. (2000). Visual hallucinations in recovery from cortical blindness: imaging correlates. *Arch. Neurol.* 57, 61–565.

Zangemeister, W.H., Oechsner, U., and Freska, C. (1995). Short-term adaptation of eye movements in patients with visual hemifield defects indicates high level control of human scanpath. *Optometry Vis. Sci.* 72, 467–77.

Zeki, S. (1993). *A vision of the brain*. Blackwell Scientific, Oxford.

Zihl, J. (1981). Recovery of visual functions in patients with cerebral blindness: effect of specific practice with saccadic localisation. *Exp. Brain Res.* 44, 159–69.

Zihl, J. (1994). Rehabilitation of visual impairments in patients with brain damage. In *Low vision. Research and new developments in rehabilitation* (ed. A.C. Kooijman *et al.*), pp. 287–95. IOS, Amsterdam.

Zihl, J. (1995a). Visual scanning behavior in patients with homonymous hemianopia. *Neuropsychologia* 33, 287–303.

Zihl, J. (1995b). Eye movement patterns in hemianopic dyslexia. *Brain* 118, 891–912.

Zihl, J. (2000). *Rehabilitation of visual disorders after brain injury*. Psychology Press, Hove, East Sussex.

Zihl, J. and Kerkhoff, G. (1990). Foveal photopic and scotopic adaptation in patients with brain damage. *Clin. Vision Sci.*, 5 185–95.

Zihl, J. and von Cramon, D. (1979). Restitution of visual function in patients with cerebral blindness. *J. Neurol. Neurosurg. Psychiatry* 42, 312–22.

Zihl, J. and von Cramon, D. (1985). Visual field recovery from scotoma in patients with postgeniculate damage. *Brain* 108, 335–65.

Zoccolotti, P., Antonucci, G., Judica, A., Montenero, P., Pizzamiglio, L, and Razzano, C. (1989). Incidence and evolution of the hemineglect disorder in chronic patients with unilateral right brain damage. *Int. J. Neurosci.* 47, 209–16.

Index

Note: References to figures are indicated by 'f' after the page number.